The Unequal Burden of Cancer

An Assessment of NIH Research and Programs for Ethnic Minorities and the Medically Underserved

M. Alfred Haynes and Brian D. Smedley, *Editors*

Committee on Cancer Research Among Minorities and the Medically Underserved

Health Sciences Policy Program

Health Sciences Section

INSTITUTE OF MEDICINE

NATIONAL ACADEMY PRESS
Washington, D.C.   1999

NATIONAL ACADEMY PRESS • 2101 Constitution Avenue, N.W. • Washington, DC 20418

NOTICE: The project that is the subject of this report was approved by the Governing Board of the National Research Council, whose members are drawn from the councils of the National Academy of Sciences, the National Academy of Engineering, and the Institute of Medicine. The members of the committee responsible for the report were chosen for their special competences and with regard for appropriate balance.

The Institute of Medicine was chartered in 1970 by the National Academy of Sciences to enlist distinguished members of the appropriate professions in the examination of policy matters pertaining to the health of the public. In this, the Institute acts under both the Academy's 1863 congressional charter responsibility to be an adviser to the federal government and its own initiative in identifying issues of medical care, research, and education. Dr. Kenneth I. Shine is president of the Institute of Medicine.

Support for this project was provided by funds from the National Institutes of Health (Contract No. N01-OD-4-2139). The views presented in this report are those of the Committee on Cancer Research Among Minorities and the Medically Underserved and are not necessarily those of the funding organization.

Library of Congress Cataloging-in-Publication Data

The unequal burden of cancer : an assessment of NIH research and programs for ethnic minorities and the medically underserved / M. Alfred Haynes and Brian D. Smedley, editors ; Committee on Cancer Research among Minorities and the Medically Underserved, Health Sciences Policy Program, Health Sciences Section, Institute of Medicine.

p. cm.

Includes bibliographical references (p.) and index.

ISBN 0-309-07154-2 (hard)

1. Cancer—Research—Government policy—United States. 2. Minorities—Diseases—Research—Government policy—United States. 3. Poor—Diseases—Research—Government policy—United States. 4. National Institutes of Health (U.S.) I. Haynes, M. Alfred. II. Smedley, Brian D. III. Institute of Medicine (U.S.) Committee on Cancer Research among Minorities and the Medically Underserved.

RC267 .A77 1999

362.1′96994′008900973—dc21 99-6105

The Unequal Burden of Cancer: An Assessment of NIH Research and Programs for Ethnic Minorities and the Medically Underserved is available for sale from the National Academy Press, 2101 Constitution Avenue, N.W., Lock Box 285, Washington, DC 20055. Call (800) 624-6242 or (202) 334-3313 (in the Washington metropolitan area), or visit the NAP's on-line bookstore at: **www.nap.edu.**

For more information about the Institute of Medicine, visit the IOM home page at **www2. nas.edu/iom.**

Printed in the United States of America

The serpent has been a symbol of long life, healing, and knowledge among almost all cultures and religions since the beginning of recorded history. The image adopted as a logotype by the Institute of Medicine is based on a relief carving from ancient Greece, now held by the Staatliche Museen in Berlin.

COMMITTEE ON CANCER RESEARCH AMONG MINORITIES AND THE MEDICALLY UNDERSERVED

M. ALFRED HAYNES (*Chair*), Former President and Dean, Drew Postgraduate Medical School, and Former Director, Drew-Meharry-Morehouse Consortium Cancer Center, Rancho Palos Verdes, California

REGINA BENJAMIN, Physician, Bayou La Batre Rural Health Clinic, Inc., Bayou La Batre, Alabama

CHARLES L. BENNETT, Director of Outcomes Research, Robert Lurie Cancer Center, Northwestern University, and VA Chicago Health Care Systems

BARUCH S. BLUMBERG, Fox Chase Distinguished Scientist, Fox Chase Cancer Center, Philadelphia

MOON S. CHEN, JR., Professor and Chair, Division of Health Behavior and Health Promotion, School of Public Health, College of Medicine and Public Health, Ohio State University

GILBERT FRIEDELL, Director for Cancer Control, University of Kentucky

ANNA R. GIULIANO, Assistant Professor of Epidemiology, Arizona Prevention Center, Director, Minority Cancer Prevention and Control Program, Arizona Cancer Center, University of Arizona

JAMES W. HAMPTON, Medical Director, Troy and Dollie Smith Cancer Center at Integris Baptist Medical Center, Clinical Professor of Medicine, University of Oklahoma College of Medicine, and Cancer Care Associates, Oklahoma City

VICTOR A. McKUSICK (*Vice Chair*) University Professor of Medical Genetics, Johns Hopkins Hospital, Johns Hopkins University School of Medicine

LAWRENCE MIIKE, Director, Department of Health, State of Hawaii, Honolulu

SARAH MOODY-THOMAS, Associate Director, Stanley S. Scott Cancer Center, and Professor, Department of Psychiatry, Louisiana State University Medical Center, New Orleans

LARRY NORTON, Associate Professor of Oncology, Mount Sinai School of Medicine, and Head, Breast Disease Management Team, Memorial Sloan-Kettering Cancer Center, New York

MADISON POWERS, Senior Research Scholar, Kennedy Institute of Ethics, Georgetown University

SUSAN C. SCRIMSHAW, Dean, School of Public Health, and Professor, Community Health Sciences and Anthropology, University of Illinois at Chicago

FERNANDO M. TREVINO, Professor and Chairman, Department of Public Health and Preventive Medicine, Health Science Center at Forth Worth, University of North Texas

Committee Liaisons

ADA SUE HINSHAW, Dean, School of Nursing, University of Michigan
AMELIE G. RAMIREZ, Associate Professor and Associate Director, Center for Cancer Control Research, Baylor College of Medicine

Study Staff

BRIAN SMEDLEY, Study Director
YVETTE BENJAMIN, Research Associate (through 10/98)
THELMA COX, Senior Project Assistant

Consultant

TED CRON

Copy Editors

MICHAEL EDINGTON
MICHAEL HAYES

Section Staff

CHARLES H. EVANS, JR., Head, Health Sciences Section
ANDREW M. POPE, Director, Health Policy Program
LINDA DEPUGH, Administrative Assistant
JAMAINE TINKER, Financial Associate (through 10/98)

Reviewers

This report has been reviewed in draft form by individuals chosen for their diverse perspectives and technical expertise, in accordance with procedures approved by the NRC's Report Review Committee. The purpose of this independent review is to provide candid and critical comments that will assist the institution in making the published report as sound as possible and to ensure that the report meets institutional standards for objectivity, evidence, and responsiveness to the study charge. The review comments and draft manuscript remain confidential to protect the integrity of the deliberative process. We wish to thank the following individuals for their participation in the review of this report:

Mary Ellen Avery, M.D., Harvard Medical School;
Lester Breslow, M.D., M.P.H., University of California at Los Angeles School of Public Health;
H. Jack Geiger, M.D., City University of New York Medical School;
Reginald C. S. Ho, M.D., Straub Clinic and Hospital, Honolulu, Hawaii;
Frederick P. Li, M.D., Harvard Medical School;
Sandra Millon-Underwood, Ph.D., R.N., University of Wisconsin School of Nursing;
Geraldine Padilla, Ph.D., Jonsson Comprehensive Cancer Center, University of California at Los Angeles;
Frank Talamantes, Ph.D., Sinsheimer Laboratories, University of California at Santa Cruz; and
Richard Warnecke, Ph.D., School of Public Health and College of Urban Planning and Public Administration, University of Illinois at Chicago.

While the individuals listed above have provided constructive comments and suggestions, it must be emphasized that responsibility for the final content of this report rests entirely with the authoring committee and the institution.

Preface

In 1971, President Richard M. Nixon signed the National Cancer Act and assigned the leadership for the "War on Cancer" to the National Cancer Institute (NCI). Since that time, NCI has vigorously supported research that has broadened our understanding of the mechanisms of carcinogenesis and has led the way to advances in prevention, control, and treatment of a disease for which there is increasing demand for a "cure." Congress, and the public at large, are deeply indebted to NCI for its outstanding research leadership, and the results of those efforts are beginning to be more widely recognized.

However, Congress has from time to time requested assurance that all segments of the population are benefiting from the results of this research, in accordance with the mission of the National Institutes of Health (NIH) to conduct research to improve the health of all Americans. This study was prompted by a concern for ethnic minority and medically underserved populations that often experience a greater burden of cancer. The committee began its work in late January 1998, and completed its report in the fall of that year. In the process, we received presentations from the director of NCI and several members in leadership positions within the institute. The committee also reviewed numerous documents from NCI and other NIH institutes. To better understand how NIH's work has been received by important constituencies, the committee also conducted a survey of researchers involved in relevant research and heard from a number of community organizations with specific interests in cancer among these populations.

Our findings and recommendations are provided in this report, which is organized as follows:

- a brief history of the nation's struggle against cancer (Chapter 1);
- information on the burden of cancer among ethnic minorities and the medically underserved, and recommendations addressing the quality and scope of the data on which cancer research for these populations is based (Chapter 2);
- a review of research and training programs and activities on ethnic minorities and medically underserved populations at NIH and recommendations on how these programs and activities could be improved (Chapters 3 through 6); and,
- an annual reporting mechanism on the status of cancer research among ethnic minorities and the medically underserved at NIH, and recommendations on what these reports should contain (Chapter 7).

The committee was impressed by the momentum around these issues at NCI. In fact, some of the recommendations were already in the process of being implemented before the report was completed. The committee has felt free to make its recommendations always with the best interests of the populations concerned in mind and with the hope that the already excellent leadership provided by NCI will become even better.

The committee deeply appreciates the cooperation received from NCI and the other institutes at NIH in providing information we requested, and then subsequently providing still more information as the first set led to further requests. These efforts were graciously coordinated by Dr. Otis Brawley of NCI. Dr. Delores Parron of the National Institute of Mental Health served as the study's project officer and was instrumental in facilitating the project's timely completion. The committee is also grateful to the National Center for Health Statistics for documenting the methodology and caveats of an alternative method for assessing progress by considering the potential reduction of cancer deaths if the best rate among all ethnic groups were used as a reference. Finally, we were fortunate to receive the active input and contributions of Dr. Amelie Ramirez, a member of the Institute of Medicine and National Research Council's National Cancer Policy Board.

The work of the committee was a pleasure because of the enthusiasm and commitment of its members, greatly facilitated by an outstanding project director and a dedicated staff. All that is now necessary to complete our feeling of satisfaction is for the recommendations to continue to be implemented in a timely fashion so that all ethnic groups of our one race, the human race, are able to benefit from a reduction in what promises to be the leading cause of death in the twenty-first century.

M. Alfred Haynes, M.D.
Chair

Contents

The Unequal Burden of Cancer

Executive Summary

Cancer is second only to cardiovascular disease as the leading cause of death among Americans. One in four deaths in the United States is attributable to cancer, and one in three Americans will eventually develop some form of cancer. Furthermore, it is expected to be the leading cause of death in the United States in the next century (National Cancer Institute, 1998a). With the expansion of federal research efforts, however, the scientific understanding of cancer control, prevention, detection, and treatment has improved significantly, leading recently to the first overall decline in the cancer mortality rate in the United States in decades (Wingo et al., 1998).

Despite scientific gains, not all segments of the U.S. population have benefited to the fullest extent from advances in the understanding of cancer. Although many ethnic minority groups experience significantly lower levels of some types of cancer than the majority of the U.S. white population, other ethnic minorities experience higher cancer incidence and mortality rates. African-American males, for example, develop cancer 15 percent more frequently than white males (Miller et al., 1996). The rate of breast cancer among African-American women is not as high as that among white women, but the former group are more likely to die from the disease once it is detected (Bacquet and Ringen, 1986). Similarly, some specific forms of cancer affect other ethnic minority communities at rates up to several times higher than national averages (e.g., stomach and liver cancers among Asian-American populations, colon and rectal cancer among Alaska Natives, and cervical cancer among Hispanic and Vietnamese-American women [Miller et al., 1996]). Many ethnic minorities also experience poorer cancer survival rates than whites. American Indians, for example, experience the lowest cancer survival rates of any U.S. ethnic group (Gilliland et al., 1998).

In addition, individuals of all ethnic backgrounds who are poor, lack health insurance, or otherwise have inadequate access to high-quality cancer care typically experience high cancer incidence and mortality rates and low rates of survival from cancer (American Cancer Society, 1990). Many low-income white populations have cancer diagnosis rates as high as or higher than those for ethnic minority groups most affected by the disease. In Appalachian Kentucky, for example, a region characterized by high rates of poverty, the incidence of lung cancer among white males was 127 per 100,000 in 1992, a rate higher than that for any ethnic minority group in the United States during the same period (Gilbert Friedell, Director of the Kentucky Cancer Registry, personal communication, August 8, 1998).

These disparities in the burden of cancer prompted the U.S. Congress in 1997 (P.L. 104-208) to request a review of the programs of research at the National Institutes of Health (NIH) relevant to ethnic minority and medically underserved populations. An Institute of Medicine (IOM) committee was impaneled in 1998 and was charged with the following:

- reviewing the status of cancer research relative to minorities and medically underserved populations at the various Institutes, Centers, and Divisions of NIH to evaluate the relative share of resources allocated to cancer in minorities (including a review of NIH's ability to prioritize its cancer research agenda for minorities and medically underserved groups and the role of minority scientists in decision making on research priorities);
- examining how well research results are communicated and applied to cancer prevention and treatment programs for minorities and medically underserved populations, and the adequacy of understanding of survivorship issues that uniquely affect minority and underserved communities; and,
- examining the adequacy of NIH procedures for equitable recruitment and retention of minorities in clinical trials.

The committee was also asked to make recommendations on an annual reporting mechanism on the status of cancer research at NIH among minority and medically underserved populations.

NIH, as the nation's leading federal agency supporting research to improve the nation's health, and the National Cancer Institute (NCI), as the principal unit of NIH charged with conducting cancer research and information dissemination services, served as the focal points of the committee's inquiry, along with other institutes and centers (ICs) of NIH that collaborate with NCI on cancer-related research. Although NCI holds the lead role in the development and implementation of the National Cancer Program, other federal agencies, such as the Centers for Disease Control and Prevention (CDC), the U.S. Department of Veterans Affairs (VA), the U.S. Department of Defense, and others perform related cancer prevention, control, and information collection and dissemination services, and therefore share responsibility with NIH for making improvements in the nation's health. The work of these other agencies lies outside of the purview of this committee, but they are critical components of the National Cancer Program and need to be incorporated into the National Cancer Plan.

FINDINGS AND RECOMMENDATIONS

To address the study charge, the committee reviewed extensive information provided by NIH and NCI staff, and received input from outside of NIH via a panel of community representatives and a survey of researchers interested in cancer among ethnic minority and medically underserved populations. The committee's recommendations are listed in Box 1.

Determining the Burden of Disease: Cancer Surveillance and Risk Factor Research

The development of sound cancer prevention and control strategies begins with an all-encompassing cancer surveillance effort. Differences in rates of cancer among various population groups detected by cancer surveillance efforts can lend clues to etiologic factors (e.g., environmental exposures, genetic susceptibility, and dietary patterns) and can therefore point to intervention and prevention strategies. In addition, disparities in cancer survival rates can lend clues to inequities in health care service accessibility and delivery, or cultural factors affecting individuals' attitudes toward the health care system. Studies of differences in the cancer experiences of various groups also have the potential to benefit the entire U.S. population, as policies and practices associated with groups that are at lower risk for cancer may be applied to those populations at greater risk.

NCI's data collection and surveillance efforts are shaped by Directive No. 15 of the U.S. Office of Management and Budget (OMB), which stipulates that the U.S. population be classified according to one of four basic "racial" categories (American Indian or Alaska Native, Asian or Pacific Islander, black or African American, or white) and one of two ethnic groups (Hispanic or non-Hispanic). Although these classifications carry

BOX 1
Committee Recommendations

Chapter 2:
The Burden of Cancer Among Ethnic Minorities and Medically Underserved Populations

Recommendation 2-1: NIH should develop and implement across all institutes a uniform definition of "special populations" with cancer. This definition should be flexible but should be based on disproportionate or insufficiently studied burdens of cancer, as measured by cancer incidence, morbidity, mortality, and survival statistics.

Recommendation 2-2a: To further enhance the excellent data provided in the Surveillance, Epidemiology, and End Results (SEER) program database, adequate resources should be provided to expand SEER program coverage beyond the existing sites to include high-risk populations for which SEER program coverage is lacking. This expansion should address a wider range of demographic and social characteristics by using consistent nomenclature and a uniform data set and by reflecting the diverse characteristics of the current U.S. population.

Recommendation 2-2b: NCI should continue to work with the North American Association of Central Cancer Registries and other organizations to expand the coverage and enhance the quality of the 45 non-SEER program state cancer registries, with the intent of ultimately achieving—together with the SEER program state registries—two goals: (1) a truly national data set obtained through a system of longitudinal population-based cancer registries covering the entire country, and (2) a reliable database for each state to serve as the basis for both the development and the evaluation of cancer control efforts in that state.

Recommendation 2-3: Annual reporting of cancer surveillance data and population-based research needs to be expanded to include survival data for all ethnic groups, as well as for medically underserved populations.

Recommendation 2-4: The committee recommends an emphasis on ethnic groups rather than on race in NIH's cancer surveillance and other population research. This implies a conceptual shift away from the emphasis on fundamental biological differences among "racial" groups to an appreciation of the range of cultural and behavioral attitudes, beliefs, lifestyle patterns, diet, environmental living conditions, and other factors that may affect cancer risk.

Recommendation 2-5: The committee commends the proposed NCI program of expanded behavioral and epidemiologic research examining the relationship between cancer and cancer risk factors associated with various ethnic minority and medically underserved groups and recommends that these studies be conducted both across and within these groups.

**Chapter 3:
Overview of Programs of Research on Ethnic Minority and Medically Underserved Populations at the National Institutes of Health**

Recommendation 3-1: The Office of Research on Minority Health should more actively serve a coordinating, planning, and facilitative function regarding research relevant to cancer among ethnic minority and medically underserved populations across relevant institutes and centers of NIH. To further this goal, the Office of Research on Minority Health should

- make criteria for Minority Health Initiative project support explicit;
- coordinate with other specialty offices (e.g., the Office of Research on Women's Health) by participating in NIH-wide coordination efforts such as the Research Enhancement Awards Program; and
- ensure that Minority Health Initiative funding does not supplant funding from institutes and centers for research and programs relevant to ethnic minority and medically underserved populations.

Recommendation 3-2: Research and research funding relevant to cancer among ethnic minority and medically underserved populations should be more adequately assessed (as per Recommendation 3-3) and should be increased.

Recommendation 3-3: NIH should improve the accuracy of its assessment of research that is relevant to ethnic minority and medically underserved groups by replacing the current "percent relevancy" accounting method with one that identifies studies whose purpose is to address a priori research questions uniquely affecting ethnic minority and medically underserved groups.

Recommendation 3-4: The newly established program of behavioral and social science research at NCI addresses an area of research that has been neglected in the past. The committee urges that this program of research identify as one of its highest priorities a focus on the cancer prevention, control, and treatment needs of ethnic minority and medically underserved groups.

Continued

BOX 1 ***Continued***

Recommendation 3-5: Collaborations between NIH and research and medical institutions that serve ethnic minority and medically underserved populations should be increased to improve the study of cancers that affect these groups and to increase the involvement of such entities and populations in scientific research.

Recommendation 3-6: NIH should increase its efforts to expand the number of ethnic minority investigators in the broad spectrum of cancer research to improve minority health research. These efforts should (1) assess relevant areas of research needs and ensure that trainees are representative of these disciplines and areas of inquiry, (2) determine guidelines for the quality and expected outcomes of training experiences, and (3) maintain funding for a sufficient period of time to assess the impact of training programs on the goal of increasing minority representation in cancer research fields.

Chapter 4:
Evaluation of Priority Setting and Programs of Research on Ethnic Minority and Medically Underserved Populations at the National Institutes of Health

Recommendation 4-1: NCI should develop a process to increase the representation of ethnically diverse researchers and public representatives serving on all advisory and program review committees so that the makeup of these committees reflects the changing diversity of the U.S. population. NCI should develop an evaluation plan to assess the effect of increased and more diversified ethnic minority community and researcher input on changes in NCI policies and priorities toward ethnic minority cancer issues.

Recommendation 4-2: The research needs of ethnic minority and medically underserved groups should be identified on the basis of the burden of cancer in these populations, with an assessment of the most appropriate areas of research (i.e., behavioral and social sciences, biology, epidemiology and genetics, prevention and control, treatment, etc.).

Recommendation 4-3: For NCI to address the needs of ethnically diverse and medically underserved populations effectively, the Office of Special Populations Research (or some other designated entity or entities) must possess the authority to coordinate and leverage programs and resources across the divisions and branches of NCI to stimulate research on ethnic minority and medically underserved populations. This authority can be established by providing such an office with:

• special resources to fund programs specifically targeted to these populations, or

• accountability for the institution-wide allocation of program resources.

Recommendation 4-4: Investigator-initiated research must be supplemented to ensure that the cancer research needs of ethnic minority and medically underserved populations are addressed.

Chapter 5:
Advancing State-of-the-Art Treatment and Prevention

Recommendation 5-1: NIH and other federal agencies (particularly the Health Care Financing Administration) should coordinate to address funding for clinical trials, particularly to address the additional diagnostic and therapeutic costs associated with prevention trials and third-party payment barriers associated with clinical treatment trials.

Recommendation 5-2: NCI should continue to work with other appropriate federal agencies and institutional review boards to explore creative approaches to improving patients' understanding of research and encouraging them to provide consent to participate in research. These approaches should address cultural bias, mistrust, literacy, and other issues that may pose barriers to the participation of ethnic minority and medically underserved groups.

Recommendation 5-3: NCI should report on the accrual and retention of ethnic minority and medically underserved populations in clinical trials using a consistent definition for medically underserved populations, including such characteristics as rural versus urban population, insurance status, socioeconomic status, and level of literacy.

Recommendation 5-4: NCI should continue to assess its dissemination practices to identify effective cancer information delivery strategies among ethnic minority and medically underserved populations, revise and implement the strategic dissemination plan on the basis of the results of that research, and institute an ongoing system of monitoring to assess its effectiveness.

Chapter 6:
Cancer Survivorship

Recommendation 6-1: NCI should establish a strategic plan to address the cancer survivorship needs of ethnic minority and medically under-

Continued

Box 1 *Continued*

served groups, including coordination of an overall research agenda on survivorship and a more structured framework for monitoring knowledge, attitudes, and behavior regarding cancer survivorship.

Chapter 7:
Monitoring and Reporting

Recommendation 7-1: The committee recommends a regular reporting mechanism to increase NIH accountability to the U.S. Congress and public constituencies. Such reports should

- report on data on progress against cancer using the nomenclature "ethnic groups" rather than "racial" groups and include data on medically underserved populations with ethnic group data;
- provide data on the incidence of cancer at several cancer sites, including those cancers that disproportionately affect ethnic minority and medically underserved populations;
- consider as one alternative reporting of mortality data in terms of "potential reduction of deaths," a statistic that is based on the lowest mortality rate among U.S. ethnic groups and that emphasizes the need for cross-cultural studies to ascertain optimal strategies for cancer prevention, treatment, and control;
- link research findings to reductions in cancer incidence and mortality and identify any gaps that may occur in this linkage; and
- report on "process" developments, such as the number and type of research programs specifically targeted to ethnic minority and medically underserved groups and the contributions of ethnic minority scientists and community groups to the research priority-setting process.

important historical, social, and political significance in the United States, they are of limited utility for purposes of health research because the concept of race rests upon unfounded assumptions that there are fundamental biological and behavioral differences among racial groups (American Anthropological Association, 1998; Cooper, 1984; President's Cancer Panel, 1997; Williams et al., 1994). In reality, human biodiversity cannot be adequately summarized according to the broad, presumably discrete categories assumed by a racial taxonomy. Furthermore, "racial" groups as defined by OMB are not discernible on the basis of genetic information (American Anthropological Association, 1998; President's Cancer Panel, 1997). The committee considers the term "ethnic group" as a more appropriate descriptor for human population groups, as it appropriately places emphasis on the range of cultural and behavioral factors, beliefs, lifestyle patterns, diet, environmental living conditions, and other factors that may affect cancer risk.

NCI's Surveillance, Epidemiology, and End Results (SEER) program was established to provide data on the incidence of cancer in selected geographic areas that may be generalized to the total U.S. population. At this time, the SEER program provides high-quality data that are the best approximation of a national cancer database. The SEER program, however, does not fully describe the burden of cancer for many U.S. ethnic minority and medically underserved populations. It lacks the necessary database concerning the disproportionate cancer incidence, mortality, and survival rates among ethnic minorities and medically underserved groups that would permit NCI to develop and evaluate effective cancer control strategies for these populations. These groups include lower-income or poverty-level whites, particularly those living in rural areas such as Appalachia; African Americans living in rural communities, particularly in the South; culturally diverse American-Indian populations; and Hispanics of national origins not currently included.

In addition, the SEER program, as with other NCI programs, fails to consistently collect and report on data for medically underserved populations. These groups, as noted above, suffer from cancer incidence and mortality rates that are disproportionately high and from low cancer survival rates. Medically underserved populations may be defined as low-income individuals, those without medical insurance, those who lack access to quality cancer care, or by other definitions. The committee, however, found no consistent definition of this population in the SEER program or in other NCI programs. A clear, consistent definition of what constitutes the medically underserved population is needed, and cancer surveillance reports should regularly include data on cancer incidence, mortality, and survival rates among the people who make up this population.

NIH Portfolio of Research Relevant to the Study of Cancer Among Ethnic Minority and Medically Underserved Populations

The committee finds that NIH, and particularly NCI, has funded an impressive array of research projects and training initiatives that may have a demonstrable impact in addressing the burden of cancer among ethnic minority and medically underserved populations. The committee concludes, however, that no blueprint or strategic plan to direct or coordinate this research activity appears to exist. As a result, model programs in one or more institutes are not replicated by other ICs where indicated, some areas of research emphasis receive greater attention than others, and overall funding to address the needs of ethnic minority and medically underserved populations is inadequate.

In addition, the committee believes that NCI and NIH should improve the accuracy of their assessment of the amount of resources allocated to addressing the needs of ethnic minority and medically underserved groups. NIH calculates the amount of money allocated to research on minority health programs on the basis of the percentage of ethnic minority individuals in NIH study populations. While the committee wishes to encourage NIH to continue to support the inclusion of diverse study populations in all the research it sponsors, such "percent relevancy" accounting methods are inappropriate as means of indicating overall expenditures for research on ethnic minority health. Diverse study populations do not, in and of themselves, address the research needs of ethnic minority and medically underserved populations unless meaningful research questions relevant to these groups can be posed a priori and answered based on the appropriateness (i.e., diversity and generality) of the study population. Estimates of expenditures on minority health research should therefore be determined by summing research expenditures associated with studies that address a priori research questions focused on the particular needs of ethnic minority and medically underserved communities. Therefore, while NCI reports that $124 million was allocated to research and training programs relevant to ethnic minority and medically underserved populations in fiscal year 1997 (based on percent relevancy accounting methods), the committee believes that the actual figure allocated for these groups is only slightly more than $24 million, or approximately 1 percent of the total NCI budget. Funds allocated to cancer-related minority health research and training programs by other NIH ICs are also small relative to their respective overall budgets. The committee finds these resources are insufficient relative to the burden of disease among ethnic minority and medically underserved communities, the changing U.S. demographics, and the scientific opportunities inherent in the study of diverse populations. Moreover, the committee found no evidence that NIH calculates total expenditures for research on medically underserved groups, apart from calculations derived from data for ethnic minority populations.

Although the committee found evidence that NCI sponsors significant behavioral and social science research aimed at examining the range of behavioral, psychosocial, dietary, and other factors that enhance or decrease the risk for cancer or poor cancer survival among ethnic minority and medically underserved groups, behavioral and social science research should be expanded, particularly with respect to prevention and outreach efforts. The agenda for such research should be based on an analysis of the prevalence of particular cancers in these populations and their preventability. Particularly for ethnic minority populations, research is needed to investigate ethnically appropriate interventions, including culturally competent and linguistically appropriate approaches.

Finally, while the committee found evidence of a significant portfolio of training programs designed to increase the numbers of ethnic minority investigators in cancer-related research fields, there is little evidence that NCI or NIH has undertaken a thorough assessment of training programs to determine whether these programs are producing adequate numbers of ethnic minority researchers in all appropriate cancer research fields (e.g., behavioral and social sciences, epidemiology, genetics, and cell biology), and to determine whether training programs have resulted in the increased representation of ethnic minorities in cancer research fields. Further, there is little evidence that guidelines or other training criteria have been established by NCI or NIH to ensure that all trainees receive high-quality instruction and mentoring. Such efforts would improve the planning and implementation of future training programs.

Research Priority Setting

Establishing priorities among areas of research and scientific inquiry is a complex process that has been addressed in greater detail in a prior IOM study authored by the Committee on the NIH Research Priority-Setting Process (Institute of Medicine, 1998). In general, the present committee supports the recommendations of that previous committee. In particular, the committee supports the recommendations that diversity and public representation on NIH's advisory panels should be increased. The presence of such diverse viewpoints can yield great benefits for NIH, as well as for the public at large (e.g., greater public support for scientific programs, and greater attention to the needs of medically underserved populations).

The establishment of the NCI Director's Consumer Liaison Group represents an important step toward this goal, for which NCI should be commended. The committee finds, however, that there has been inconsistent progress in increasing the numbers of scientists, consumers, and community members from and representing ethnic minority and medically underserved communities on NCI advisory panels and committees. Such representation is a critical component of larger efforts to increase constituency input in priority setting and public accountability at NCI. Inclusion of members and representatives of ethnic minority and medically underserved groups on decision-making panels, however, is not sufficient in and of itself to ensure that the concerns of these groups are addressed within NCI. The impact of ethnic minority and medically underserved groups on the advisory and priority-setting process should be evaluated to ensure that policy changes follow from increased representation.

As noted above, many factors influence the setting of research priorities at NIH. Priority setting for research on ethnic minority and medically underserved populations, however, is complicated by differences in philosophy regarding how best to address the needs of these groups. NCI's leadership, for example, appears to take the position that research on "special" populations, like other areas of scientific inquiry, cannot be directed or planned and that issues for these groups may be addressed within the larger portfolio of population research (Richard Klausner, director of the National Cancer Institute, presentation to the study committee, June 12, 1998). There is significant evidence to support the position that research often proceeds because of the opportunities presented, and that in many instances, scientific opportunities have resulted in breakthroughs that offer tremendous benefits for ethnic minority and medically underserved communities, as well as for the nation as a whole. For example, the discovery of the role of the hepatitis B virus in the etiology of primary liver cancer, which disproportionately affects Southeast Asian populations, was linked with the development of a vaccine for the prevention of hepatitis B virus infection.

The committee finds, however, that the research priority-setting process at NCI and NIH fails to serve the needs of ethnic minority and medically underserved groups. Assessment of the burden of cancer among ethnic minority and medically underserved populations and consideration of these factors within the larger framework of scientific opportunity should be key aspects of the research priority-setting process. This conclusion is also supported in a recommendation made by the NCI Special Action Committee in its 1996 report (National Cancer Institute, 1996a), which advocated a data-driven review of the cancer burden among ethnic minority and medically underserved populations as a means of identifying priority research areas.

Two offices serve as logical focal points for the development of a strategic plan to address cancer among ethnic minority and medically underserved populations and assess progress toward that goal. One, the NIH Office of Research on Minority Health (ORMH), serves to coordinate research across NIH institutes on broad ethnic minority health research topics. One of the office's major functions is to stimulate research on minority populations at relevant NIH ICs by providing research supplements to leverage IC resources. ORMH has only recently, however, created a standing advisory panel to help guide the establishment of research priorities (this function had previously been assumed by an ad hoc panel), and it does not participate in the Research Enhancement Awards Program with other specialty offices at NIH to coordinate funding proposals and priorities. Its criteria for program funding and research priorities have therefore been less open to public scrutiny. In addition, ORMH program funding appears to have supplanted rather than leveraged NCI resources for important research and program activities in many instances.

Much of the authority within NCI for establishing research priorities among ethnic minority and medically underserved populations would logically fall to the NCI Office of Special Populations Research (OSPR). Currently, however, OSPR lacks the institutional advantages that would ensure that an NCI commitment to research among special populations has a chance to be successful. It has no independent resources to fund a separate portfolio of initiatives for special populations research, has no clear criteria or guidance for recommending the priorities for such initiatives that are dependent on the resources of other parts of NCI, and holds no official position on any of the NCI advisory committees responsible for setting major intramural or extramural priorities. Rather, OSPR serves as the "eyes and ears" to the NCI director regarding research on ethnic minority and medically underserved populations, as it monitors program activities and provides guidance and advice. For the reasons stated above, the committee finds that this model is insufficient to address the needs of ethnic minority and medically underserved populations. These conditions must be rectified or other lines of authority must be established for NCI to benefit from a coordinated program of research on cancer among ethnic minority and medically underserved populations.

Finally, the committee is doubtful that the incentives present in the scientific research marketplace will encourage efforts to address critical research questions among the most heavily burdened populations. To increase and improve the quality of research on cancer among ethnic minority and medically underserved populations, NCI must expand requests for applications and other funding mechanisms, especially in areas where critical gaps exist.

Clinical Trials and Cancer Information Dissemination

The inclusion of ethnic minority and medically underserved individuals in clinical trials and the dissemination of information to their communities and health care providers are critical links connecting scientific innovation with improvements in health and health care delivery. Enhancement of these links is clearly within the purview of NCI and NIH. Although many factors pose challenges to such improvements (e.g., mistrust of the scientific establishment among many members of ethnic minority communities), without a concerted effort to enhance this process, ethnic minority and medically underserved communities will continue to lag behind the American majority in benefiting from the tremendous recent scientific advancements and medical breakthroughs in cancer prevention, treatment, and control.

The committee finds that overall, the level of accrual of ethnic minorities in NCI-sponsored treatment trials is proportionate to the disease burden among these populations, with a few exceptions for specific cancer sites. NCI-sponsored prevention trials, however, suffer from poor accrual of ethnic minorities. The recently concluded trials of the chemopreventive agent tamoxifen, for example, demonstrated that the drug successfully prevented breast cancers in thousands of women at high risk for the disease. Only 2 percent of the overall study sample, however, were African American, and even smaller percentages of individuals from other ethnic groups were entered into this study. Such poor accrual raises significant questions regarding the generality of these findings to the total U.S. population.

Many factors may affect researchers' ability to recruit ethnic minority and medically underserved populations into prevention trials. One of the most significant challenges lies in the lack of funding for associated follow-up costs. In cancer screening trials, for example, NIH in most instances does not provide funding to cover costs of care for indigent populations with positive test results (Peter Greenwald, acting director, Division of Cancer Prevention, National Cancer Institute, presentation to the study committee, June 12, 1998). The committee considers the federal government's failure to provide follow-up care to needy, uninsured patients to be unethical and urges greater coordination among federal agencies to address the problem.

Another factor that may limit the participation of ethnic minority and medically underserved populations in clinical trial research is the complexity of the informed-consent process. Informed consent is the first step in establishing a bond of trust between researchers and research subjects; yet too often informed-consent forms are long, technical, difficult to administer, and not well understood by patients. The committee urges NIH to work with other agencies to explore alternative means of obtaining patient consent (e.g., oral consent) that respect patient autonomy and that do not compromise the informed-consent process.

NCI has developed several sophisticated mechanisms for the dissemination of information to cancer patients, clinicians, and others. Much of this effort has been guided by consumer research and an effective marketing plan. Relatively little attention, however, has been devoted to the specific needs of ethnic minority and medically underserved populations. Despite the presence of cancer information materials that have been translated into Spanish and other products targeted to ethnic minority communities, no strategic plan regarding information dissemination to these groups and their health providers appears to exist. Furthermore, the committee did not find evidence of any evaluations of the effectiveness of dissemination practices in ethnic minority and medically underserved communities. Such efforts are necessary to ensure that individuals in these communities, who may be more likely to hold fatalistic attitudes toward cancer and inaccurate beliefs regarding its preventability, are being adequately served.

Cancer Survivorship in Ethnic Minority and Medically Underserved Communities

Cancer survivors are, in the committee's view, perhaps the most underutilized resource in the War on Cancer. This is especially true among ethnic minority and medically underserved populations, who face numerous cultural, socioeconomic, and institutional barriers to cancer prevention and treatment services. Cancer survivors in these communities are often painfully aware of the lack of services and information that might assist neighbors, friends, and relatives either to avoid or to cope with a cancer diagnosis. Perhaps more important, however, they possess critical expertise on how to reach members of their communities with cancer education and services information. This expertise should be tapped to its fullest.

NCI, to its credit, has established an impressive infrastructure of research programs and resources to assist cancer survivors. Greater attention must be paid, however, to the unique needs of ethnic minority and medically underserved communities. As indicated above, the committee did not find evidence of a strategic plan that addresses the needs of these communities and has offered a number of specific recommendations for the establishment of such a plan.

Monitoring and Measuring Results

To assess progress toward reducing the disparities in the cancer burden among U.S. ethnic and socioeconomic groups, it is important that the U.S. Congress and the public receive regular information regarding NIH activities that include objective performance indicators. The progress that has been achieved toward this goal can be assessed at three levels: (1) reductions in cancer incidence and mortality rates and increased cancer survival rates; (2) changes in cancer risk behavior among affected populations, such as reductions in tobacco use or efficiency of vaccination programs against hepatitis B as a means of reducing risk for primary cancer of the liver; and (3) process-related changes at NIH that reflect new organizational standards, policies, and priorities designed to better address the needs of ethnic minority and medically underserved communities. It is assumed that changes at the organizational level will result in positive outcomes in the behavior of risk groups, which in turn will result in reductions in cancer incidence and mortality and increases in cancer survival.

1

The Struggle Against Cancer

At the beginning of the 20th century, cancer was eighth among the leading causes of death. Infectious diseases were prominent, with pneumonia, influenza, tuberculosis, and gastrointestinal diseases being responsible for one-third of all deaths. Life expectancy at birth was 49 years. As the century progressed, however, people survived to older ages and chronic noninfectious diseases became much more common, such that by the middle of the century, the leading causes of death were heart disease, cancer, and stroke. At the beginning of the century, cases of lung cancer was so rare that it was shown to medical students as a condition that the students were unlikely to see again during their medical practices. By the 1940s, however, lung cancer was becoming quite common (Weinberg, 1996). As a result of these changes in the causes of mortality, important changes in national health policy began to take place.

In 1937 the National Cancer Institute Act established the National Cancer Institute (NCI) within the U.S. Public Health Service (P.L. 75-244). The Act directed the Surgeon General to promote the coordination of research conducted by the Institute and similar research conducted by other agencies, organizations, and individuals. To reduce the rate of mortality from the major causes of death, however, it was necessary to do more than conduct research. The federal government initiated a concerted effort to increase the training of qualified practitioners capable of managing these diseases, as well as to make knowledge regarding cancer prevention and treatment generally available to the public. The U.S. Congress was considering a planned attack against these problems and favored a decentralized approach involving the largely private nonprofit medical centers and community hospitals. The heart disease, cancer, and stroke amendments to the Public Health Service Act of 1965, for example, provided grants-in-aid for the support of regional medical programs (RMPs) for research and training, as well as for the diagnosis and treatment of these major diseases. The RMPs were centered at medical schools and their affiliated hospitals. The intent was to encourage a linkage between the medical centers and the community hospitals, thereby improving the quality of care for these conditions (Bodenhimer, 1969). The President's Commission on Heart Disease, Cancer, and Stroke had also recommended the development of a network of regional comprehensive cancer centers (President's Commission on Heart Disease, Cancer, and Stroke, 1964). These centers were to focus on cancer control programs and conduct studies at the various regional centers. The centers were to be at the forefront of the struggle against cancer, but these recommendations were not realized until later, and in 1974 the RMPs were absorbed into the National Health Planning and Resources Development Act (see Box 1-1 for a timeline of significant events in the War on Cancer, and Box 1-2 for a listing of recent developments in NCI efforts regarding ethnic minority and medically underserved populations).

THE FOCUS ON CANCER

The greatest impetus to the effort against cancer came with the enactment of the National Cancer Act of 1971 (P.L. 92-218). The National Panel of Consultants on the Conquest of Cancer (the Yarborough Commission) had emphasized the need for a coherent and systematic attack on the complex problems of cancer and urged the development of a comprehensive national plan to conquer cancer as soon as possible. This was to be the beginning of the real War on Cancer. The National Cancer Act of 1971 increased funding for NCI and made major changes to previous efforts against cancer. It provided for greater authority of the NCI director, who became a presidential appointee and who could submit a budget request directly to the president. It established the President's Cancer Panel and the National Cancer Advisory Board. The Act also called for a National Cancer Program under the leadership of the NCI director, who was to coordinate not only the cancer research programs within the Institute but also the efforts of related federal and nonfederal programs. It also authorized the first cancer centers and an information dissemination program.

Beginning of the War on Cancer

The War on Cancer was launched with great expectations and with

BOX 1-1
Highlights of National Cancer Program Events Relevant to Ethnic Minority and Medically Underserved Populations (years are calendar years)

1937 National Cancer Institute Act signed into law [P.L. 75-244]. Appropriation limit of $700,000 for each fiscal year is authorized.

1964 Surgeon General's report on Tobacco and Health is released.

1971 President Richard Nixon signs into law the National Cancer Act of 1971 (P.L. 92-218).

1973 Surveillance, Epidemiology, and End Results (SEER) program is established.

1975 Cooperative Minority Biomedical Program is established, providing funds to train research students at historically black colleges and universities.

1984 "Heckler Report" outlines disparities in health between ethnic minority and non-minority Americans

1984 Comprehensive Minority Biomedical Program is established.

1985 Cancer Prevention Awareness Program for Black Americans becomes first NCI prevention campaign directed toward a high-risk population.

1987 National Cancer Advisory Board announces establishment of the National Black Leadership Initiative on Cancer.

1987, 1988
Director of NIH and the Advisory Committee to the Director hold a series of regional meetings on underrepresentation of minorities in biomedical and behavioral research. It is concluded that NIH must increase opportunities for underrepresented minority scientists.

1988 First minority-focused Consortium Cancer Center is established with three historically black medical schools: Charles R. Drew University of Medicine and Science in Los Angeles, Meharry Medical College in Nashville, and Morehouse School of Medicine in Atlanta.

1989 NCI initiates mechanism of supplementing research grants to encourage recruitment of minority scientists and science students into extramural research laboratories. The mechanism is later expanded to include science students, women, and people with disabilities.

1990 Office of Research on Minority Health is established by the Director of the National Institutes of Health (NIH).

Office of Research on Women's Health is established.

Network for Cancer Control Research in American Indian and Alaska Native populations is established by NCI Division of Cancer Prevention and Control.

1992 Hispanic Leadership Initiative on Cancer, Appalachia Leadership Initiative on Cancer is established.

The SEER Program expands coverage to better represent minority, elderly, and rural populations.

The Minority Health Initiative is established.

1993 National Institutes of Health Revitalization Act of 1993 signed into law. It encourages NCI to expand and intensify efforts in breast cancer and other cancers affecting women. Authorizes increased appropriations with similar language for prostate cancer.

Office of Research on Minority Health is authorized by Congress in P.L.103-43 as part of the National Institutes of Health Revitalization Act of 1993.

1994 Notice of NIH Guidelines on the Inclusion of Women and Minorities as Subjects in Clinical Research appears in *Federal Register.*

Notice of Outreach Notebook appears in *Federal Register.* Notebook is published later same year.

Office of Protection from Research Risks Reports: Memorandum to Institutional Officials and Institutional Review Board on Inclusion of Women and Minorities in Research.

Office of Research on Minority Health holds meeting with 350

Continued

BOX 1-1 *Continued*

members of the minority biomedical community: National Conference on Minority Health Research and Research Training.

Sowing Seeds in the Mountains, publication of the Appalachian Leadership Initiative on Cancer.

1995–1996
NCI leadership initiates major reorganization based on recommendations of the Ad Hoc Working Group of the National Cancer Advisory Board and NCI.

1996 Office of Research and Minority Health holds four meetings, one for each of the four racial and ethnic groups identified in U.S. Office of Management and Budget Directive No. 15: African American, Hispanic American, Native American, and Asian and Pacific Islanders.

1997 NCI Director's Consumer Liaison Group is formed.

1998 En Accion Training Manual, a community-centered health communications manual drawn from successful experiences of the 5-year research and demonstration project of the National Hispanic Leadership Initiative on Cancer, is published.

BOX 1-2
Chronology of Recent Events Relevant to Cancer Research Among Ethnic Minority and Medically Underserved Populations

January 1996
National Conference on the Recruitment and Retention of Minority Participants in Clinical Cancer Research.

April 1996
Women and Minority Recruitment: Small Grant (CA-96-003) and Women and Minority Recruitment: Intervention Testing (CA-96-004) funding opportunities announced.

May 1996

Report of NCI Special Action Committee released internally.

Minorities in Medical Oncology (CA-96-006) and Minority Enhancement Awards (CA-96-007) funding opportunities announced.

September 1996

Senate Subcommittee on Labor, Health and Human Services Appropriations cites IOM to perform study of NIH research on cancer among minorities and the medically underserved.

Minority-Based Community Oncology Program (CA-96-016) funding opportunity announced.

October 1996

Four programs receive grants to develop model cancer survivorship programs for minority populations—Celebration of Living (African American); People Living Through Cancer (PLTC—American Indian); Sisters Network (African American); Women Achieving Victory & Esteem (WAVE—African American)

December 1996

Aging, Race, and Ethnicity in Prostate Cancer (PA-97-019) funding opportunity announced.

January–December 1997

NCI funds or co-funds 22 conferences and meetings related to cancer research among minorities, including 12 meetings on increasing minority participation in clinical cancer research.

March 1997

NCI/MARC Summer Training Supplement (PAR-98-016) announced.

April 1997

President's Cancer Panel meeting, "The Meaning of Race in Science—Considerations for Cancer Research" held in New York City.

May 1997

Mentored Career Development Award (CA-97-003) announced.

July 1997

Barbara K. Rimer, Dr.P.H., appointed to newly created NCI Division of Cancer Control and Population Science (DCCPS). The focus of DC-

Continued

BOX 1-2 *Continued*

CPS will be on populations, behavior, surveillance, special populations, outcomes, and other aspects of cancer control.

September 1997
Report of the NCI Cancer Control Review Group released.

October 1997
NCI DCCPS reorganization initiated.

November 1997
NCI selects members of new Director's Consumer Liaison Group (DCLG).

Minority-Based Community Clinical Oncology Program (CA-97-016) announced.

December 1997
Mentored Career Development Award (CA-97-023) announced.

January–November 1998
NCI funds or co-funds 17 conferences and meetings related to cancer research among minorities.

January 1998
IOM Committee on Cancer Research Among Minorities and the Medically Underserved holds first meeting.

February 1998
Program Announcement, "Diet, Lifestyle, and Cancer in U.S. Special Populations" released (PA-98-028).

July–September 1998
NCI Office of Cancer Control Cervical Cancer Screening Campaign for Minority Women initiated (radio announcements to promote participation in cancer screening)

August 1998
Health Communications in Cancer Control (CA-98-0114) funding opportunity announced.

September 1998
Minority-Based Community Clinical Oncology Program (CA-98-021) announced.

increased funding just before Christmas of 1971. Some enthusiastically expected that it would come to a swift and successful end. To complicate matters, however, the war had a series of commanders, each adding his or her own perspective to the overall strategy and how it should be implemented. Despite warnings to the contrary, it appeared reasonable for some to assume that if there were enough money and sufficient commitment, scientists could quickly solve this problem, at least by the 200th anniversary of the founding of the nation in 1976. After all, scientists had developed the atomic bomb and had successfully landed a man on the moon. There was no quick result, however, in the War on Cancer.

What did happen in 1976 was a revolution in thinking about cancer genes. That revolution was triggered by a publication in the journal *Nature* by Stehelin, Varmus, Bishop, and colleagues (Stehelin et al., 1976). It was the beginning of the concept that a gene from a normal cell could be converted to a cancer-causing gene. The significance of this fundamental finding was not fully appreciated until later. Rather, the expectation of quick results continued, and might have been strengthened when NCI announced the goal of reducing the incidence of cancer by 50 percent by the year 2000.

Mechanisms of Development of Cancer

Although the Panel of Consultants had placed great emphasis on a national plan, such planning was contrary to the tradition of the National Institutes of Health (NIH), which had always acted on the basis that the greatest progress occurs when independent investigators are allowed to pursue their interests. Many argued that research could not be planned at all, and in the case of cancer, about which so little was known, directed research would have been inappropriate. It would be better for the Institute to focus on understanding the underlying mechanisms of the development of cancer. To make matters worse, some of the demonstration programs were premature and did not yield the expected results. They did, however, demonstrate that the Institute did not know how to effect change among either practicing physicians or the lay public. As a result, NCI placed most of its emphasis on doing and supporting what it does best: basic research.

There was a period when the overwhelming evidence for the relationship between tobacco and lung cancer was known but the mechanism of the development of cancer was not understood. Until then there was a struggle between those who believed that cancer was caused by environmental exposures to carcinogens and those who believed that the cause was a viral infection. To add to the confusion, the tobacco industry and its supporters did not accept the "environmental exposure" concept. Later legislation called for expansion of research for the prevention of cancer caused by occupational or environmental exposures to carcinogens. The focus on viral infections in cancer research did a great deal to promote virology, but the mechanisms by which viruses caused cancer remained unclear. As a result, the War on Cancer was a strange war, one in which it was not quite clear who the enemy was, nor was there an effective method of defeat.

Soldiers in the War on Cancer

The cancer centers played a major role in the War on Cancer. They were the focal point for clinical and nonclinical research, and from these centers the latest and best methods for the treatment, prevention, and control of cancer were discussed with professionals and the lay public. These centers grew in number, and the level of funding that they received grew as well, but the efforts were not coordinated into a national plan. The greatest emphasis was on trying to understand the underlying mechanisms of cancer development.

The National Cancer Act also mandated the collection, analysis, and dissemination of information that would be useful in the prevention, diagnosis, and treatment of cancer. This resulted in the development of the Surveillance, Epidemiology, and End Results (SEER) program in 1973. The rationale for the establishment of the SEER program was that data collection could be useful in the effort to understand the cancer problem, especially when the rates of cancer are significantly different in various groups of the population. In fact, the data pointed to wide disparity in the rate of mortality from cancer among the African-American population, compared with that among the white population. Race or poverty was often stated as an explanation for this disparity, but a completely satisfactory answer was not available. The data pointed to a need for special attention to cancer in the African-American population and may have been a major factor in approving the development of the Drew-Meharry-Morehouse Consortium Cancer Center in 1988. Other initiatives also focused on what the Institute called "special populations." These included the Black Leadership Initiative on Cancer, the Hispanic Leadership Initiative, and the Appalachian Leadership Initiative. The last initiative was formed in recognition of the fact that rural, poor whites experienced the same burden of cancer as ethnic minority groups. A Leadership Initiative for American Indian and Alaska Native populations or other groups was never formed. These efforts were stimulated by the groups involved and were supported by the Institute, but they were not the result of an Institute strategy to reduce the burden of disease in these populations.

Legislation established the position of Associate Director for Prevention in NCI and added to the mission of the Institute research on the continuing care of patients with cancer and their families. In 1993, the NIH Revitalization Act (P.L. 103-43) required that the Institute intensify and expand its research on breast and women's cancers and prostate cancer. It also required a set-aside for cancer control activities.

PROGRESS REPORTS

The U.S. Congress had given NCI special consideration since the beginning of the War on Cancer, as evidenced by increased levels of funding and authority. In 1993, however, the nation, through its elected representatives in the House and the Senate, appeared to be unhappy with the progress of the War, although it was impressed by the breakthroughs in molecular biology.

Progress Report 1

In 1993 the Institute prepared a report on the progress that had taken place between 1982 and 1992 in the scientific understanding of cancer (National Cancer Institute, 1993). Six expert panels provided evidence of substantial progress in a variety of areas. Perhaps the most fundamental progress, according to this report, was in understanding of the multistep process of genetic changes by which cancer is initiated and promoted. Cancer had come to be recognized as a genetic disease or a category of diseases caused by the accumulation of mutations. Most of the mutations are somatic and occur only in an individual's cancer cells, but about 1 percent of all cancers are associated with a hereditary syndrome, and individuals with these hereditary syndromes carry the mutation in every cell of their body (Fearon, 1997). Advances in biotechnology had enabled scientists to identify normal genes that stimulate cell proliferation. These genes undergo mutation as a result of exposure to carcinogens, and the disruption in their function results in abnormal cell growth. In addition to these genes, which are called *oncogenes*, suppressor genes suppress the growth of tumors. Mutation or damage to these genes also causes abnormal growth.

Much of the new knowledge about the prevention, diagnosis, and treatment of cancer had resulted from the study of cells at the genetic level and had become possible through the use of new technologies such as the polymerase chain reaction. New technologies included nuclear magnetic resonance imaging and computer modeling. In addition, the ability to identify genetic markers had contributed to the ability to detect inherited susceptibility to cancer, and some marker genes such as the *BRCA1* gene had been identified.

Progress in the detection of cancer had been affected by new or improved imaging technologies such as mammography for the detection of breast cancer. Instead of using open surgical techniques, it had become possible to use image-guided procedures that would allow biopsy needles to precisely collect minute tumor samples. In general, it became possible to use less invasive procedures to obtain more reliable results.

In the area of treatment, the greatest improvements were achieved against the cancers that occur during childhood. Improvements in bone marrow transplantation techniques had also taken place. The quality of life for cancer survivors had improved through advances in treatment involving better conservation of function. Improvements in the use of counseling, support groups, and behavioral techniques had also taken place.

In the area of prevention, progress had occurred on a number of fronts. For example, there had been progress in understanding the relationship between environmental secondhand smoke and lung cancer. As a result, increasing prohibitions against smoking in public places and the work site had taken place. The observed reduction in smoking rates (from 50 percent in 1950 to 26 percent in 1993) was expected to have a significant impact on rates of death, not only deaths due to lung cancer but also those due to cancers of the mouth, pharynx, esophagus, and bladder. The reduction in the smoking rate would also reduce the numbers of deaths from heart disease. However, the NCI warned that the rate of progress in reducing the numbers of deaths would be slow.

Progress in prevention occurred in other areas as well. Research had strengthened the evidence of a connection between diet, nutrition, and cancer, but the preventive effects of dietary change were expected to be measurable only over a period of many years. In addition, the Women's Health Initiative Hormone Trial investigated the impact of combined estrogen and progesterone therapy and its association with breast cancer. Further, on the cutting edge of prevention research were early attempts to use biomarkers and intermediate endpoints as a means of identifying individuals who were likely to develop cancer and for whom justifiable interventions exist. The use of such markers would shorten the time and the number of patients needed to complete an intervention trial.

With respect to environmental carcinogens, new knowledge concerning the synergistic effects of multiple environmental exposures such as cigarette smoke and asbestos had been gained, and many of the known workplace carcinogens had been removed from common use. However, the scientific evidence that could be used to connect particular environmental risks to specific diseases had not yet been well developed.

Whereas cancer prevention research sought to establish the efficacies of preventive interventions, cancer control sought to develop effective strategies that could be used to translate them into practice. The Institute's progress report included specific advances in several areas, including the following:

- control of tobacco use;
- development of information dissemination programs about screening for the detection of breast and cervical cancers;
- development of strategies to reach special populations at high risk; increased public interest and activism in reducing cancer risk and participating in screening and early-detection programs;
- improving the quality for life of cancer survivors;
- recognition of the importance of population-based health care providers in the dissemination of state-of-the-art cancer prevention and treatment; and
- educational efforts to inform individuals about reducing their risk of cancer through dietary modification.

This was an impressive record of accomplishments, and it was accompanied by statistics that showed that there had been progress against some cancers, little change in progress against other cancers, and significantly increasing public health problems posed by still other cancers.

Progress Report 2

A different assessment of the War on Cancer was best expressed by John Bailar, the first director of cancer prevention research at NCI, although it was also held by others. His view was that the War on Cancer had been a failure. This was not a new conclusion for Bailar and colleagues (Bailar and Gornik, 1997; Bailar and Smith, 1986), and the overall mortality statistics supplied by the Institute were consistent with his conclusion. Despite the War on Cancer, the numbers of deaths from cancer had increased, and different interpretations had been made to explain the increase. The largest contribution to the increase was due to lung cancer. Those rates were beginning to fall for men but were still rising for women. When one excluded lung cancer from the statistics, the conclusions allowed one to be optimistic, but the reason for excluding lung cancer was recognition of the fact that deaths from lung cancer would decrease only over a period of many years, even if the rate of smoking were sharply reduced. The greatest impact would come from an emphasis on smoking prevention rather than smoking cessation. Bailar and colleagues concluded that the Institute needed to change its strategy if it wanted to win the War. It needed to emphasize prevention.

Progress Report 3

The view of Bailar and colleagues was not as negative as that held by a small segment of the public, especially those who are more favorably disposed to the use of "natural" remedies. Their view is that there is a conspiracy among researchers and the pharmaceutical industry to suppress a cure for cancer because it is a lucrative business. Cancer treatments are expensive for patients but rewarding for those who devote their careers or their investments to cancer treatment. In their view, there is no incentive to find a real cure. This is not a scientific perspective, but the perception should not be ignored.

FINALLY, SOME GOOD NEWS

In 1998 there was finally some good news about the rate of mortality from cancer, the kind of news that suggested that the War on Cancer is being won. The American Cancer Society, along with NCI, the Centers for Disease Control and Prevention, and the National Center for Health Statistics (NCHS), released a report card to the nation (Wingo et al., 1998) indicating that for the period from 1990 to 1995 death rates from cancer for all sites of cancer combined decreased 0.5 percent per year, after increasing 0.4 percent per year between 1973 and 1990. This was a significant change in direction. The declines per year for all sites of cancer combined were significant among African Americans (–0.8 percent), whites (–0.4 percent), and Hispanics (–0.6 percent). For Asians and Pacific Islanders the death rates from cancer for all sites combined were not changed because the rate increased for females and decreased for males. Cancer remains the leading cause of death among women of Asian and Pacific Islander decent; this is not the case among any other ethnic or gender group. Among males, the rate of mortality from prostate cancer increased 1.6 percent per year during the same period. Among white and African-American females, rates of lung cancer increased 1.7 and 1.0 percent per year, respectively (Wingo et al., 1998).

These data would be even more impressive if the reasons for the declines were understood. In the case of lung cancer the decrease is clearly related to the smoking rate reductions that have taken place over the past 30 years, suggesting the effectiveness of previous cancer control programs. The reasons for the decrease in the rate of mortality from prostate cancer remain unclear. The decline in the rate of mortality from breast cancer among white females is most likely due to the increased use of mammography, but there was no decrease in the rate of mortality from breast cancer among black females, despite the increased use of mammography by that group. The decline in colorectal cancer among all ethnic groups is also not satisfactorily explained.

The report was immediately challenged by the Intercultural Cancer Council (ICC) on the grounds that the database from which the statistics were drawn had major blind spots that leave nearly half of the U.S. population, especially minority and poor individuals, undercounted (Intercultural Cancer Council, 1998). ICC urged that the director of NCI follow his commitment to place a high priority on achieving better statistics on the rate of cancer among these populations.

The director of NCI, Richard Klausner, presented a more optimistic note to Congress. He pointed out that the problem of cancer among ethnic minority populations is not monolithic but varies by ethnic group, gender, and disease site, with some ethnic groups having lower rates of some cancers than the overall population. When questioned by Representative Louis Stokes about the disparity in the rate of mortality from cancer among African Americans, Klausner noted that there had been a decline in mortality among African Americans. When questioned about the Institute's ability to make good use of increased funds, Klausner stated, "We know cancer is a complicated puzzle, but I actually believe we know what we need to do to push us much farther to knowing what the puzzle looks like. I don't know how long it will take to finish, and I don't know what we will find, but we really do know what to do" (The Cancer Letter, 1998, p. 4).

THE HEALTHY PEOPLE 2000 REVIEW

Another way of assessing progress is on the basis of the Healthy People 2000 cancer objectives. NCI organized the progress review for a meeting chaired by the Surgeon General on April 17, 1998. That review focused on the 17 objectives in the *Healthy People 2000* cancer priority area (U.S. Public Health Service, 1991). In 1995, the year 2000 target for overall death rates from all forms of cancer was achieved with the finding of a rate of 130 cases reported per 100,000 population. In 1995, the death rate among African Americans had exceeded the year 2000 target of 175 by reaching 172 per 100,000 population. Deaths from cervical cancer, however, were continuing to rise among African-American and Hispanic women to levels of 5.2 and 3.1 per 100,000 population, respectively, whereas the death rate from cervical cancer for all females was 2.5 per 100,000 population in 1995. This increase was disturbing, given that with the present state of knowledge, death from this form of cancer is practically preventable. The decrease in deaths from colorectal cancer exceeded the year 2000 target. Smoking rates among African Americans, Hispanics, and American Indians and Alaska Natives ages 18 years and older decreased to 26, 18, and 25 percent, respectively, but the smoking rate among African-American adolescents had begun to rise. Among Vietnamese males the smoking rate had decreased sharply from the 1984 to 1988 baseline of 55 percent to 35 percent in 1990. The average daily intake of vegetables, fruits, and grain products was moving toward the year 2000 target, with the daily intake of grain products exceeding the target of 6.0 servings. The proportion of primary care providers who routinely counsel patients about tobacco use cessation had exceeded the year 2000 target of 75 percent. In 1994, 56 percent of all females ages 50 years and older had received a clinical breast examination and mammogram. For African-American females the rate was 56 percent, whereas for Hispanics and low-income females the rates were 50 and 38 percent, respectively. The year 2000 target is 60 percent for all groups. In 1994, 94 percent of females reported having received a Pap smear. The proportion of Hispanic females ages 18 years and over who had ever received a Pap smear had increased from 75 percent in 1987 to 91 percent in 1994. The year 2000 target is 95 percent. Death rates from oral cancer were decreasing, but the rate among African Americans was still about twice as high as that among the general population.

MORE GOOD NEWS

There was more good news in 1998, especially relating to the prevention and treatment of breast cancer. In April of 1998, NCI announced results of the Breast Cancer Prevention Trial, which demonstrated that tamoxifen was effective in preventing breast cancer (National Cancer Institute, 1998a). The data showed a 45 percent reduction in breast cancer incidence among the high-risk participants who took tamoxifen. In addition, herceptin was shown to be effective in targeting the abnormal gene *HER-2/neu*. This gene occurs in 30 percent of patients with breast cancer. As in other cases, these announcements reflect the fact that there is a substantial investment in research over many years before success is finally achieved.

THE FUNDAMENTAL QUESTIONS

The fundamental questions being asked by members of the public and their elected representatives can be expressed in simple terms: Is there a strategic plan for reducing the numbers of deaths from cancer, and when can measurable results be expected? Progress Report 1 did not provide satisfactory answers to these questions because the strategic plan, if it existed, appeared to place a high priority on understanding the mechanisms of the development and spread of cancer, and there was no evidence that there was an overall reduction in the number of deaths from cancer.

Progress Report 2, an assessment performed independently of NCI, stated that the wrong strategy was pursued and suggested that a prevention strategy would yield the desired results. These are only partial answers to the questions. Knowing and removing the cause of disease can often achieve substantial results without providing an understanding of the underlying mechanisms, but even then, change does not always occur quickly. Lung cancer is highly preventable and the relationship between tobacco use and cancer has been known since 1950, but the rates of mortality from lung cancer have only recently begun to decline and the rate among women is still rising. Furthermore, cancer is not a single disease affecting one organ, but rather, it is a complex of diseases related to a variety of factors. Prevention efforts are long term and require a broad spectrum of disciplines, and individuals trained to work in these disciplines are in short supply.

Progress Report 3 is partially the result of a failure to provide an adequate answer to the fundamental question.

The 1998 report card (Wingo et al., 1998), based on data from the NCI SEER program and NCHS, provides more evidence that progress is actually occurring, but notes that not all populations have benefited equally from advances against cancer. It also suggested that progress will be slow. The *Healthy People 2000* report (U.S. Public Health Service, 1991) indicates that progress has exceeded expectations in some areas but has been disappointing in others. Good news about prevention (tamoxifen) and treatment (herceptin) might emphasize the need to continue vigorous efforts on both fronts.

Following publication of the reports of the panels on Measuring the Progress Against Cancer (Extramural Committee to Assess Measures of Progress Against Cancer, 1990), a special National Cancer Advisory Board Committee concluded that much of the cause of the failure to achieve the desired results was beyond the domain of NCI. It clearly defined three research categories: basic research (the foundation and engine), translational research (the bridge between basic research and application), and applications research (in which the participants were neither researchers nor the funding agencies). The NCI-designated cancer centers were to be the primary bodies conducting the research, along with the community clinical oncology programs and the clinical trials cooperative groups. The centers and related programs were to participate in public information programs, community outreach activities, and training programs for community-based physicians. The committee offers a more thorough discussion of the cancer centers in Chapter 3.

The current director is reorganizing NCI, giving special attention to the Division of Cancer Control and Population Science, and is reportedly interested in improving the quality of care provided to poor, ethnic minority, and elderly populations with cancer.

The fundamental questions mentioned above will continue to be asked in a variety of ways. From the perspective of this committee, however, the question can be framed as follows: *Is there a strategic plan for reducing the numbers of deaths from cancer among poor and minority individuals, and when can results be expected?*

2
The Burden of Cancer Among Ethnic Minorities and Medically Underserved Populations

This chapter focuses on the burden of cancer among ethnic minorities and medically underserved populations. These deceptively simple terms conceal the degree of complexity involved in defining the populations and the disease. The chapter therefore discusses the problems associated with defining "minorities" and "underserved individuals," the complexity of the disease commonly known as cancer, the findings that describe the burden of cancer in these groups, and the conclusions derived from those data. The limitations of current federal cancer surveillance data are then discussed, followed by recommendations for the improvement of cancer surveillance among ethnic minority and medically underserved populations. Finally, a discussion of surveillance needs for cancer risk factor and control research is presented, with recommendations for National Institutes of Health (NIH) programs.

DEFINING THE POPULATIONS

Federal Definitions of Race and Ethnicity

The simplest way of defining ethnic minority groups would be to use the census counts for the distribution of the total U.S. population, but it would first be necessary to have an appropriate method of classifying the various groups in the population. Herein lies the first problem. The existing federal classification by race and ethnicity was established by the U.S. Office of Management and Budget (OMB) in its Statistical Policy Directive No. 15, "Race and Ethnic Standards for Federal Statistics and Administrative Reporting" (U.S. Office of Management and Budget, 1997; see Box 2-1). Directive No. 15 requires that all federal agencies collect and report demographic data according to a limited number of racial and ethnic categories, despite criticism that such a classification scheme fails to recognize the increasing ethnic diversity of the U.S. population (U.S. Bureau of the Census, 1998a).

Definitions of race, ethnicity, or origin are not included within the Directive, although the categories and inclusion criteria for the categories are given. OMB specifies four minimum categories for race, which include American Indian or Alaska Native, black or African American, white, and Asian or Pacific Islander. The two categories for data on ethnicity are Hispanic or Latino and Not Hispanic or Not Latino. The latest revisions to the Directive separated the Asian or Pacific Islander populations into two categories, and the term "Hispanic" was changed to "Hispanic or Latino." OMB recommends that these new revisions of the categories be adopted by other federal programs as soon as possible, but the official deadline for adoption of the requirement is January 1, 2003. Modifications to Directive No. 15 were made at the recommendation of the Interagency Committee for the Review of the Racial and Ethnic Standards, which suggested that changes are needed to reflect the nation's population (U.S. Bureau of the Census, 1998a).

A number of scientific and professional organizations have criticized the Directive, stating that the standards lack scientific utility and do not encompass the diverse range of peoples in the United States. For example, the American Anthropological Association (AAA) has commented that OMB has noted the absence of "scientific or anthropological" foundations in developing its categories (American Anthropological Association, 1997). However, the race and ethnicity categories of the Directive are regularly used in federally sponsored scientific research and the interpretations of the findings are often based on the variables of race and ethnicity. (The scientific utility of the concept of race and its use in epidemiologic and health research will be discussed later in this chapter.) AAA also criticized the fact that Directive No. 15 did not explain what is meant by "race" or "origin" or the difference between the two concepts.

In addition, it is not clear whether the race or origins of people were to be chosen by the individual respondent (self-identification) or by others such as interviewers. Many discrepancies in these two methods may arise in the process of sampling populations, although the Bureau of the Census department disagrees (Sink, 1997). In the U.S. census, respondents are allowed to self-identify their racial and ethnic background. In other health research, however, both methods may be used. Further, it is unclear what the impact will be for the reporting of health statistics for population groups of the policy change in the year 2000 census allowing respondents to report more than one category of racial and ethnic background. Many federal agencies, including the National Cancer Institute (NCI), are attempting to address these challenges to identify populations accurately and trace any possible risk factors affecting their health.

Robert Hahn of the Centers for Disease Control and Prevention (CDC) points out the varying and conflicting definitions of race and ethnicity used by federal agencies, and noted the difficulty this situation creates for comparing populations. He notes four assumptions that must be confronted and redressed to operationalize such an effort (Hahn, 1992). These four assumptions have allowed for an ambiguity about terms that define or characterize racial and ethnic groups. Too often, he argues, it is assumed that:

1. Government agencies have no conflicting classifications of denominator for disease rates, that classifications do not vary by region, sub-group, or individual, and do not change over time;
2. Racial and ethnic categories are understood by the populations questioned and that understanding does not vary by region, sub-group, or individual;
3. Survey enumeration, participation, and response rates are high and similar for all racial and ethnic populations;
4. Individual responses to questions of racial and ethnic identity are consistent in different surveys and at different times.

These assumptions lead to inaccurate data by miscounting or misunderstanding both the base population denominator and the numerator (Scrimshaw and McMiller, 1996).

Defining Ethnicity and Race

Anthropologists and other social scientists view "race" and "ethnicity" differently from the federal definitions of population groups noted above. In fact, the federal definitions as currently applied mix and confuse the concepts of race and ethnicity, thereby reinforcing the outmoded concept of race, failing to allow the important concept of ethnicity to be fully functional, and failing to acknowledge recent advances in our understanding of the role that genetics plays in illness and susceptibility to illness. Ethnicity is a recent term that involves how one sees oneself and how one is "seen by others as part of a group on the basis of presumed ancestry and sharing a common destiny with others on the basis of this background" (Zenner, 1996, p. 393). Common threads that may tie one to an ethnic group include skin color, religion, language, customs, ancestry, and occupational or regional features. In addition, persons belonging to the same

BOX 2-1
OMB Directive No. 15 (adopted May 12, 1977): Excerpts from Race and Ethnic Standards for Federal Statistics and Administrative Reporting

This directive provides standard classifications for recordkeeping, collection, and presentation of data on race and ethnicity in Federal program administrative reporting and statistical activities. These classifications should not be interpreted as being scientific or anthropological in nature, nor should they be viewed as determinants of eligibility for participation in any Federal program. They have been developed in response to needs expressed by both the executive branch and the Congress to provide for the collection and use of compatible, nonduplicated, exchangeable racial and ethnic data by Federal agencies.

1. Definitions

The basic racial and ethnic categories for Federal statistics and program administrative reporting are defined as follows:

A. **American Indian or Alaskan** [sic] **Native**.* A person having origins in any of the original peoples of North America, and who maintains cultural identification through tribal affiliations or community recognition.
B. **Asian or Pacific Islander.** A person having origins in any of the original peoples of the Far East, Southeast Asia, the Indian subcontinent, or the Pacific Islands. This area includes, for example, China, India, Japan, Korea, the Philippine Islands, and Samoa.
C. **Black**. A person having origins in any of the black racial groups of Africa.
D. **Hispanic.** A person of Mexican, Puerto Rican, Cuban, Central or South American or other Spanish culture or origin, regardless of race.
E. **White.** A person having origins in any of the original peoples of Europe, North Africa, or the Middle East.

2. Utilization of Recordkeeping and Reporting

To provide flexibility, it is preferable to collect data on race and eth-

*This population is currently referred to as "Alaska Native."

nicity separately. If separate race and ethnic categories are used, the minimum designations are:

a. **Race:**
— American Indian or Alaskan [sic] Native
— Asian or Pacific Islander
— Black
— White

b. **Ethnicity:**
— Hispanic origin
— Not of Hispanic origin

When race and ethnicity are collected separately, the number of White and Black persons who are Hispanic must be identifiable, and capable of being reported in that category.

If combined format is used to collect racial and ethnic data, the minimum acceptable categories are:

American Indian or Alaskan [sic] Native
Asian or Pacific Islander
Black, not of Hispanic origin
Hispanic
White, not of Hispanic origin.

The category which most closely reflects the individual's recognition in his community should be used for purposes of reporting on persons who are of mixed racial and/or ethnic origins.

In no case should the provision of this Directive be construed to limit the collection of data to the categories described above. However, any reporting required which uses more detail shall be organized in such a way that the additional categories can be aggregated into these basic racial/ethnic categories.

SOURCE: U.S. Office of Management and Budget (1997).

ethnic group share a unique history different from that of other ethnic groups (American Anthropological Association, 1997; Zenner, 1996). Usually, a combination of these features identifies an ethnic group. For example, physical appearance alone does not consistently identify one as belonging to a particular ethnic group; individuals belonging to certain ethnic groups may vary widely in physical appearance (e.g., skin color and hair texture), but they share a common ethnic identity. In the U.S., there are "macro" ethnic groups, such as Latinos or Hispanics, which have many sub-groups, such as Mexicans, Mexican Americans, Cubans, Puerto Ricans, and so on. "Race," in contrast, represents a social or cultural construct of human variability based on perceived differences in biology, physical appearance, and behavior (American Anthropological Association, 1997; Smedley, 1999). The problems with the concept of race for purposes of health research will be discussed later in this chapter.

It is useful in medical and epidemiologic research to distinguish ethnic groups from one another, provided that researchers are clear on the nature and source of human variation (e.g., cultural and behavioral patterns, environmental influences) and their relationship to health outcomes. Membership in an ethnic group may be associated with behavioral and environmental factors which may increase or decrease the likelihood of illness. Thus, the availability of pertinent information for a diversity of ethnic groups would assist both those involved in health research and the population as a whole by indicating if any ethnic differences need to be further explored. Such research, however, can be accomplished only by clearly identifying population groups and understanding that human identity is not static or mutually exclusive. Ethnicity can be a product of interaction between people of different origins and identities. The "boundaries" of ethnic identity, however, are still unclear. Some may identify themselves as belonging to a particular group in one context, and to another group in a different context. "Identities thus become circumstantial" (Zenner, 1996, p. 394). Ethnicity is more flexible, fluid, or perceived, than rigid or fixed. This has been compounded by the increased number of mixed ethnicity families in this country, where individuals may claim two or more ethnicities, or give different ethnic identifications at different times or for different purposes. This makes the proposed revisions for the year 2000 census all the more important, as federally sponsored health research will need to account for individuals who identify themselves as from diverse backgrounds.

Medically Underserved Populations

In the study of cancer, considerable attention has been given to "minorities" as a group, but medically underserved individuals make up a separate group that cuts across all ethnic groups. The term "medically underserved" is sometimes used to include underinsured or uninsured people; those with low levels of education; rural and inner-city populations; unemployed people; or those with low socioeconomic status (SES). As noted below, no consistent definition of "medically underserved" populations appears in the NIH descriptions of this construct.

Socioeconomic Status

Social class is traditionally measured through socioeconomic indicators such as education, income, and occupation (Adler et al., 1994). Many problems have been linked to low SES such as crime (Reiman, 1997), ill health (Pincus and Callahan, 1995), poor education (Levine and Nidiffer, 1996) and inadequate access to health care. Criticism and controversy have existed over which indexes have appropriately or inappropriately assessed SES to characterize social determinants of health. Schneider (1986) criticizes the use of common measures of SES such as Hollingshead's Four Factor Index of Social Status and Duncan's Socioeconomic Index for all occupations, noting the paucity of information on household patterns, social relationships, and the historical context of people's lives, all of which are factors that may mediate social status. Schneider advocates the use of an index that includes race or ethnicity, a detailed work history, autonomy, and decision-making authority. Lillie-Blanton and LaVeist (1996) agree that these factors in one's social environment (including power arrangements such as political empowerment and individual and community control and influence) are related to one's physical and mental health. A person may be working or living in an environment that exposes him or her to toxins that directly affect health, yet social relations and the conditions of one's neighborhood and work environment can also affect health. The latter experiences may shape the sense of "self worth, influence linkages to social structure and develop adaptive skills" (Lillie-Blanton and La Viest, 1996, p. 85).

Many researchers have made the mistake of attributing the health disparities between groups to race or ethnicity without paying close attention to socioeconomic variability. Lillie-Blanton and LaVeist (1996) explain the social context of health by describing an individual's SES as an "expression of the educational and economic opportunities available in one's social environment" (p. 84). They suggest that SES may be more relevant than race or ethnicity in assessing one's socioeconomic context or social environment. This approach not only incorporates the individual, but also incorporates the social forces that also affect individuals and their health.

Socioeconomic Status and Cancer

A number of factors have been implicated in the relatively poor cancer outcomes for populations of lower SES. Disparities in cancer incidence by SES can be explained by differential levels of exposure to environmental carcinogens, differences in personal health habits (e.g., cigarette smoking, poor diet, and lack of education regarding health risks), and other sociocultural factors. Some negative health behaviors are more prevalent among people of lower SES, but these behaviors should not be considered only as matters of purely personal choice. One's social environment can pose barriers to awareness and to making changes in behavior. Individuals living in poverty, for example, have poorer access to information regarding cancer risks and health behavior, to nutritious foods that may diminish cancer risk, and to role models in the form of cancer survivors who can relay information regarding help-seeking. On the other hand, individuals living in poverty "tend to concentrate on day-to-day survival and often develop a sense of hopelessness and powerlessness and become socially isolated" (Freeman, 1990, p. 18), all of which may contribute to negative health behaviors and decreased survival.

Poverty or low SES has not been implicated as a direct cause for a higher incidence of cancer, although research has found that it has an adverse relationship to survival rates. The American Cancer Society estimates that cancer survival rates of poor individuals are 10 to 15 percent lower than those of other Americans (American Cancer Society, 1990). For example, more affluent women have a higher incidence of breast cancer, yet their survival rates surpass those for women living under disadvantaged socioeconomic conditions. Some of the proposed reasons for the disparities in survival rates between the groups are that women of lower SES are diagnosed or seek treatment at later stages of the disease, compared to women in higher income brackets. The results of the 1990 U.S. National Health Interview Survey show that "poorer" women (i.e., those whose annual income was less than $15,200) were significantly less likely to receive Pap smears and mammograms within the previous year than women whose income was at least $46,500. The survey reported that the upper-income women were twice as likely to have received a Pap smear and almost three times as likely to have had a mammogram within the previous year compared with women of low SES. It is suggested that poorer people have fewer opportunities to seek preventive care because of life obstacles, such as difficulties in finding a job or having job security, arranging child care, and arranging transportation (Harvard Center for Cancer Prevention, 1996).

Friedell, Linville, and Hullet (1998), in discussing cancer control efforts among low-income women, note that

> some barriers to increasing participation in cancer control exist at all socioeconomic levels, e.g., lack of information about cancer and about both the availability and the benefit of cancer screening. Fear of what might be found during such an examination mitigates against women either gaining information about cancer or doing something with the information once it is obtained. Other barriers . . . are more prevalent in low-income, medically underserved populations (Friedell, Linville, and Hullet, 1998, p. 1869).

These barriers are noted in Table 2-1.

Even after the diagnosis of cancer, not all groups of people are given the opportunity to receive the same quality of treatment. In one study reviewing lung cancer treatment patterns for more than 1,800 patients in New England hospitals, researchers found that more educated and privately insured individuals received more aggressive therapy than those without these attributes. In addition, people of lower SES seek health care more often in emergency room settings because they are underinsured or uninsured, which diminishes the continuity of care (Harvard Center for Cancer Prevention, 1996). This lack of proper and continuous care for individuals of lower SES subjects many to higher cancer mortality rates.

Tracing cancer disparities between groups of different SES continues

TABLE 2-1 Barriers to Optimal Cancer Screening, Diagnosis, and Treatment

- Poverty
- Isolation
  - Geographic
  - Transportation
  - Literacy
  - Age
  - Cultural
    - "Fatalism"
    - Male dominance
    - Putting the family's needs above one's own
- Fear
  - Fear that cancer will be diagnosed
  - Fear of the exam (e.g., mammogram and proctoscopy)
- Acceptability of the service provided
  - Physical arrangements, visiting time
  - Hours of service
  - Staff attitudes
  - Language barriers
  - Cultural understanding by staff
- Lack of continuity of care

SOURCE: Friedell et al. (1998), with additions by the study committee.

to prove to be complex when integrating other factors such as psychological responses to illness. Exposure to psychological stresses and a lack of coping skills or resources also affect survival from cancer. Individuals of lower SES are less likely to have social networks and support than those of higher SES, because the former may lack employment or other social resources in their communities. Such social supports contribute to a sense of connection to others, aiding in one's ability to deal with an illness such as cancer (Harvard Center for Cancer Prevention, 1996). Increased research support in this area may demonstrate that strengthening social support for those with cancer in disadvantaged communities can help to lower mortality rates when the many components of lower SES prove less amenable to intervention.

In summary, poverty "is a proxy for other elements of living, including lack of education, unemployment, substandard housing, poor nutrition, risk-promoting lifestyle and behavior, and diminished access to health care" (Freeman, 1990, p. 18), all of which affect an individual's chances of developing cancer and surviving it.

NCI does not define SES in its report to this committee (National Cancer Institute, 1998b), although it does consider individuals of low income as "special populations," without further defining that group. Nevertheless, studies are underway at NCI to evaluate the extent to which racial and ethnic disparities in cancer incidence may be related to SES factors (see Chapter 3). As noted above, however, the term "low SES" could imply the existence of a number of cancer risk factors, yet for the low-income group within the NCI's "special populations" portfolio the focus seems to be only on the lack of monetary resources. It is therefore unclear what populations are referred to, or what needs should be addressed first (i.e., education, income, insurance status, or social environment) to reduce the risk of cancer.

Ethnicity, Socioeconomic Status and Health

Unfortunately, differences in SES among U.S. ethnic groups exist. When examined collectively, African Americans and Hispanics are three times as likely as whites to be poor, according to U.S. Census Bureau (as reported by the National Center for Health Statistics, 1998; see Table 2-2). Such gaps have been related to inequalities in the levels of educational and economic attainment associated with racial barriers (Gimenez, 1989; Lillie-Blanton and LaVeist, 1996; Harvard Center for Cancer Prevention, 1996). Low SES and ethnic minority status are not synonymous, but many members of ethnic minority groups who also have low income comprise an important proportion of underserved populations in the United States. Low-income ethnic minorities are least likely to have a regular source of

TABLE 2-2 Percentage of People Below Poverty Level, 1996

Race and Hispanic Origin	Percent Below Poverty Level
All races	12.8
White	10.0
Black or African American	30.7
Asian or Pacific Islander	14.1
Hispanic origin	26.2
American Indian	31.2

SOURCE: U.S. Bureau of the Census, as reported by the National Center for Health Statistics (1998).

TABLE 2-3 Percent and Number of Individuals Below Poverty Level, by Ethnicity and Metropolitan Region, 1987

	Metropolitan		Non-Metropolitan	
Ethnicity	Percent	Number	Percent	Number
White	9.6	13.3 million	13.7	6.6 million
African American	30.7	7.3 million	44.1	2.2 million
Hispanic	27.6	3.9 million	35.6	0.6 million

SOURCE: U.S. Congress, Office of Technology Assessment (1990).

primary care (i.e., family doctor or clinic; Giachello, 1994). Many of these ethnic minority group members do not know where to go when they get sick (Robert Wood Johnson Foundation, 1997). When a regular source of care is reported, it tends to be a public health care facility, a hospital outpatient clinic, or an emergency room (Giachello, 1994; Robert Wood Johnson Foundation, 1997). Members of ethnic minority groups are also least likely to have insurance coverage. Approximately one-third of the Hispanic population does not have health insurance coverage, and the problem is most severe among Mexican Americans and Central Americans (Giachello, 1993; Naranjo, 1992; Valdez et al., 1993).

Conversely, the largest numbers of low-SES persons are white, and many of them have the same health care access problems as do members of minority groups (Friedell, Linville, and Hullet, 1998). Nearly 20 million white Americans lived below the poverty line in 1987, as depicted in Table 2-3, with many of these living in non-metropolitan, rural areas.

Special Populations

NCI states that several ethnic minority populations have "disturbingly" high cancer incidence and mortality rates for cancers at some sites. These disparities, they state, may be genetically triggered, although the incidence more likely reflects differences in environmental exposures, risk behaviors, and utilization of prevention, screening, treatment, and rehabilitation services (National Cancer Institute, 1998b). These and other "underserved" populations have inadequate access to or reduced rates of utilization of high-quality cancer-related services or cancer programs. NCI refers to these groups as "special populations." In its report, *NCI Initiatives for Special Populations, 1998,* the Institute writes:

> The term "special populations" encompasses those ethnic and racial groups designated by the U.S. government (namely Alaska Natives, American Indians, Native Hawaiians, Pacific Islanders, Asians, Hispanics or Latinos, and Blacks or African Americans). In many instances, these groups experience higher cancer incidence and/or mortality rates, or have been relatively underserved in terms of cancer programs. The National Cancer Institute (NCI) working definition of "special populations" also includes the elderly, low-income and low-literate individuals. The term "underserved" is meant to refer to populations that have inadequate access to, or reduced utilization of, high quality cancer prevention, screening and early detection, treatment, and/or rehabilitation services. (National Cancer Institute, 1998b, p. 1)

The NCI report did not define low-income individuals or groups with low levels of literacy. One could be led to believe that low-income groups could be interchanged with groups living under the poverty level, given that NCI follows OMB's recommendations, as well as those of the U.S. Bureau of the Census, which reports estimates of the numbers of people in the United States living under the poverty level. The low-income group, which is part of the "special populations" group, could possibly include some of the 15.6 percent of Americans who did not have health insurance during all of 1996. It was unclear if the low-income group includes some of the 14.4 million people in 1996 who had incomes of less than half of the poverty level, up from 13.9 million in 1995 (U.S. Bureau of the Census, 1997). NCI notes that the nomenclature for these groups is not standardized across the NIH.

Among the changes being considered within NCI's new Division of Cancer Control and Population Science (DCCPS) is the use of the term "special populations." According to Division Director Barbara Rimer, "the definition of 'special' should emerge from data and will change over time" (Barbara Rimer, National Cancer Institute, communication with the study committee, June 12, 1998). The committee agrees with this statement, and recognizes the difficulty of trying to classify a heterogeneous group, but the statement did not suggest the kind of data that would prompt a change in name. One way of interpreting this would be to assume that the emphasis would be on risk and that "special populations" would include those populations at highest risk. On the other hand, understanding the factors related to cancer would involve a careful study of the differences between those who are at highest risk and those who are at lowest risk. In the end, it does not matter so much who is defined as "special" as that there be consistency within NCI—and within NIH in general—with respect to how the term is defined.

Defining populations under study is a critical first step to adequately addressing needs of groups most burdened by cancer. The committee therefore offers the following recommendation:

> **Recommendation 2-1: NIH should develop and implement across all institutes a uniform definition of "special populations" with cancer. This definition should be flexible but should be based on disproportionate or insufficiently studied burdens of cancer, as measured by cancer incidence, morbidity, mortality, and survival statistics.**

A consistent definition of "special populations" would therefore result from a thorough assessment of cancer burden among specific groups, including data on cancer incidence, mortality, survival, and access to and utilization of cancer services or cancer programs. Where these data are lacking, special efforts should be made to increase data collection and availability. Presumably, these definitions will change as groups at greatest risk for or experiencing disproportionate cancer burden are identified.

THE BURDEN OF CANCER AMONG ETHNIC MINORITIES AND MEDICALLY UNDERSERVED POPULATIONS

Cancer was the eighth leading cause of death in the United States at the beginning of the 20th century. Today it is the second leading cause of death. Current estimates indicate that cancer is responsible for one of every four deaths in the United States, second only to cardiovascular disease. The combined national cost of cancer is estimated to be $104 billion, with costs attributed to loss of productivity, medical care, and mortality (National Cancer Institute, 1996c).

Cancer can take the form of more than 100 different diseases, each of which is characterized by the uncontrolled growth of abnormal cells. Researchers have discovered that changes in the genetic material of cells initiate the abnormal growth. Some of the causes of these genetic changes are known, such as tobacco smoke, but others remain elusive. However, the study of the distribution of cancer within the population has led to important developments in cancer prevention and control. The identification of factors associated with an increased risk of cancer (e.g., smoking and lung cancer) allows health professionals and public health experts to target areas for interventions and future research.

In studying cancer in relationship to different population groups, one focuses on those forms that are most prevalent in each group and that are associated with the highest rate of mortality. This means that the same forms of cancer may not be of equal importance for all groups. Because there are so many different forms of cancer and because changes in the prevalence of the disease occur slowly, it is neither practical nor necessary to report routinely on all possible forms of cancer. In addition, because of the complexity of classifying groups, because of the different ways of identifying people within groups at the numerator (i.e., the number of specific cases counted) or denominator (i.e., the number of individuals in a defined group) levels, and because small groups with only a few cases of individuals with cancer will result in unreliable rates, one must be aware of the limitations of data analysis and avoid drawing conclusions beyond what is justified by the quality of the data.

Assessing the Burden of Cancer Among U.S. Population Groups

The responsibility within NIH for assessing the burden of cancer among various groups lies with the NCI, and specifically with the Surveillance, Epidemiology and End Results (SEER) program. The goals of the SEER program are as follows (National Cancer Institute, 1998c):

1. Determine the incidence of cancer in selected geographic areas of the United States with respect to demographic and social characteristics of the population and provide information relevant to the generalizability of the rates to the total U.S. population.
2. Using data from the National Center for Health Statistics, provide cancer mortality rates for the total U.S. as well as by county and state.
3. Monitor trends in cancer incidence and mortality associated with specific forms of cancer with respect to geographic area and demographic, social, ethnic, and biological characteristics of the population.
4. Monitor trends in cancer patient survival with respect to specific forms of cancer, extent of disease, demographic and socioeconomic variables of prognostic importance, and patterns of care.
5. Identify factors related to the length and quality of patient survival through special studies of treatment patterns and other aspects of medical care.

6. Provide a basis for cancer control interventions through the identification of subgroups of the population at high risk of cancer. These groups may be defined by geographic location, demographic variables, variables reflecting socioeconomic status, environmental and occupational exposures, biological characteristics, and factors which measure the effects of host and environment interactions.

7. Conduct surveys of selected subgroups of the covered populations which provide data on the prevalence of cancer risk factors and screening, knowledge, and attitudes related to cancer control.

8. Promote research studies measuring progress in cancer control and that link information from the biomedical and social sciences.

9. Conduct studies of multiple primary cancers with particular emphasis on the identification of iatrogenic cancers.

10. Encourage specialty training in epidemiology, biostatistics, and tumor registry methodology, operation, and management.

Data collection for the SEER program began in 1973 and included the entire states of Connecticut, Iowa, New Mexico, Utah, and Hawaii, and the metropolitan areas of Detroit and San Francisco-Oakland. These seven areas were selected both because of their diverse ethnic subgroups and because of ongoing registration activities. The Commonwealth of Puerto Rico was also included as a participant to "monitor cancer incidence in an industrially developing area with overall low cancer risk" (National Cancer Institute, 1998c, p. 35). Coverage of the SEER program was expanded in 1974 to include representation from southern (New Orleans, Louisiana) and northwestern (Seattle-Puget Sound in Washington state) regions of the country which were not covered in the initial program. The program was further expanded in 1975 to include the metropolitan area of Atlanta, Georgia, which increased coverage of the African-American population, and was expanded again in 1979 to include 10 rural counties in Georgia to provide coverage of a rural, African-American population of 50,000. In 1983, a four-county area of New Jersey was added to increase coverage of African Americans and Hispanics. New Orleans and New Jersey were subsequently dropped from the program for "technical reasons" (National Cancer Institute, 1998c).

In early 1988, an extramural panel of epidemiologists, clinical oncologists, and pathologists was convened to review the accomplishments of the SEER program and make recommendations for the future. They recommended that the scope be expanded to cover a much wider range of surveillance. Specifically, the committee recommended that the "registration areas should be expanded to achieve adequate coverage of those populations—such as ethnic groups, rural dwellers, and the economically deprived—that are not yet sufficiently represented" (National Cancer Institute, 1998c, p. 36). In response to these recommendations, the SEER program was expanded in 1992 to include the county of Los Angeles and the San Jose-Monterey area of California to further increase representation of Hispanics and other ethnic groups of interest. This resulted in a 46 percent increase in the overall, population covered by the SEER program, and increases of 41 percent for African Americans and 223 percent for Hispanics. The relative increases for other groups were also substantial. The current coverage areas of the 11 SEER program contractors are shown in Table 2-4.

In 1997, the NCI Cancer Control Review Group also recommended that SEER program coverage "be expanded to include several populations not adequately represented: Appalachia; the rural south (with emphasis

TABLE 2-4 Areas Covered by the 11 SEER Program Contractors

Registry Location	Year of Entry	First Full Year of Data	Coverage Area
Utah	1973	1973	Entire state
Connecticut	1973	1973	Entire state
Iowa	1973	1973	Entire state
New Mexico	1973	1973	Entire state
Hawaii	1973	1973	Entire state
Detroit, Michigan	1973	1973	Macomb, Oakland, and Wayne counties
San Francisco-Oakland, California	1973	1973	Alameda, Contra Costa, Marin, San Francisco, and San Mateo counties
Seattle, Washington	1974	1975	Clallam, Grays Harbor, Island, Jefferson, King, Kitsap, Mason, Pierce, San Juan, Skagit, Snohomish, Thurston, and Whatcom counties
Atlanta, Georgia	1974	1975	Clayton, Cobb, DeKalb, Fulton, and Gwinnet counties
Rural Georgia	1978	1979	Glasock, Greene Hancock, Jasper, Jefferson, Morgan, Putnam, Taliaferro, Warren, and Washington counties
San Jose-Monterey, California	1992	1993	Monterey, San Benito, Santa Clara, and Santa Cruz counties
Los Angeles, California	1992	1993	Los Angeles County

SOURCE: Miller et al. (1996).

on African Americans); Native Americans; and Hispanics from Cuban, Puerto Rican, and similar ancestries" (National Cancer Institute, 1997a, p. 22–23). To date, this recommendation has not been fully implemented, although it is under study by NCI.

Representation of Ethnic Minorities and Underserved Populations in the SEER Program

With regard to the current sampling configuration, it is apparent that the ethnic minority populations are not equally distributed across the SEER program regions (Miller et al., 1996). For example, most of the SEER program Hispanic population lives in California (69 percent), and Mexican Americans account for the majority of the Hispanic population in that area. Therefore, results from the SEER program may not reflect the lifestyle, environment, or cancer burden among Hispanic groups in other geographic areas such as the Northeast and Florida. Similarly, two-thirds of the Chinese population covered by the SEER program lives in California, as does 54 percent of the Korean population. Half of the SEER program's Japanese population lives in Hawaii, and 40 percent lives in areas of California. The SEER program's urban African-American population is more evenly distributed across the country, with 28 percent in Los Angeles, 25 percent in Detroit, 19 percent in Atlanta, 12 percent in San Francisco, and 8 percent in Connecticut. However, current representation of African Americans in rural areas is limited primarily to the 10 rural counties in Georgia. Numbering approximately 50,000, these African Americans are poorer and less well-educated than whites in the same counties. The majority of the American Indians in the SEER program registry live in New Mexico and Arizona, although the American Indian population resides primarily in other regions of the United States.

The overall percentage of people living below the poverty level and the number of high school graduates in the SEER program registry are similar to those among adults in the United States (13 percent and 78 percent, respectively). Ethnic minority groups are intentionally overrepresented in the SEER program to ensure adequate numbers for statistical purposes (i.e., to allow the enumeration of cancer rates). The populations covered by the SEER program areas, based on the 1990 Census, are shown in Table 2-5 (Miller et al., 1996).

However, even with this expanded coverage, the data for smaller populations are less precise than those for larger groups and must be viewed with caution. Another difficulty in interpreting information from the SEER program is the manner in which racial or ethnic group membership is determined. SEER program data on cancer cases are based on informa-

TABLE 2-5 Populations Covered by the 11 SEER Program Areas

Racial or Ethnic Group	U.S. Population Size	Percent Covered by SEER Program
Total	248,710,000	13.9
White	199,686,000	12.5
Black	29,968,000	12.3
Hispanic	22,354,000	24.9
Native American	1,959,000	27.2
Chinese	1,645,000	43.0
Filipino	1,407,000	49.2
Japanese	848,000	59.9
Korean	799,000	33.8
Vietnamese	615,000	30.7
Hawaiian	211,000	77.6

SOURCE: Miller et al. (1996).

tion in medical records or death certificates, whereas the U.S. Census uses self-designation of race or ethnicity. Surname lists were used to improve the identification of several groups (Hispanic, Chinese, Filipino, Japanese and Korean patients with cancer). These sources of error, however, indicate that "the cancer rates are best used to identify general racial/ethnic patterns of cancer" (Miller et al., 1996, p. 8).

Measuring Progress Against Cancer

The SEER program registry reports on three important pieces of information for selected populations: (1) the occurrence of cancer (incidence); (2) rate of death from cancer (mortality), as reported by the National Center for Health Statistics (NCHS); and (3) the length of survival following cancer diagnosis (survival rate). Incidence measures the frequency of cancer in a group or population. Decreases in cancer incidence can indicate successful efforts in the prevention of cancer. For example, the incidence of cervical cancer has decreased in the United States since the advent of the Pap smear in the 1940s, which detects cervical lesions for treatment before they become cancerous. Conversely, an increase in the prevalence of smoking among women has been reflected in increasing rates of lung cancer in this group. Typically, as in the case of lung cancer among women, increased incidences of cancer precede an increase in mortality (Extramural Committee to Assess Measures of Progress Against Cancer, 1990).

Mortality rates remain the most important measure of the overall progress against cancer. Decreasing rates of death from cancer reflect improvements in both prevention and treatment. Rates of mortality from cancer were steadily increasing in the United States since they were first measured by the SEER program in 1973. However, the recent "Report Card to the Nation" on progress against cancer indicates that this trend was reversed for the first time during 1991–1995, when a decrease in overall cancer mortality in the United States could be shown (Wingo et al., 1998). However, this may not reflect trends in the cancer burden experienced by ethnic minorities and underserved groups.

SEER program data are the major source for cancer survival statistics in the United States, and one of the biggest accomplishments of the War on Cancer has been the ability to measure improvements in the rate of survival among patients with some cancers (American Cancer Society, 1997). Advances in diagnosis and treatment have improved the overall rate of survival among these populations from one in four cancer patients in 1930 to one in two patients today.

Today, no single database provides information on incidence, mortality, and survival data on all cancer cases in the United States. Therefore, SEER program data are frequently used as an estimate of cancer rates in this country. Data from the SEER program are used by legislators, health professionals, advocacy groups, educators, patients, and the public to guide cancer prevention and control efforts, and to allocate funds for research and treatment based on the assumption that SEER program data can be extrapolated to geographic areas and populations not covered by the SEER program. Unfortunately, this assumption does not hold for ethnic minorities and medically underserved populations. It is important that cancer surveillance information truly reflect the national populations for which programs are to be developed if the War on Cancer is to be effective.

Cancer Burden Among Ethnic Minority and Underserved Populations—Existing SEER Program Data

Cancer can strike persons of any age, race, gender or SES. However, the occurrence of cancer, mortality rates, and length of survival can vary from group to group. In fact, research suggests that the cancer experience of ethnic minorities and underserved populations is very different than that of the majority of Americans. Data collected by the SEER program were used to target cancer prevention and control efforts in minorities beginning in 1985, when then Secretary of Health and Human Services Margaret M. Heckler noted a "stubborn disparity" in the cancer experience of minorities in comparison to the nation as a whole (U.S. Department of Health and Human Services, 1985). The SEER program registry does not currently provide reports regarding SES and cancer. Therefore, the discussion in this section is limited to patterns of disease according to the prevailing racial and ethnic classifications.

Cancer Incidence Among Ethnic Minorities

In the United States, African American males experience cancer approximately 15 percent more frequently than white men, according to SEER program data, and have the highest overall incidence of cancer among all racial groups (Miller et al., 1996). This trend is consistent when major sites of cancer (colon and rectum, lung and bronchus, prostate, and stomach) are examined (see Table 2-6). However, it is noteworthy that the incidence of lung cancer in 1992 among white men in Kentucky (111 per 100,000) was almost the same as that reported for African American men in the SEER program data. In Appalachian Kentucky, a region characterized by high poverty, the incidence of lung cancer among white males in 1992 was 127 per 100,000 (Gilbert Friedell, Director for Cancer Control, Kentucky Cancer Program, personal communication, 1998).

TABLE 2-6 Cancer Incidence at Selected Sites Among U.S. Men by Racial or Ethnic Group, Age Adjusted to 1970 U.S. Standards[a]

	Incidence per 100,000 Population				
Racial or Ethnic Group	Stomach	Colon and Rectum	Lung and Bronchus	Prostate	All Sites
Alaska Native	27.2	79.7	81.1	46.1	372
American Indian (New Mexico)	[b]	18.6	14.4	52.5	196
Black	17.9	60.7	117.0	180.6	560
Chinese	15.7	44.8	52.1	46.0	282
Filipino	8.5	35.4	52.6	69.8	274
Hawaiian	20.5	42.4	89.0	57.2	340
Japanese	30.5	64.1	43.0	88.0	322
Korean	48.9	31.7	53.2	24.2	266
Vietnamese	25.8	30.5	70.9	40.0	326
Hispanic (total)	15.3	38.3	41.8	89.0	319
White, non-Hispanic[c]	9.6	57.6	79.0	137.9	481

[a]SEER program estimates are from 1988 to 1992.

[b]SEER program does not calculate incidence when fewer than 25 cases are reported.

[c]Includes medically underserved white, non-Hispanic males among whom the cancer incidence differs from that among the majority white, non-Hispanic population.

SOURCE: Miller et al. (1996).

In general, other ethnic minority groups among the U.S. population have an overall cancer incidence rate that is lower than that of white, non-Hispanic Americans. However, examination of cancer incidence by site of diagnosis and ethnic group suggests several areas of concern. All ethnic minority groups have higher rates of stomach cancer than the majority of white Americans. Korean males, for example, experience up to a fivefold increased incidence of stomach cancer compared to the majority of white Americans (Table 2-6). Similarly, disproportionate rates of cancer of the cervix are observed in many minority women (Table 2-7). For example, African-American and Hispanic women are twice as likely as white women to receive a diagnosis of cervical cancer. However, it is noteworthy that the incidence of cervical cancer among white women in Appalachian Kentucky (14.9 per 100,000) was almost twice as high as the incidence among white women and almost the same as the incidence among African-American women in the United States, according to SEER program data (Friedell, 1992). The rate of cervical cancer among Vietnamese women is an alarming 43.0 per 100,000, whereas it is 7.5 per 100,000 among U.S. white women.

Mortality Among Ethnic Minorities

Among all ethnic groups in the United States, African-American males have the highest overall rate of mortality from cancer (Miller et al., 1996; see Table 2-8). Rates of mortality from prostate cancer are notably high at two to five times higher than the level seen among other groups. Rates of mortality from lung cancer are also high among African-American males (30 percent higher than that among white males).

Examination by site of cancer and ethnic group indicates that ethnic minorities have the highest rate of mortality from stomach cancer. Rates of mortality from cancer of the cervix are also elevated among many groups of ethnic minority women (see Table 2-9). Cancer mortality rates for Native Americans were not reported because of a low incidence (fewer than 25 cases), and information on rates among Koreans and Vietnamese were also not available.

Cancer Survival Among Ethnic Minorities

Examination of survival data from the SEER program (1978 to 1981) gives a dismal picture of progress against cancer in ethnic minorities (Bacquet and Ringen, 1986). Although overall incidence and rates of mortality from cancer for many ethnic minority groups are low in comparison to those for the majority of Americans, survival from cancer is consistently poorer in these groups (Table 2-10). Today, half of all whites with cancer

TABLE 2-7 Cancer Incidence at Selected Sites Among U.S. Women by Racial or Ethnic Group, Age Adjusted to 1970 U.S. Standards[a]

Racial or Ethnic Group	Incidence per 100,000 Population					
	Stomach	Colon and Rectum	Lung and Bronchus	Breast	Cervix Uteri	All Sites
Alaska Native	[b]	67.4	50.6	78.9	15.8	348
American Indian (New Mexico)	[b]	15.3	[b]	31.6	9.9	180
Black	7.6	45.5	44.2	95.4	13.2	326
Chinese	8.3	33.6	25.3	55.0	7.3	213
Filipino	5.3	20.9	17.5	73.1	9.6	224
Hawaiian	13.0	30.5	43.0	105.6	9.3	321
Japanese	15.3	39.5	15.2	82.3	5.8	241
Korean	19.1	21.9	16.0	28.5	15.2	180
Vietnamese	25.8	27.1	31.2	37.5	43.0	273
Hispanic (total)	15.3	24.7	19.5	69.8	16.2	243
White, non-Hispanic[c]	9.6	39.2	43.7	115.7	7.5	354

[a]SEER program estimates are from 1988 to 1992.

[b]SEER program does not calculate incidence when fewer than 25 cases are reported.

[c]Includes medically underserved white, non-Hispanic males among whom the cancer incidence differs from that among the majority white, non-Hispanic population.

SOURCE: Miller et al. (1996).

TABLE 2-8 Cancer Mortality at Selected Sites Among U.S. Men by Racial or Ethnic Group, Age Adjusted to 1970 U.S. Standards[a]

Racial or Ethnic Group	Deaths per 100,000 Population: Stomach	Colon and Rectum	Lung and Bronchus	Prostate	All Sites
Alaska Native	*b*	27.2	69.4	*b*	225
American Indian (New Mexico)	*b*	*b*	*b*	16.2	123
Black	13.6	28.2	44.2	53.7	319
Chinese	10.5	15.7	25.3	6.6	139
Filipino	3.6	11.4	17.5	13.5	105
Hawaiian	14.4	23.7	43.0	19.9	239
Japanese	17.4	20.5	15.2	11.7	133
Korean	NA	NA	16.0	NA	NA
Vietnamese	NA	NA	31.2	NA	NA
Hispanic (Total)	8.4	12.8	19.5	15.3	129
White, non-Hispanic[c]	6.0	23.4	43.7	24.4	217

[a]SEER program estimates are from 1988 to 1992.

[b]SEER program does not calculate mortality when fewer than 25 cases are reported.

[c]Includes medically underserved white, non-Hispanic males among whom the cancer mortality differs from that among the majority white, non-Hispanic population.

SOURCE: Miller et al. (1996).

TABLE 2-9 Cancer Mortality at Selected Sites Among U.S. Women by Racial or Ethnic Group, Age Adjusted to 1970 U.S. Standards[a]

	Incidence per 100,000 Population					
Racial or Ethnic Group	Stomach	Colon and Rectum	Lung and Bronchus	Breast	Cervix Uteri	All Sites
Alaska Native	*b*	24.0	45.3	*b*	*b*	179
American Indian (New Mexico)	*b*	*b*	*b*	*b*	*b*	99
Black	5.6	20.4	31.5	31.4	6.7	168
Chinese	4.8	10.5	18.5	11.2	2.6	86
Filipino	2.5	5.8	10.0	11.9	2.4	63
Hawaiian	12.8	11.4	44.1	25.0	*b*	168
Japanese	9.3	12.3	12.9	12.5	1.5	88
Korean	NA[b]	NA	NA	NA	NA	NA
Vietnamese	NA	NA	NA	NA	NA	NA
Hispanic (total)	4.2	7.3	10.8	15.0	3.4	85
White, non-Hispanic	2.7	15.6	32.9	27.7	2.5	143

[a]SEER program estimates are from 1988 to 1992.
[b]SEER program does not calculate mortality when fewer than 25 cases are reported.

SOURCE: Miller et al. (1996).

TABLE 2-10 Five-Year Relative Survival Rates by Selected Sites Among Racial or Ethnic Groups in the United States[a]

Racial or Ethnic Group	Colon and Rectum	Lung and Bronchus	Female Breast	Cervix Uteri	All Sites
Native American	37	5	53	67	34
Black	44	11	63	63	38
Chinese	50	15	78	72	44
Filipino	41	12	72	72	46
Hawaiian	51	16	76	73	44
Japanese	58	14	85	72	51
Korean	NA[b]	NA	NA	NA	NA
Vietnamese	NA	NA	NA	NA	NA
Hispanic (total)	46	11	72	69	47
White, non-Hispanic	51	12	75	68	50

[a]Percentage (both sexes) surviving 5 years following cancer diagnosis; SEER program estimates are from 1978 to 1981.

[b]SEER program does not calculate incidence when fewer than 25 cases are reported.

SOURCE: Miller et al. (1996).

will be alive 5 years from the time of diagnosis. In contrast, 5-year survival rates among African Americans and Native Americans are considerably reduced (38 percent and 34 percent, respectively). Similar patterns are seen, for example, for breast cancer among females and cancers of the colon and rectum. The 5-year breast cancer survival rate among U.S. white women is 75 percent, whereas the rates are 63 percent among African Americans and 53 percent among Native American women. Survival rates for cancer of the colon and rectum are 51 percent among U.S. whites, 41 percent among Filipinos, and 37 percent among Native Americans. Updated survival rates (1960 to 1992), which are available only for African Americans, support the suggested picture of poor survival among ethnic minority populations.

Thus, the effort to improve survival rates appears to have been least effective for members of ethnic minority groups. This has largely been attributed to late stage at diagnosis, perhaps in part due the limited use of early-detection services and access to state-of-the-art treatment.

Other Data Sources

Information from sources other than the SEER program, such as other national databases, special collaborative reports, or the results of independent researchers, serve as valuable resources in assessing the cancer burden among members of ethnic minority and medically underserved groups. The discussion in this section highlights some of the major information available and compares the findings to those of the SEER program when appropriate.

National Center for Health Statistics

NCHS collects all vital health statistics in the United States and has virtually complete data on all causes of death, including cancer. Using NCHS data, Frey et al. (1992) compared the rate of mortality from cancer among SEER programs registry participants to that among the total U.S. population and found that in most cases the SEER program provides an accurate picture of rates of mortality from cancer for the entire U.S. population. However, SEER program data failed to identify statistically significant trends in rates of mortality from cancer among ethnic minorities and in the rates of mortality from relatively rare cancers due to the small numbers of cases such types of cancer. For example, the SEER program failed to identify significant increases in mortality from cancers of the colon and rectum among African-American males.

The most disturbing highlight of this study was the lack of a consistent pattern of nonrepresentativeness of the SEER program data:

> These results should be reviewed in the context of the underlying issue that motivated these analyses. In particular, the fact that SEER data are frequently used in lieu of national estimates for cancer incidence, survival, and in some cases mortality has created a need for a systematic understanding of the degree of representativeness in the SEER data. This need is especially acute insofar as the SEER data are used not just to provide a summary of experiences, but also to establish baselines and projections for future trends. (Frey et al., 1992, p. 876)

Future work in understanding the differences between the SEER program data and the actual data for the U.S. population may be used to adjust SEER program data to ensure that they accurately describe the national cancer burden.

State Tumor Registries

The National Program of Cancer Registries (NPCR) was established by the U.S. Congress in 1992 to enable states to enhance existing cancer registries or to establish new cancer registries through funding and technical assistance from the CDC (Centers for Disease Control and Prevention, 1998). At this time some states have excellent registries, but 10 states did not begin registries until 1990 and half the states have had one for less than 10 years. Most of these registries currently collect and report incidence, tumor diagnosis and stage, and first course of treatment, but several have become or are becoming longitudinal registries collecting follow-up information regarding subsequent treatment and survival.

These registries complement and cooperate with other national databases, primarily through the North American Association of Central Cancer Registries (NAACCR). Sponsoring members of NAACCR include NCI, CDC, the American Cancer Society, the American College of Surgeons, the American Joint Committee on Cancer, Laboratory Centre for Disease Control Health Canada, Statistics Canada, and the National Cancer Registrars Association. Dr. Brenda Edwards of NCI serves as permanent Secretary and as an ex-officio member of the Board of Directors of NAACCR. All SEER program registries and all other central cancer registries in the U.S. are members of NAACCR. Cancer statistics from the non-SEER program state cancer registries are published annually by NAACCR together with those of the five SEER program-supported state registries. This is the closest approximation to a national cancer registry report available in the United States. Published data, however, are limited to only African American and white racial classifications, and no survival data are included in these reports. The usefulness of this aggregate information from NAACCR is limited, but this database—including information from both the SEER program and NPCR-supported state registries—will become increasingly useful as more state registries improve the completeness and quality of their data collection and analysis.

Through a separate activity NAACCR is now responsible on a voluntary basis for quality assurance review of state supported cancer registries. After extensive consideration, NAACCR has established an annual program of certification based on the completeness, timeliness, and quality of data collection and reporting. In its first year of operation 36 U.S. and Canadian registries, including all SEER program registries, applied for certification. Twenty-seven were awarded certificates. Every registry is encouraged to submit data annually for review. The intent of NAACCR and NPCR is to have all state-funded (and SEER program) registries be certified annually by NAACCR. All registries are also encouraged to become longitudinal registries in time. When that happens, a truly national picture of cancer incidence, mortality, and survival will be available in the U.S.

Data collected by state cancer registries highlight some important regional differences in cancer rates that are not ascertained by the SEER program and illustrate the need to have state-specific data in order to develop and evaluate cancer control programs in each state. SEER data cannot be used for this purpose, except for the states included in the

TABLE 2-11 Age-Adjusted Cancer Incidence in Kentucky for Selected Sites, 1992 to 1995

	Incidence per 100,000 Population				
Year	Colon and Rectum	Lung and Bronchus	Female Breast	Cervix Uteri	All Sites
1992	49.1	75.2	103.1	11.3	385.7
1993	47.3	78.0	103.0	10.5	390.5
1994	48.4	84.6	109.8	11.4	403.7
1995	50.1	86.7	109.7	12.2	415.7

SOURCE: Gilbert Friedell, Director for Cancer Control, Kentucky Cancer Center, Personal communication, 1998.

SEER program. For example, the cancer incidence rate reported for Kentucky, a state that does not participate in the SEER program and that has a large, rural white population and a high prevalence of poverty (19.0 percent versus a 13.7 percent rate of poverty nationally), suggests that overall rates of cancer in Kentucky are somewhat higher than estimates of the rates for the U.S. population as a whole (see Table 2-11). Specifically, the incidences of colorectal, lung, and cervical cancer are higher among the population in Kentucky than among the non-Hispanic white rate U.S. population, according to SEER program data. Of additional concern is the increasing cancer incidence trend suggested by the data for Kentucky. This is in contrast to the decrease in cancer incidence noted nationally among non-Hispanic whites for the same time period according to SEER program data.

Coordinated National Effort

The American Cancer Society, SEER, NCHS, and CDC combined efforts to produce a report card covering over 20 years of cancer experience in the United States, *Cancer Incidence and Mortality, 1973–1995: A Report Card for the United States* (Wingo et al., 1998), using data drawn from SEER and NCHS databases. Rates of cancer for several ethnic minority groups (African Americans, Asians, Pacific Islanders, and Hispanics) were included. However, cancer rates for Native Americans were notably absent. Also notably absent from this report were survival rates.

The report card confirmed the disparate cancer burdens among members of different ethnic minority groups, illustrated by SEER program data from 1988 to 1992. Additionally, data from this coordinated effort suggested an increasing trend in the incidence of and mortality from all major cancers among Asians and Pacific Islanders, but statistical significance was not attained due to the small numbers of cases in these groups. As noted in the report of the NCI Cancer Control Review Group, SEER program incidence data do not cover Appalachia or the rural South (National Cancer Institute, 1997b).

Cancer Incidence Among Native Americans

Four facts are consistently found in studies examining cancer among American Indian populations. They are:

- cancer is the second leading cause of death;
- American Indians have the lowest 5-year survival rate for all cancers when compared to other populations;
- American Indians have the highest percentage of disseminated and ill-defined cancers; and,
- very little is known about prevention and treatment patterns for cancer in American Indians.

SEER program information on cancer incidence, mortality and survival in Native Americans is only available for American Indians living in New Mexico and Arizona (the Southwestern American Indians), and Alaska Natives (Miller et al., 1996). As indicated in Table 2-12, the five foremost

TABLE 2-12 Five Most Frequently Diagnosed Cancers Among Alaska Native and American Indian (New Mexico) Men, 1988 to 1992, Age Adjusted to 1970 U.S. Standard Population*

	Incidence per 100,000 Population				
Group	Lung and Bronchus	Colon and Rectum	Prostate	Stomach	Kidney and Renal Pelvis
Alaska Native	81.1	79.7	46.1	27.2	19.0*
	Prostate	Colon and Rectum	Kidney and Renal Pelvis	Lung and Bronchus	Liver and Intrahepatic
American Indian (New Mexico)	52.5	18.6	15.6	14.4	13.1*

*The rate is based on fewer than 25 cases and may be subject to greater variability than the other rates, which are based on larger numbers.

SOURCE: SEER program (Miller et al., 1996).

TABLE 2-13 Five Most Frequently Diagnosed Cancers Among Alaska Native and American Indian (New Mexico) Women, 1988 to 1992, Age Adjusted to 1970 U.S. Standard Population*

	Incidence per 100,000 Population				
Group	Breast	Colon and Rectum	Lung and Bronchus	Kidney and Renal Pelvis	Cervix Uteri
Alaska Native	78.9	67.4	50.6	16.7*	15.8
	Breast	Ovary	Colon and Rectum	Gallbladder	Corpus Uteri
American Indian (New Mexico)	31.6	17.5	15.3	13.2	10.7

*The rate is based on fewer than 25 cases and may be subject to greater variability than the other rates, which are based on larger numbers

SOURCE: SEER program (Miller et al., 1996).

cancers in Alaska Native men are lung, colon and rectum, prostrate, stomach, and kidney, whereas the leading sites for Southwestern American Indian men are prostrate, colon and rectum, kidney, lung, and liver. Colorectal cancers among Alaska Native men and kidney cancer among Southwestern American Indian men are higher than those for any other racial or ethnic group. The high incidence of liver cancer in Southwestern American Indian men may not be very accurate due to the reporting of fewer than 25 cases.

Among Alaska Native women, the leading cancer sites are breast, colon and rectum, lung, kidney, and cervix, while among Southwestern American Indian women the leading incidence sites are breast, ovary, colon and rectum, gallbladder, and corpus uteri (see Table 2-13). Alaska Native women have higher rates of colorectal cancer and lung cancer than any other ethnic group. Southwestern American Indian women, in contrast, have very high incidence rates of ovarian and gallbladder cancers.

Mortality data provided by SEER indicate a disparity in the two Native American groups studied (see Tables 2-14 and 2-15). Cancer mortality rates for Alaska Native women from 1988 to 1992 exceeds that for white non-Hispanic women (45.3 compared to 32.9). Mortality rates for Alaska Native women from colorectal cancer also exceeded white non-Hispanic women (24 compared to 15.6). Whereas Alaska Native men had higher

TABLE 2-14 Five Most Common Causes of Cancer Deaths Among Alaska Native and American Indian (New Mexico) Men, 1988 to 1992, Age Adjusted to 1970 U.S. Standard Population*

	Incidence per 100,000 Population				
Group	Lung and Bronchus	Colon and Rectum	Stomach	Kidney and Renal Pelvis	Nasopharynx
Alaska Native	69.4	27.2	18.9*	13.4*	11.6*
	Prostate	Stomach	Liver and Intrahepatic	Lung and Bronchus	Colon and Rectum
American Indian (New Mexico)	16.2	11.2*	11.2*	10.4*	8.5*

*The rate is based on fewer than 25 deaths and may be subject to greater variability than the other rates which are based on larger numbers.

SOURCE: SEER program (Miller et al., 1996).

TABLE 2-15 Five Most Common Causes of Cancer Deaths Among Alaska Native and American Indian (New Mexico) Women, 1988 to 1992, Age Adjusted to 1970 U.S. Standard Population*

	Incidence per 100,000 Population				
Group	Lung and Bronchus	Colon and Rectum	Breast	Pancreas	Kidney and Renal Pelvis
Alaska Native	45.3	24.0	16.0*	15.5*	7.4*
	Gallbladder	Breast	Cervix Uteri	Pancreas	Ovary
American Indian (New Mexico)	8.9*	8.7*	8.0*	7.4*	7.3*

*The rate is based on fewer than 25 deaths and may be subject to greater variability than the other rates which are based on larger numbers.

SOURCE: SEER program (Miller et al., 1996).

mortality rates due to cancer of lung and colon and rectum, Southwestern American Indian men experienced their highest mortality due to prostate cancer for that same period.

In general, the cancer incidence and mortality rates are not necessarily lower for all Native American populations and the data from the Southwest cannot be extrapolated to all American Indian and Alaska Native populations. Mortality statistics in state tumor registries are subject to underreporting of Indian ethnicity and hence all of this data must be interpreted with caution. Data on the larger cross-section of the American Indian population are needed to more accurately evaluate the cancer status of American Indians. SEER has established a tumor registry among the Cherokee Nation of Oklahoma to provide accurate statistics on this tribe.

Although the Indian Health Service (IHS) is generally viewed as the overseer of medical care for American Indian/Alaska Native populations, involvement is limited to the 33 "reservation states" (Mahoney and Michalek, 1998). Contrary to popular impression, about two-thirds of American Indians reside in urban areas while fewer than 40 percent reside on federal reservations. Urban Indian health care programs account for just 2 percent of the IHS budget. IHS does not assume sole responsibility for American Indian and Alaska Native health care and attempts to incorporate support from federal and states agencies to assist in these programs.

IHS data for cancer incidence and mortality among American Indian and Alaska Native women demonstrated marked regional differences (Valway, 1990). These data document a high incidence of lung cancer among Alaska Native men (85 per 100,000 compared to 79 per 100,000, the overall average rate for U.S. men), and a high incidence of colorectal cancer among Alaska Native women (90.2 per 100,000 compared to 39.2 per 100,000 for U.S. women). In addition, IHS data reveal a higher incidence of lung cancer in American Indian men of the Northern Plains area, as well as a high incidence of breast cancer in American Indian women of that region.

Valway (1990), reporting on regional differences in cancer mortality among Native Americans, indicates that reporting statistics on one region of American Indians did not adequately describe cancer mortality for all Native Americans. Mortality statistics for Native Americans in the Southwest were lower than those living in the Northern Plains (North and South Dakota, Wisconsin, Michigan, Minnesota and Montana). This study confirmed the increasing American Indian mortality rates from cancer from 1968 to 1987, which was subsequently observed by Mahoney et al. (1998) from 1973 to 1993.

Special Studies

Studies by independent researchers who used data from agencies, hospitals, and state health departments provide additional insight into the cancer burden among members of ethnic minority and medically underserved groups. In many cases, as discussed below, these studies highlight important differences between regional data and national estimates provided by the SEER program.

A study that used hospital discharge data from IHS during the period between 1980 and 1987 provides estimates of cancer incidence and mortality for the 11 IHS regions (Nutting et al., 1993). A high degree of variation in the occurrence of cancer was seen among Native Americans in different geographic regions (see Tables 2-16 and 2-17). For example, the incidence of cancer among American Indian males in the Billings, Montana, area was nine times higher than that among American Indian males of the Phoenix area (56.4 per 100,000 population, in contrast to 6.3 per 100,000 population). Female breast cancer incidence also varied widely according to geographic region. The incidence in the Phoenix area was 18.8 per 100,000 population, in comparison to 51.5 per 100,000 population among Alaska Natives.

The IHS data for cancer incidence among American Indian women also illustrated large regional differences not shown by the SEER program estimates. For example, the incidence of cancer of the cervix in the Albuquerque, New Mexico area was approximately two- to threefold higher than seen in Portland, Bemidji, and Oklahoma.

A second study was initiated to determine the extent of racial misclassification of American Indians in the Washington State Cancer Registry when compared to data obtained from the Portland Area Indian Health Service and tribal specific cancer data (Sugarman et al., 1996). The estimated age-adjusted cancer incidence among American Indians in Washington state increased from 153.5 per 100,000 population before record linkage to 267.5 per 100,000 after linkage. This study found that most cases of cancer in American Indian individuals were identified by the IHS registry and a few additional cases were identified using the tribal rolls. More than one quarter of American Indians classified as full heritage (100 percent blood quantum) were not coded as American Indians in the tumor registry, again suggesting that true misclassification frequently occurs.

Cancer Survival Among Ethnic Groups

Special studies that use data from the SEER program are also a source of important information regarding the incidence of cancer among mem-

TABLE 2-16 Cancer Incidence Among American Indian, Alaska Native, and Non-Hispanic White Males, Age Adjusted to 1970 U.S. Standard

	Incidence per 100,000 Population					
Data Source and Region	Stomach	Colon and Rectum	Lung and Bronchus	Prostate	Gall-bladder	All Sites
IHS						
Aberdeen	10.7	20.2	46.2	30.9	2.9	174.8
Alaska	24.4	50.6	85.2	33.2	3.5	324.3
Albuquerque	20.1	6.9	14.4	34.3	6.1	170.8
Bemidji	5.9	58.0	42.3	33.1	5.2	227.7
Billings	7.2	17.1	56.4	43.0	1.6	174.7
Navajo	10.3	8.2	12.3	25.6	3.8	30.0
Oklahoma	4.0	11.8	28.4	20.5	0.5	107.7
Phoenix	8.6	8.9	6.3	14.4	3.8	93.2
Portland	9.4	14.2	12.8	27.0	1.5	104.6
All IHS regions	9.5	15.0	27.8	25.8	2.4	142.1
SEER Program (non-Hispanic whites)	9.6	57.6	79.0	137.9	0.8	481

NOTE: IHS estimates are from 1980 to 1987. SEER program estimates are from 1988 to 1992.

SOURCE: Miller et al. (1996).

TABLE 2-17 Cancer Incidence Among American Indian, Alaska Native, and Non-Hispanic White Women, Age Adjusted to 1970 U.S. Standard

	Incidence per 100,000 Population						
Data Source and Region	Stomach	Colon and Rectum	Lung and Bronchus	Breast	Cervix Uteri	Gall-bladder	All Sites
IHS							
Aberdeen	9.0	16.4	32.1	46.7	23.5	4.6	212.7
Alaska	8.9	90.2	58.4	51.5	29.5	14.4	355.6
Albuquerque	18.6	22.0	12.1	19.5	31.3	6.7	214.9
Bemidji	6.8	57.7	52.3	20.4	10.8	5.3	214.9
Billings	5.0	19.2	37.8	42.2	32.3	2.8	232.0
Navajo	9.5	9.5	4.1	26.0	24.4	9.6	170.3
Oklahoma	3.9	18.5	12.1	30.9	11.4	3.0	124.1
Phoenix	5.6	13.1	10.9	18.8	20.5	16.1	167.5
Portland	1.5	19.7	10.3	20.1	8.8	5.6	132.2
All IHS regions	6.8	20.8	16.8	30.2	19.5	7.1	173.2
SEER program (non-Hispanic whites)	3.9	39.2	43.7	115.7	7.5	1.4	354

NOTE: IHS estimates are from 1980 to 1987. SEER program estimates are from 1988 to 1992.

SOURCE: Nutting et al. (1993).

TABLE 2-18 Five-Year Survival Rates by Selected Cancer Sites and Ethnic Group

	Percent			
Group	Colon	Lung	Female Breast	Cervix (invasive)
Non-Hispanic white	64	11	85	94
Hispanic	58	10	76	94
Native American	48	10	75	90

SOURCE: Gilliland, Hunt, and Key (1998).

bers of ethnic minority groups. For example, a study using the New Mexico (a SEER program state) tumor registry data from 1983 to 1994 found significant differences in the rate of survival from cancer among Hispanic, Native American, and white patients (Gilliland, Hunt, and Key, 1998). The study found that whites had the highest 5-year survival rates, that the rates among Hispanics were intermediate, and that Native Americans had the poorest rates of survival (see Table 2-18).

Similarly, Samet et al. (1987) in an earlier study found that the diagnosis of cancer at a late stage was correlated with poor survival rates (see Table 2-19), supporting the rationale for increased early detection services in special populations.

Gilliland and Key (1998), in a study of prostate cancer among American Indians in New Mexico from 1969 to 1994, also point to late stage at diagnosis as a factor in disproportionate mortality rates in relation to incidence rates. For example, among American Indian men, 23.3 percent of prostate cancers were diagnosed after distant spread, whereas among non-Hispanic white men 11.6 percent of prostate cancer were diagnosed after distant spread (Gilliland and Key, 1998). Other studies of cancer survival rates for this population (covering 1973 to 1992) supports the findings that American Indian women have poorer survival rates than non-Hispanic whites (Frost et al., 1996). For example, survival was poorer among American Indian women during both the period from 1973 to 1982 and the period from 1983 to 1992 . Survival among Hispanic women was also notably poor during the latter time period. The authors note that the lower survival rates among this population is amplified by increasing breast cancer incidence rates among New Mexico Hispanics and American Indians (Frost et al., 1996).

In addition to early detection, cancer survival is highly dependent upon effective treatment. Evidence indicates that there are ethnic differ-

TABLE 2-19 Stage of Cancer at Diagnosis by Selected Cancer Site and Ethnic Group

	Percent			
Stage of Cancer and Ethnic Group	Colon	Lung	Female Breast	Cervix (invasive)
In Situ				
Non-Hispanic white	2.5	0.2	5.0	81.0
Hispanic	1.3	0.0	3.9	72.7
Native American	3.6	0.0	2.2	76.1
Local				
Non-Hispanic white	28.4	32.0	52.3	12.3
Hispanic	29.3	32.5	43.8	15.2
Native American	29.1	23.2	33.3	11.3
Regional				
Non-Hispanic white	43.1	24.7	36.3	4.8
Hispanic	40.7	21.9	42.9	8.5
Native American	42.7	25.3	48.4	9.2
Distant				
Non-Hispanic white	26.0	43.1	6.5	1.9
Hispanic	28.7	45.6	9.5	3.6
Native American	24.5	51.5	16.1	3.3

SOURCE: Samet et al. (1987).

ences in the aggressiveness of treatment of cancer. For example, one study found that African-American women with advanced breast cancer were less likely than white women to receive surgery, and mortality was higher among African-American women than in white women with advanced disease (Breen and Ching, 1995). Similarly, SEER program data were used to evaluate prostate cancer treatment, and the proportion of African-American men who receive prostatectomy was lower than that of white men (Harlan et al., 1995). This trend appears to be consistent over the time period of evaluation (1984 to 1991).

Socioeconomic Status and Cancer Surveillance

No national database or agency reports the relationship between SES and cancer. Over the last 40 years, many studies have supported the conclusion that SES is somehow related to cancer. However, differences in the measures of SES (education, income, residence, occupation, or a calculated composite value) between studies have resulted in difficulties in examining this relationship in its entirety (Greenwald et al., 1996). Differences in the types of cancers studied may also affect the interpretability of the results. For example, studies of disease in which early detection through screening is a determinant of survival (such as breast cancer) may indicate that income level is a predictor of outcome because this measures the level of access to health care. Conversely, a cancer that is largely affected by lifestyle choices (such as colon cancer, which is associated with poor diet) may show a stronger relationship to education than to income.

Further complicating the issue is the fact that many members of ethnic minority groups are also among the most poor citizens of the population. This is more true in some regions of the country than others, as shown in Table 2-20.

Other Measures of Progress Against Cancer

Beyond the measurement of cancer outcomes such as survival and mortality, efforts have been made to measure a number of attributes related to cancer, such as levels of screening for cancer and the incidence of risk factors for cancer such as smoking and diet, and to assess differences among members of ethnic minority groups and medically underserved individuals in these attributes. These measures are important in cancer prevention and control efforts.

Primary prevention measures related to behavioral risk factors have the greatest potential for reducing the incidence of and mortality from cancer in the United States. For example, smoking and diet have been shown to significantly influence the rate of death from cancer (estimated to cause 30 percent and 35 percent of deaths from cancer, respectively). Smoking is a well-established etiologic agent in lung cancer and has been associated with cancers of the cervix, stomach, pancreas, and colorectal system. High-fat, high-calorie, low-fiber diets often lead to obesity and have been associated with cancers of the breast, prostate, and digestive system. Excessive alcohol consumption increases the risk of cancers of the mouth and esophagus when combined with smoking, and has also been linked to breast and prostate cancers. Regular monitoring of the prevalence of these behavioral factors is an important tool in the national effort because it identifies segments of the population at high risk of developing cancer and permits the targeting of research and intervention efforts.

In addition to lifestyle changes, increasing levels of participation in cancer screening programs among high-risk groups can effectively reduce the burden of cancer. Early detection improves the rate of survival. For example, studies indicate that regular mammography can reduce the mortality rate from breast cancer by 35 percent among U.S. women ages 50 to 69 years (Harris et al., 1992). The introduction of the Pap smear in the 1940s effectively reduced the incidence of cervical cancer by 90 percent

TABLE 2-20 Distribution of Racial or Ethnic Minority Groups, by State and Percentage of Population with Incomes Below the Poverty Level

State (% below poverty level)	Non-Hispanic White	Hispanic	Black	American Indian	Pacific Islander/ Asian
Alabama (18.3)	73.3	0.6	25.2	0.5	0.5
Alaska (9.0)	74.0	3.3	3.9	15.5	3.3
Arizona (15.8)	71.8	18.6	2.9	5.2	1.4
Arkansas (19.1)	82.2	0.8	15.1	0.6	0.5
California (12.5)	57.4	25.4	7.1	0.7	9.2
Colorado (11.7)	80.9	12.7	3.9	0.7	1.7
Connecticut (6.8)	84.0	6.2	8.0	0.2	1.5
Delaware (8.7)	79.4	2.3	16.6	0.3	1.3
District of Columbia (16.9)	27.4	5.2	65.3	0.2	1.8
Florida (12.7)	73.3	12.0	13.2	0.3	1.1
Georgia (14.7)	70.2	1.6	26.8	0.2	1.1
Hawaii (8.3)	31.4	7.1	2.3	0.4	58.5
Idaho (13.3)	92.3	5.1	0.3	1.3	0.9
Illinois (11.9)	75.0	7.7	14.7	0.2	2.4
Indiana (10.7)	89.6	1.7	7.7	0.3	0.7
Iowa (11.5)	96.1	1.1	1.7	0.3	0.9
Kansas (11.5)	88.6	3.6	5.7	0.9	1.2
Kentucky (19.0)	91.7	0.6	7.1	0.2	0.5
Louisiana (23.6)	65.8	2.2	30.6	0.5	0.9
Maine (10.8)	97.9	0.6	0.4	0.5	0.6
Maryland (8.3)	69.6	2.5	24.7	0.3	2.8
Massachusetts (8.9)	88.0	4.6	4.6	0.2	2.3
Michigan (13.1)	82.4	2.0	13.8	0.6	1.1
Minnesota (10.2)	93.9	1.1	2.1	1.1	1.7
Mississippi (25.2)	63.1	0.6	35.5	0.3	0.5
Missouri (13.3)	87.0	1.2	10.6	0.4	0.8
Montana (16.1)	91.9	<0.1	0.2	5.8	0.5
Nebraska (11.1)	92.6	2.2	3.6	0.8	0.8
Nevada (10.2)	78.8	10.1	6.4	1.5	3.1
New Hampshire (6.4)	97.3	1.0	0.6	0.2	0.8
New Jersey (7.6)	74.2	9.3	12.8	0.2	3.4
New Mexico (20.6)	50.6	38.1	1.8	8.5	0.9

Continued

TABLE 2-20 *Continued*

State (% below poverty level)	Non-Hispanic White	Hispanic	Black	American Indian	Pacific Islander/ Asian
New York (13.0)	69.4	12.0	14.5	0.3	3.7
North Carolina (13.0)	75.1	1.0	21.9	1.2	0.7
North Dakota (14.4)	94.3	0.7	0.5	3.9	0.5
Ohio (12.5)	87.1	1.2	10.6	0.2	0.8
Oklahoma (16.7)	81.1	2.7	7.3	7.9	1.0
Oregon (12.4)	90.8	3.9	1.6	1.4	2.3
Pennsylvania (11.1)	87.8	1.9	9.0	0.1	1.1
Rhode Island (9.6)	89.5	4.4	3.4	0.4	1.7
South Carolina (15.4)	68.6	0.8	29.7	0.3	0.6
South Dakota (15.9)	91.2	0.8	0.4	7.1	0.5
Tennessee (15.7)	82.6	0.6	15.9	0.3	0.6
Texas (18.1)	60.8	25.3	11.7	0.4	1.8
Utah (11.4)	91.3	4.8	0.6	1.4	1.9
Vermont (9.9)	98.0	0.7	0.4	0.4	0.5
Virginia (10.3)	76.0	2.5	18.7	0.3	2.5
Washington (10.9)	86.9	4.2	3.0	1.6	4.2
West Virginia (19.7)	95.9	0.4	3.1	0.2	0.4
Wisconsin (10.7)	91.4	1.8	5.0	0.8	1.1
Wyoming (11.9)	91.1	5.5	0.7	2.1	0.6

SOURCE: Statistics are from the U.S. Bureau of the Census (1997a).

because the procedure can detect abnormal cells before they become cancerous (U.S. Public Health Service, 1991). Other cancer screening tests such as fecal occult blood testing are readily available.

Existing data demonstrate that the rates of late stage at diagnosis and poor cancer survival rates are disproportionately higher among ethnic minorities. Similarly, the available information indicates that the rate of participation in cancer screening programs is lower among ethnic minorities and low SES individuals (Breen and Figueroa, 1996; Breen et al., 1996; Hoffman-Goetz et al., 1998). For example, recent trends in breast cancer mortality indicate that the mortality rate for U.S. white women decreased during the period from 1980 to 1988, whereas the rate for African-American women increased significantly. This difference in trends was largely attributed to late stage at diagnosis (Chevarley and White, 1997). Increasing levels of participation in screening programs by groups at high risk of death from cancers can lead to earlier detection, greater treatment efficacy, and better survival rates.

Behavioral Risk Factor Surveillance: Existing Mechanisms

The purpose of the Behavioral Risk Factor Surveillance Survey (BRFSS) is to collect data regarding the prevalence of behavioral risk factors among U.S. adults to be used to establish and monitor progress toward public health objectives. The data are collected by telephone by using responses to surveys that are administered by the states in coordination with the CDC (Sugarman et al., 1992). Use of telephone responses limits the generalizability of the results of BRFSS, since many low-income households lack telephone service. For example, only approximately a third of all households on northern Arizona reservations (e.g., that of the Hopi tribe) have telephones (National Cancer Institute, 1994). Special studies with the results of BRFSS have been conducted among Native Americans in attempts to address some of these concerns. Oklahoma developed its own Native-American Supplement, which was administered in 1994 (Smith et al., 1995). Additionally, BRFSS data from 1,055 Native American respondents obtained from 1985 to 1988 were evaluated for their usefulness in monitoring the progress of this population toward achieving year 2000 national health objectives (Sugarman et al., 1992). The conclusion of that report was that BRFSS data may be useful in the surveillance of Native Americans if they are combined with community-specific household-based surveys. Similar conclusions may be appropriate for other distinct geographic, cultural, and ethnic groups. For example, in several counties of eastern Kentucky, 20 percent or more of the households do not have telephones (U.S. Bureau of Census, 1997b).

National Health and Nutrition Examination Survey

In 1967, the U.S. Congress mandated that appropriate federal and state officials conduct a comprehensive survey in response to concerns about hunger, malnutrition, and health. In 1969, the initial 10-state effort was expanded by President Richard Nixon to cover the entire United States. NCHS added a nutritional assessment component to health status measurements already being collected in the National Health Examination Survey, and the first National Health and Nutrition Examination Survey (NHANES) was conducted between 1971 and 1974.

The purpose of NHANES is to periodically assess the nutritional and health status of the U.S. population and to monitor trends over time. Nutritional status is evaluated through interviews and direct physician examinations. During interviews a 24-hour diet recall, a food frequency questionnaire, and a medical history are obtained. Physical examinations include anthropometric and biochemical measurements and physical and dental examinations.

A multistage probability cluster sampling plan is used to ensure a representative sample of U.S. households. For example, the second NHANES, (NHANES II; 1976 to 1980) had a sample size of 27,805, with 91 percent of these agreeing to participate in the survey. Oversampling of subgroups at high risk of malnutrition (such as households in areas with high levels of poverty) was conducted to ensure their adequate representation. In addition, a special survey of Hispanics in five southwestern states, Cubans in Dade County, Florida, and Puerto Ricans in the New York City metropolitan area was conducted from 1982 to 1984. To date, the routine collection of nutrition and health information has systematically excluded people in the military, institutionalized individuals, and individuals living on Native American reservations.

National Health Interview Survey

In addition to NHANES, NCHS administers the annual National Health Interview Survey (NHIS) to collect information on the health of civilian, noninstitutionalized Americans. NHIS collects information on the occurrence of injuries, acute illnesses, chronic conditions, and disabilities and the utilization of health care serves among people in the United States who are 17 years of age and older. NHIS consists of a two-part questionnaire that requests basic health and demographic information and a supplemental survey of several health related topics. For example, information on cancer-related risk factors such as participation in screening programs, diet, and family history of cancer were collected in 1987 and 1992.

African Americans and Hispanics have been oversampled in NHIS to improve estimates for these populations. However, Americans Indians and other ethnic minority groups with smaller numbers of individuals have historically been surveyed in insufficient numbers to draw conclusions about these populations. For example, 0.0006 percent ($n = 135$) of respondents to the 1987 Cancer Control Supplement were American or Alaska Natives. This percentage of respondents was poor in comparison to the proportions of indigenous peoples in the United States, which were estimated to be 0.6 percent in 1980 and 0.8 percent in 1990.

TABLE 2-21 Percentage of U.S. Women Who Reported Ever Having a Mammogram or Pap Smear, by Racial or Ethnic Group

	Percent of U.S. Women Who Have Had the Following:	
Racial or Ethnic Group	Mammogram	Pap Smear
White, non-Hispanic[a]	38.9	91.0
Black[a]	29.6	88.1
Hispanic[a]	26.2	74.8
American Indian[b]	14.8	82.6

SOURCE: [a]National Health Interview Survey for 1987; [b]National Medical Expenditure Survey for 1987.

National Medical Expenditure Survey

A special survey of American Indians and Alaska Natives was conducted in 1982 by using the National Medical Expenditure Survey. Some of its findings regarding the use of mammography and Pap smear screening techniques are summarized in Table 2-21. There are several major concerns with the validity of the results of this survey. These concerns were related to the cultural appropriateness of the survey instrument and the possibility of misinterpretation of responses by researchers who are not American Indians or Alaska Natives (Burhansstipanov, 1995). However, the results of this survey indicate that American Indian women, like other minorities, received screenings less often than the non-Hispanic white population (Coyne et al., 1992).

National Survey of Family Growth

The National Survey of Family Growth (Wilcox and Mosher, 1993) was based on a national sample of 8,450 reproductive age (15 to 44 years) U.S. women who participated in NHIS between October 1985 and March 1987. The NHIS data were used to compare women who had received screening in the previous year to those who had not received an annual screening. Results indicated that women with little education or low income, Native American women, Hispanic women, and women of Asian or Pacific Islander descent were less likely to receive regular screenings (see Table 2-22).

TABLE 2-22 Percentage of U.S. Women Who Reported Annual Breast Examination or Pap Smear, by Racial or Ethnic Group, Education, and Income

	Percent of U.S. Women Who Have Reported Having the Following:	
Racial or Ethnic Group	Breast Examination	Pap Smear
White, non-Hispanic	67.3	67.1
Black	74.2	76.3
Hispanic	62.9	63.6
American Indian	53.3	50.0
Asian or Pacific Islander	56.7	54.2
Education (in years)		
<12	62.9	65.5
12	69.9	70.8
13–15	74.3	73.7
≥16 or more	77.5	77.1
Income as percentage of poverty level		
<150	60.7	61.8
150–299	63.7	64.8
300–399	67.8	66.8
≥400	73.2	72.9

SOURCE: National Survey of Family Growth.

FUTURE DIRECTIONS IN ASSESSING THE BURDEN OF CANCER AMONG ETHNIC MINORITY AND MEDICALLY UNDERSERVED GROUPS

Cancer Surveillance Among Ethnic Minorities and Medically Underserved Individuals

Data on the incidence of cancer among ethnic minorities and medically underserved individuals indicate that not all of these groups are at higher risk of cancer than members of the majority population, and that the rates of some cancers among white Americans who are medically underserved are not very different from the highest rates among some ethnic minority groups. On the other hand, cancer mortality rates are significantly higher and cancer survival rates are lower among many ethnic minority populations, a fact attributed in several studies to late stage of diagnosis and inferior treatment in the health care system. Further, many cancer risk behaviors are more prevalent among ethnic minority and medically underserved groups, portending an increase in cancer mortality.

It is important that the reasons for the differences in cancer incidence, mortality, survival rates, and risk behaviors be understood, because this understanding may be crucial to reducing the rates of cancer among the entire population. Studying groups of people of different cultures, behaviors, environmental exposures, and patterns of cancer in different geographic settings is a critical step in identifying factors related to risk of disease. However, before the reasons for the differences can be understood, it is necessary to have reliable and valid data for the groups under consideration. For reasons beyond the control of the agencies collecting these data, the available data are not always valid. For example, as noted earlier, the identification of both "race" and ethnicity in the U.S. census may cause confusion among respondents and inconsistent self-reporting. Federal health data are also distorted because of the persistent problem of census "undercounting," which is more prevalent among ethnic minority and underserved groups. Statistical sampling to correct this undercount, which has been debated extensively in Congress, would help to yield more reliable data regarding cancer incidence and mortality rates. Another methodological challenge is posed by the various methods that data collectors, providers, interviewers, and others used to identify the "race" or ethnicity of individuals. The lack of consistency in definitions among various government agencies also raises questions about the reliability of some of the data.

Accurate classification of groups and enumeration of their cancer experience are therefore critical to ensuring the effectiveness of future cancer prevention and control efforts. It is clear from the review of data collection from the government sector that several agencies are involved in this activity, including NCI, CDC (including the NCHS), state tumor registries, and the IHS, but that data collection activities are inconsistent. These agencies all acknowledge that there are ethnic minority and medically underserved populations but do not always publish or collect information in a consistent fashion that would adequately assess the burden of cancer in these groups. Some entities, for example, primarily report on rates of cancer on a racial basis and provide information only on whites and African Americans. In addition, information is not routinely collected on the basis of medically underserved status, but some information regarding these populations is available based on special studies in limited regions.

These and other problems related to cancer surveillance must be addressed in order to fully understand the burden of cancer among all segments of the U.S. population. The remainder of this chapter is therefore dedicated to illustrating and addressing significant conceptual and methodological issues that NIH (and other federal agencies) should consider in its cancer surveillance and other population-based research. In general, these issues are related to:

- the accurate enumeration of population groups, and collection and reporting of important indicators of cancer;
- the appropriate conceptualization of human diversity; and,
- consideration of the full range of cancer risk factors that should be studied among diverse populations, including socioeconomic factors, environmental factors, behavioral risk, and other factors.

Each of these issues is reviewed in greater detail below.

To its credit, NCI has already begun the process of reevaluating and improving its research and surveillance activities in each of these areas. Recent and ongoing evaluations of these programs include the report of the NCI Cancer Control Review Group (National Cancer Institute, 1997a), recommendations from which have already been implemented to improve the NCI's activities related to behavioral research and the study of ethnic minority populations; the NCI Special Action Committee Report (National Cancer Institute, 1996a), which called for improved assessment and conceptualization of the cancer research needs of ethnic minority and medically underserved groups; and the Surveillance Implementation Review Group, which is on-going and is charged with recommending improvements in NCI's cancer surveillance activities. These activities are described in greater detail below.

Enumeration of Population Groups, and Collection and Reporting of Important Indicators of Cancer

Improving SEER Program Coverage of High-Risk Populations

As discussed earlier in this chapter, the SEER program currently provides the best approximation of a national cancer database. However, its geographic coverage of minorities and medically underserved individuals must be improved. Based on findings and recommendations of the previously cited reviews of the SEER programs, coverage of high-risk populations should be improved to include lower-income or poverty-level whites, particularly those living in rural areas such as Appalachia; Hispanics of all national origins; African Americans living in rural communities, particularly in the South; and American Indian populations. The expansion of the SEER program would permit better analyses of the differences which exist among individuals within the same ethnic group, but who reside in different geographic regions of the country, such as Native Americans, African Americans, Hispanics, and non-Hispanic whites. Including states such as Florida and Texas, Appalachia, and the rural South, which have a high prevalence of poverty and large rural areas, would broaden the representation of many ethnic minority and low-income white populations in the SEER program. Hispanics, for example, represent a diverse cultural group with varying places of origin. Including other states with significant Hispanic populations would increase the representativeness of this population in the registry, as the Hispanic population in SEER reside predominantly in California. The inclusion of border areas of Texas would improve Hispanic representation in the SEER program, as would areas of the northeast such as New York or New Jersey, both of which have significant Hispanic and Asian populations. Likewise, inclusion of tribes in Oklahoma and Montana would begin to address the diversity within the American Indian population and provide a more complete assessment of the cancer experience of this population. It is not expected that a national registry will compensate for small numbers if the population under study is small.

Expansion of the SEER program can be accomplished through existing mechanisms. Standards for data collection and reporting, and a uniform data set have been established by the North American Association of Central Cancer Registries (NAACCR) for use by all of its members, including both SEER and non-SEER population-based registries. Inclusion in the SEER program of selected state registries meeting these standards might be one means of facilitating expansion of SEER coverage to areas or populations not currently covered.

Recommendation 2-2a: To further enhance the excellent data provided in the SEER program database, adequate resources should be provided to expand SEER program coverage beyond the existing sites to include high-risk populations for which SEER program coverage is lacking. This expansion should address a wider range of demographic and social characteristics by using consistent nomenclature and a uniform data set and by reflecting the diverse characteristics of the current U.S. population.

In addition to the SEER program, the federal government assists in the support of the National Program of Cancer Registries (NPCR). These non-SEER program registries are currently funded by the individual states with additional financial and technical support from the CDC through the NPCR. Some of these registries are currently only collecting data concerning incidence, stage at diagnosis, and first course of treatment. The Veterans Administration Hospital system and others are also collecting information regarding course of disease, other treatment(s) and survival. Greater collaboration and coordination of data collection efforts among these registries will ultimately provide tremendous benefits in the form of a national cancer data set.

Currently, collaborative efforts among the five SEER registries and the

45 non-SEER state registries are effectively facilitated by the NAACCR. Each of these registries has accepted NAACCR's comprehensive three-volume Standards for Data Exchange Records, Data Variable Definitions, and Completeness, Quality, and Timeliness of central registry operations. In addition, several NAACCR committees dealing with uniform data standards, data exchange, publication, certification, education, and other important issues include members from SEER, as well as from CDC and from state registries. NCI also offers significant leadership support to NAACCR, as Dr. Brenda Edwards of SEER serves as Secretary of the organization and sits on the Board of Directors. In addition, data from all SEER and non-SEER state registries are currently aggregated and published by NAACCR. Continued support for this activity should be assured.

In addition to these efforts, the National Coordinating Council for Cancer Surveillance (NCCCS), which was organized in 1995 and is currently comprised of representatives from SEER, CDC, NAACCR, NCHS, the American Cancer Society, the American College of Surgeons, and the National Cancer Registrars Association is also working to facilitate collaboration among the several surveillance agencies. As noted above, NCI should continue to support NCCCS activities.

Recommendation 2-2b: NCI should continue to work with the North American Association of Central Cancer Registries and other organizations to expand the coverage and enhance the quality of the 45 non-SEER program state cancer registries with the intent of ultimately achieving—together with the SEER program state registries—two goals: (1) a truly national data set through a system of longitudinal population-based cancer registries covering the entire country, and (2) a reliable database for each state to serve as the basis for both the development and evaluation of cancer control efforts in that state.

Medically Underserved Individuals

As discussed earlier in this chapter, medically underserved populations may be defined in many ways, including on the basis of income, insurance status, access to cancer services, or some combination of factors, such as those related to SES. The committee urges NCI to establish a consistent definition, and regularly report cancer surveillance data related to this population.

It is important that studies be undertaken to clarify whether differences in the burden of cancer are due to "racial-ethnic" or to socioeconomic factors, and the data collected on the medically underserved could help to resolve this issue. Because of the large overlap between medically underserved and ethnic minority populations, data should be cross-tabulated to reveal information on "medically underserved" and "non-medically underserved" populations within each ethnic group. Improving data collection and obtaining the necessary information can be obtained by collecting data on several indicators of SES, along with the respondent's ethnic self-identification, native language, and information on the birthplace of the respondent's parents and their ethnic identities, where possible. This more comprehensive information is especially needed for clinical and epidemiologic work. Perhaps the simplest way to begin would be to focus on access to health services (both treatment and prevention) as a data element in surveillance.

Linkage of Cancer Prevention, Screening, and Surveillance Data

One of the important pieces of information lacking in the current cancer surveillance system is the linkage of screening data or related information on cancer prevention activities to cancer incidence. Such data include access to care, which can be defined as the timely use of personal health care services to achieve the best possible health outcome. This definition relies on both the use of health care services and successful outcomes as a measure of access to care, a key aspect of cancer control among ethnic minorities and medically underserved individuals. This issue has recently been addressed by the Surveillance Implementation Group, formed by NCI in March 1998. The purpose of this group is to provide advice on proposed implementation plans, research directions, and priorities for expanding the NCI Surveillance Research Program and to recommend such plans, directions, and priorities. Defining the needed databases and surveillance systems is one of the many activities to be performed by this group in the near future.

An example of a group that links screening data to outcomes in the Breast Cancer Surveillance Consortium, which links national mammography screening data to an outcomes database (Ballard-Barbash et al., 1997). By standardizing data collection and linkage mechanisms for mammography and cancer registry data, this program will assess and improve the effectiveness of screening mammography. This important work should be continued and should serve as a model for additional programs.

Survival Data for Ethnic Groups

As noted earlier in this chapter, information on survival rates of cancer patients can help in the identification of potential problems in either access to or quality of cancer screening and treatment services. The most recently published survival data for minorities other than African Americans is from the 1978 to 1981 SEER program registry and is therefore nearly 20 years old. These data suggest that the rate of survival from cancer is much poorer among minorities and that additional follow-up is needed. The most recent SEER program monograph to addrcss racial and ethnic patterns of cancer (1988 to 1992) evaluates survival rates only among African Americans and whites. In addition, the reported SEER program data do not adequately address patterns of cancer survival among medically underserved white populations.

Recommendation 2-3: Annual reporting of cancer surveillance data and population-based research needs to be expanded to include survival data for all ethnic groups, as well as for medically underserved populations.

Human Diversity, Population Groups, and Cancer

As noted earlier in this chapter, NCI's population-based data collection efforts are shaped by Directive No. 15 of the OMB, which stipulates that the U.S. population be classified according to one of four basic "racial" categories (American Indian or Alaska Native, Asian or Pacific Islander, black or African American, or white) and one of two ethnic groups (Hispanic or non-Hispanic). Although these classifications carry important historical, social and political significance in the United States, they are of limited utility for purposes of health research because the concept of race rests upon unfounded assumptions that there are fundamental biological and behavioral differences among racial groups (Cooper, 1984; Williams, Lavizzo-Mourey, and Warren, 1994; President's Cancer Panel, 1997; American Anthropological Association, 1998) . In reality, human diversity cannot be adequately summarized according to the broad, presumably discrete categories assumed by a racial taxonomy. Furthermore, "racial" groups as defined by OMB are not discernible on the basis of genetic information (President's Cancer Panel, 1997; American Anthropological Association, 1998).

Although the four racial groups defined by OMB are broad and imprecise, and greater genetic heterogeneity exists within groups than between groups, health researchers may nonetheless benefit from understanding differences in health status between these groups. Health differences between "racial" groups may be due to many factors, including discrimination in the health care system, limited access to prevention and treatment services, poverty and socioeconomic factors, exposure to environmental toxins, and cultural factors, such as attitudes about health, beliefs, diet, and lifestyle patterns. Health is therefore a biological response to all of these conditions—conditions that are more accurately emphasized when groups are defined on the basis of ethnic background.

Ethnic groups include individuals who share a unique history different from that of other groups, in addition to other attributes, such as language, customs, ancestry, and religion. Usually, a combination of these features identifies an ethnic group. In the U.S., many groups commonly referred to as "racial groups" may be more accurately referred to as "macro-ethnic" groups. These include "white" Americans of European descent, African Americans, Asian Americans, Hispanics, and Native Americans. It is important to recognize, however, that there is considerable cultural and biological heterogeneity within these groups, and therefore the precision of population-based research can be enhanced by referring to specific subgroups. For example, within the Asian American population, there are many ethnic subgroups, including individuals of Southeast Asian, Korean, Japanese, Chinese, and Indian descent.

Distinguishing many ethnic groups from one another is therefore useful in medical and epidemiologic research, provided that researchers are clear on the nature and source of human variation (e.g., cultural and behavioral patterns, environmental influences, and genetic variation) and their relationship to health outcomes. Researchers must therefore use caution in interpreting the sources of observed differences between these groups. Ultimately, greater precision in understanding and describing human diversity is needed to distinguish genetic and environmental contributions to cancer risk and the complex effects of the gene-environment interaction. This precision can be improved with greater clarity in the conceptualization and definition of population groups.

The views of AAA are pertinent to this approach. AAA recognizes that classical racial terms may be useful for many people who prefer to use such terms about themselves with pride, but it recommends phasing out the term "race" and recommends that it be replaced with more correct terms related to ethnicity, such as "ethnic origin," which would be less prone to misunderstanding (American Anthropological Association, 1997).

Recommendation 2-4: The committee recommends an emphasis on ethnic groups rather than on race in NIH's cancer surveillance and other population research. This implies a conceptual shift away from the emphasis on fundamental biological differences among "racial" groups to an appreciation of the range of cultural and behavioral attitudes, beliefs, lifestyle patterns, diet, environmental living conditions, and other factors that may affect cancer risk.

This change should not be difficult because, under the present arrangements, the aggregations which are called "races" are really macro-ethnic groups. Scientifically speaking, there is only one race, *Homo sapiens*, but many ethnic groups and the entire population can be described within the five macro-ethnic groups we have indicated. This arrangement recognizes both the unity of the human race and the diversity of the ethnic groups, without any major disturbance in the data collection. Macro-ethnic groups can then be subdivided as indicated by the needs of cancer research to permit studies within such groups. The committee feels that it is important to study cancer within as well as across macro-ethnic groups. In this respect the diversity of the U.S. population offers an excellent opportunity to clarify issues relating to prevention and control. The study of several ethnic groups permit a better assessment of the factors contributing to cancer than studies based on "race," especially when these studies are limited to black-white differences. The racial emphasis is often associated with supposed genetic differences, but these assumptions are inconsistent with our current knowledge of the genetic diversity of the human race.

Cancer Risk Factor Research and Cancer Control

Cancer surveillance data are often used to measure the progress toward reducing the incidence of cancer that has already occurred, but the potential of those data is far greater than that. The differences in incidence, survival, and mortality rates for various ethnic groups raise critical questions about the causes of cancer and how it can best be prevented and controlled. The data suggest that many lives could be saved if more were understood about the role of behavior, the environment, socioeconomic factors, and genetic factors related to cancer and their interplay. To date, the research effort has failed to take adequate advantage of the increasing diversity of the U.S. population as a tool in understanding the interplay of cancer risk factors. Such an effort would benefit not only ethnic minorities and medically underserved individuals, but also the entire U.S. population. It requires, however, that the appropriate data be collected. This is the challenge facing the newly organized Division of Cancer Control and Population Science (DCCPS).

NCI's Cancer Control Review Group report (National Cancer Institute, 1997a) made recommendations regarding the pursuit of research opportunities most likely to accelerate reductions in the nation's cancer burden (see Appendix B for the Review Group's recommendations). One of the items highlighted in that report was the need for basic behavioral and social science research in NCI to enhance the focus on primary prevention efforts. Included in the scope of this recommendation was the need to measure risk factors and screening behaviors, especially among medically underserved individuals.

The Review Group defined cancer control research as the conduct of basic and applied research in the behavioral, social, and population sciences that, independently or in combination with biomedical approaches, reduces cancer risk, incidence, morbidity, and mortality. Thus, optimum cancer prevention and control strategies are those that combine biomedical and public health research to address the process of carcinogenesis across the life span, from prevention to screening and treatment.

The surveillance data reviewed earlier in this chapter reveal considerable gaps in the understanding of cancer risk factors among ethnic minority and medically underserved populations. Greater research is needed to illuminate risk factors both within and across population groups. Such research should address the full range of cancer risk factors, as noted above, including cultural factors affecting health attitudes, behaviors, diet, and other factors, as discussed below.

The Role of Genetics

As in the case with many other diseases such as hypertension or diabetes, large disparities in cancer incidence, mortality, and survival rates are sometimes observed between "racial" groups. These differences are sometimes assumed to be due to genetically determined differences between "races." However, it is important to understand the true nature of genetic variability both within and among "racial" groups and how evolutionary and sociocultural forces have shaped human genetic diversity to understand the meaning of the observed differences.

As noted above, assumptions that differences are due to "race" or genetics may not be justified by the evidence. Behavioral factors (e.g., smoking), environmental factors (e.g., chemical and viral exposure), and socioeconomic factors (e.g., availability, affordability, and accessibility of diagnostic, therapeutic and preventive services) are likely to be the major links responsible for a higher (or lower) incidence or prevalence of cancer in ethnic minority and medically underserved populations (or in any population). The distribution of particular genetic polymorphisms in a population may be a significant factor, however, and must also be considered in comprehensive evaluations of cancer causation. In all comprehensive population-based research on carcinogenesis, the genetic constitutions of the study subjects must be taken into account.

In a small proportion of patients with cancers of various types, mutations in a single gene can be identified as a predominant cause. In such instances, cancers of specific types show a strong tendency to run in families. Examples of genes causing hereditary breast cancer are the *BRCA1* gene on chromosome 17 and the *BRCA2* gene on chromosome 13; another example is the *p53* gene, some mutant forms of which lead to the Li-Fraumeni syndrome, which has breast cancer as one feature. These genes, however, account for no more than 3 to 5 percent of cases of breast cancer. As to the genetic factors involved in causation, most cancers are the consequence of an interplay between more than one gene collaborating with one or more environmental factors. The environmental factor may be of overwhelming importance, such as cigarette smoking in lung cancer and papillomavirus infection in cervical cancer; however, even in these instances the existence of genes that make some individuals more or less vulnerable to the environmental factors are suspected or such genes can be identified.

In general, genetic factors responsible for common disorders with multifactorial causes, such as cancers, are usually "susceptibility genes," and multiple genes are often responsible for the disorder. They represent a variable form (or allele) of a particular gene and have common variations, called *polymorphic alleles*. Alone, each variation has little effect, but in combination with other specific polymorphic alleles or nongenetic influences, these variations give rise to a particular disorder. Figure 2-1 diagrams the contrast between disorders caused by a mutation in a single gene, such as cystic fibrosis, Huntington disease, and Li-Fraumeni syndrome on the one hand and common disorders with multifactorial causation such as hypertension, manic-depressive illness, and lung cancer on the other. Each polymorphic allele occurs relatively frequently in the general "normal" population; it is present at a higher frequency (and usually in combination with other specific alleles) in people with a particular common disorder. The variable gene is a susceptibility factor, not a causative factor.

Genetic factors in common disorders with multifactorial etiology are usually investigated by allele association studies with DNA markers. These markers are sometimes variations in the sequences of specific genes that are investigated as candidate genes; because of the known functions of the genes, implication of their association in the pathogenesis of the given disorder is plausible. Alternatively, the DNA marker may be located in an "anonymous" section of the genome, that is, in a gene with an unknown function or in a noncoding region of the genome. A common variation, or "polymorphism," of a gene may alter the function of the gene product, thereby contributing to susceptibility to a disease. In such instances, the marker itself is the disease-related change. In the case of a common variation not involving the coding or gene-regulating sequence of DNA, linkage (in which genes are located close to each other on the same chromosome) is presumed to exist between the DNA variation and a specific allelic form of a susceptibility gene. Studies of associations between allelic vari-

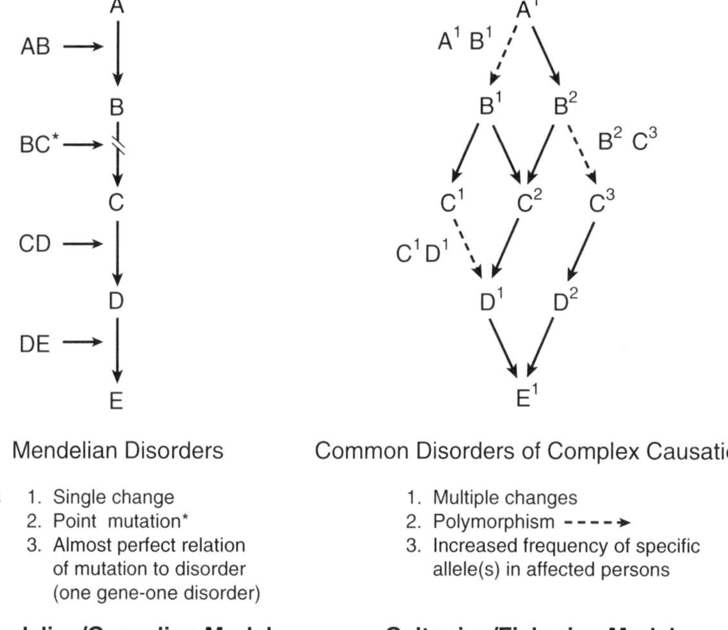

FIGURE 2-1 The contrast between disorders caused by a mutation in a single gene and common disorders with multifactorial etiology. SOURCE: Victor A. McKusick.

ants and common disorders are being undertaken with increasing frequency, in part under the stimulus of the Human Genome Project, which is identifying many genes and many polymorphisms. Caution in the interpretation of results in such studies is indicated for at least two reasons. First, population admixture, a conspicuous feature of the United States and other ethnically heterogeneous parts of the world, can cause an artifactual association if the study includes genetically distinct subpopulations, one of which coincidentally displays a higher frequency of both the disorder and the allelic variant. In such a situation, an observed association may be explained by differences in the genetic contributions of subpopulations to the case patient and control groups rather than by a physiologic effect of the genetic variant.

Consideration of the ethnic backgrounds of subjects and the study of multiple, independent populations can help avoid the subpopulation stratification problem. Also, family-based studies can provide a test of the validity of an association between an allelic variant and a disorder. In the transmission disequilibrium test, for example, if a given allele contributes to a given disease, then the probability that an affected person has inherited the allele from a heterozygous parent should vary from the expected Mendelian ratio of 50:50; association with a neutral polymorphism due to population admixture displays no such deviation in family data (Spielman at al., 1993).

A second pitfall is that testing of multiple hypotheses, aggravated by publication bias, can lead to fallacious conclusions concerning associations. Researchers who test a single genetic change (mutation) for its association with a single disorder base their statistical conclusions on a single hypothesis. Many researchers, however, seek associations using multiple genetic variants. Each test represents an independent hypothesis, but there is a tendency to publish only positive results. In fact, these may merely represent those cases expected to fall outside the 95 percent confidence limits in tests with multiple genetic variants. Statistical correction for multiple testing is possible, but such corrections result in a loss of statistical power (Altshuler et al., 1998).

The types of DNA markers used in association studies include restriction fragment length polymorphisms, variable-number tandem repeats, microsatellites (short tandem repeats), and single nucleotide polymorphisms (Collins et al., 1997). These markers are listed roughly in the order in which they have been used historically. NCI is initiating a research program to identify all variations in the human genome (Richard Klausner, Director, National Cancer Institute, personal communication, 1998). The Human Genome Diversity Project is a follow-up to the Human Genome Project. When the goals of the Human Genome Project—mapping of all human genes and determination of the sequences of all DNA in those genes—are achieved, it will still be unknown how the genes and the DNA vary among the 6 billion or 7 billion or more people who will inhabit the Earth at that time. The functions of all those genes will also still be unknown, as will how variations in the structure of the DNA and genes relate to variations in function, including variations in susceptibility to common disorders, including cancers.

The Human Genome Diversity Project proposes to identify the range of DNA variation that can be the basis for studies of genetic factors in common disorders. In the pursuit of the Human Genome Diversity Project or any DNA-based studies with special populations, including ethnic minorities and medically underserved individuals, concerns about the risks of discrimination and stigmatization have been raised. The ethical, legal, and societal implications of the project have been addressed by Knoppers et al. (1996, 1998) and by the report of a committee of the National Research Council.

The newly organized DCCPS recognizes that epidemiology and genetics represent the foundations of cancer control research. Its Epidemiology and Genetics Program has studied the following:

- Interactions of genetic and metabolic factors with lifestyle, social and behavioral factors, diet and nutrition, hormones, and medications.
- Gene prevalence-associated metabolic markers and predictive value of identified genes and markers.
- Definitions of ethnicity using molecular genetics and; application of these definitions, as well as data on behavior and lifestyle choices, to studies of the effects of migration on the incidence of cancers.
- The genetic determinants, tumor markers, and cancer risk from immune function.
- Special populations with different patterns of cancer risk.
- Means of improving estimate of exposures by direct and indirect means.

Studies of Human Behavior

NCI research in the area of human behavior has not been strong in the past, but an expanded behavioral research program is planned in DC-CPS, according to NCI officials (Barbara Rimer, National Cancer Institute, communication with the study committee, June 12, 1998). This program will place greater emphasis on the development of balanced behavioral research portfolios that include a range of research in all areas, spanning basic research, dissemination research, and policy development.

The literature from anthropology, psychology, sociology, behavioral medicine, and public health has shown that different ethnic groups vary in their attitudes, perceptions, and behaviors toward health. As noted earlier, macro-ethnic groups, such as Asian Americans, include many sub-groups, such as Chinese Americans, Japanese Americans, and Vietnamese Americans, to name only a few. For each ethnic group, culture influences their health, their attitudes toward health, and their health practices, although individual beliefs, attitudes, and behaviors may vary. Another factor is acculturation, the degree to which immigrants leave behind a culture of origin and assimilate aspects of their new culture. Some health behaviors may change within a few years of taking up residence in the U.S., while others may persist for generations. For example, newly arrived Mexican women are less likely to smoke than women of Mexican origin raised in the U.S. In addition, a study on Pap smear and mammogram screening in Mexican-American women found that the prevalence of these screenings increased with acculturation (Suarez, 1994). Given the diversity of health practices even within one ethnic group, it is essential to obtain accurate and detailed ethnic histories of people to obtain a better understanding and knowledge of differences in health practices and possible risk.

Research on the different health care practices of various ethnic minority groups has described the existence of subcultures with different values, actions, and perceptions about health and illness (e.g., Saunders, 1954; Kleinman et al., 1978; Leslie, 1976; Good and DelVecchio, 1981; Hahn, 1995). These also include behaviors such as diet and exercise patterns, and interaction with the health care system (Salazar, 1996; Crane et al., 1996). For many of these groups the family and other social networks are important in providing support during illness in and health-seeking behaviors.

During the testimony heard by this committee from representatives of several ethnic minority and community groups (see Chapter 4 for a description of this testimony), two conflicting concerns about ethnicity were raised. One was that by identifying cultural habits that increase risk or reduce the likelihood of carrying out treatment, one is "blaming the victim" by "blaming culture." In contrast, the concern was also expressed that not enough attention is paid to cultural norms, values, and concerns. Since all human beings are influenced by culture, these influences and their effects must be taken into account, but in ways which are sensitive to community concerns. It is understandable that many individuals in ethnic groups share common fears and distrust of both the medical care system and the research community, based on a history of disrespect and mistreatment of minorities by the research community. The Tuskegee syphilis experiment (summarized in greater detail in Chapter 5) is cited by African Americans and by Hispanics as a reason not to trust the government or researchers (Robinson et al., 1996). It is therefore important to understand the factual basis for this mistrust, and assess its impact on health care delivery and health behaviors among ethnic minority populations.

Summary of Cancer Risk Factor Research and Surveillance Needs

The committee finds that the newly reorganized DCCPS at NCI is well poised to address a wide range of challenges to improving our understanding of cancer risk among ethnic minority and medically underserved populations. Greater precision is needed in the definition and conceptualization of high-risk populations, and research must examine the diverse range of cancer risk both within and between ethnic groups. The committee is confident, however, that such research conducted under DCCPS's auspices will prove fruitful for the national cancer effort.

Recommendation 2-5: The committee commends the proposed NCI program of expanded behavioral and epidemiological research examining the relationship between cancer and cancer risk factors associated with various ethnic minority and medically underserved groups, and recommends that these studies be conducted both across and within these groups.

SUMMARY

In this chapter, the committee has reviewed some of the difficulties associated with understanding and defining the problem of cancer among ethnic minorities and medically underserved individuals. In a large and diverse nation such as the United States, with its many overlapping population groups that may experience differences in cancer risk as a result of a complex interplay of environmental, cultural, socioeconomic, behavioral, and other factors, the use of clear and consistent definitions of populations is imperative to understanding how cancer differentially burdens various groups among the overall population. Depending on how populations are defined, cancer incidence, mortality, and survival rates vary considerably. Some ethnic minority groups, for example, may experience lower rates of some forms of cancer relative to the white majority; others, such as African Americans, experience higher rates of cancer incidence and mortality, and lower cancer survival rates. Groups of lower SES experience cancer incidence and mortality rates that are, in many instances, as high as the highest of any ethnic minority group. Understanding why cancer differentially affects these groups offers important clues to cancer etiology and control research.

Because cancer surveillance is critical to this effort, the committee finds that greater resources must be committed to expanding upon the existing, high-quality SEER program data. Additional data must be collected to understand cancer among medically underserved groups, and SEER program coverage of other important population groups should be improved. Because the problem of defining populations is complex, the committee offers recommendations on how population groups may be conceptualized, but recognizes that the NIH has been constrained in its data collection efforts by current federal guidelines.

The following recommendations were offered:

Recommendation 2-1: NIH should develop and implement across all institutes a uniform definition of "special populations" with cancer. This definition should be flexible but should be based on disproportionate or insufficiently studied burdens of cancer, as measured by cancer incidence, morbidity, mortality, and survival statistics.

Recommendation 2-2a: To further enhance the excellent data provided in the SEER program database, adequate resources should be provided to expand SEER program coverage beyond the existing sites to include high-risk populations for which SEER program coverage is lacking. This expansion should address a wider range of demographic and social characteristics by using consistent nomenclature and a uniform data set and by reflecting the diverse characteristics of the current U.S. population.

Recommendation 2-2b: NCI should continue to work with the North American Association of Central Cancer Registries and other organizations to expand the coverage and enhance the quality of the 45 non-SEER program state cancer registries with the intent of ultimately achieving—together with the SEER program state registries—two goals: (1) a truly national data set through a system of longitudinal population-based cancer registries covering the entire country, and (2) a reliable database for each state to serve as the basis for both the development and evaluation of cancer control efforts in that state.

Recommendation 2-3: Annual reporting of cancer surveillance data and population-based research needs to be expanded to include survival data for all ethnic groups, as well as for medically underserved populations.

Recommendation 2-4: The committee recommends an emphasis on ethnic groups rather than on race in NIH's cancer surveillance and other population research. This implies a conceptual shift away from the emphasis on fundamental biological differences among "racial" groups to an appreciation of the range of cultural and behavioral attitudes, beliefs, lifestyle patterns, diet, environmental living conditions, and other factors that may affect cancer risk.

Recommendation 2-5: The committee commends the proposed NCI program of expanded behavioral and epidemiological research examining the relationship between cancer and cancer risk factors associated with various ethnic minority and medically underserved groups, and recommends that these studies be conducted both across and within these groups.

3
Overview of Programs of Research on Ethnic Minority and Medically Underserved Populations at the National Institutes of Health

The National Institutes of Health (NIH) is responsible for a broad range of basic, biomedical, behavioral, epidemiologic, and clinical research that addresses America's health needs. Research on the prevention, detection, treatment, and control of cancer is the primary responsibility of the National Cancer Institute (NCI). The National Cancer Act of 1971 (P.L. 75-244) directs NCI to plan and develop a coordinated research program that encompasses all institutes, centers, and divisions (ICDs) of NIH, as well as other federal and nonfederal research organizations, and to develop a cancer control program that demonstrates effective practices in cancer prevention and management. NCI interprets its mission as follows:

> The National Cancer Institute coordinates the National Cancer Program, which conducts and supports research, training, health information dissemination, and other programs with respect to the cause, diagnosis, prevention, and treatment of cancer, rehabilitation from cancer, and the continuing care of cancer patients and the families of cancer patients. Specifically, the Institute:
>
> - Supports and coordinates research projects conducted by universities, hospitals, research foundations, and businesses throughout this country and abroad through research grants and cooperative agreements.
> - Conducts research in its own laboratories and clinics.
> - Supports education and training in fundamental sciences and clinical disciplines for participation in basic and clinical research programs

and treatment programs relating to cancer through career awards, training grants, and fellowships.

- Supports research projects in cancer control.
- Supports a national network of cancer centers.
- Collaborates with voluntary organizations and other national and foreign institutions engaged in cancer research and training activities.
- Encourages and coordinates cancer research by industrial concerns where such concerns evidence a particular capability for programmatic research.
- Collects and disseminates information on cancer.
- Supports construction of laboratories, clinics, and related facilities necessary for cancer research through the award of construction grants (National Cancer Institute, 1998d).

Although NCI directs a large and comprehensive program of cancer research within its portfolio and collaborates with other groups on research or cosponsors other cancer research at other ICDs, the committee finds that there is little evidence of a strategic plan for cancer research relevant to ethnic minority and medically underserved populations at NIH coordinated through NCI or any other central mechanism, as noted below.

This section describes the range of ongoing cancer-related research and programs at NCI and other ICDs, summarizes cancer-related research programs at NCI and other ICDs that are relevant to ethnic minority and medically underserved populations, and reviews the funding for these programs. Particular emphasis is placed on the programs and functions of NCI, given its stated role in coordinating cancer-related research at NIH.

OVERVIEW OF NIH APPROPRIATIONS AND FUNDING FOR CANCER RESEARCH

Over the past decade, NIH and NCI have enjoyed significant increases in congressional appropriations, from periods of little to no growth in the early 1980s to steady increases in the mid-1990s (Figure 3-1). NCI experienced a slight decline in its budget from 1980 ($1 billion) to 1983 ($987.6 million), but by 1986 the Institute's budget reached $1.26 billion, and it had reached nearly $1.6 billion by the end of the decade (National Cancer Institute, 1998e). Annually, nearly 80 percent of the institute's budget is dedicated to research, whereas approximately 10 percent of the budget is allocated toward both resource development and cancer prevention and control activities. In fiscal year (FY) 1997, $1.411 billion was allocated for research grants, including $577 million for investigator-initiated grants (R01 grants) and $132 million for cancer center grants. More than $412

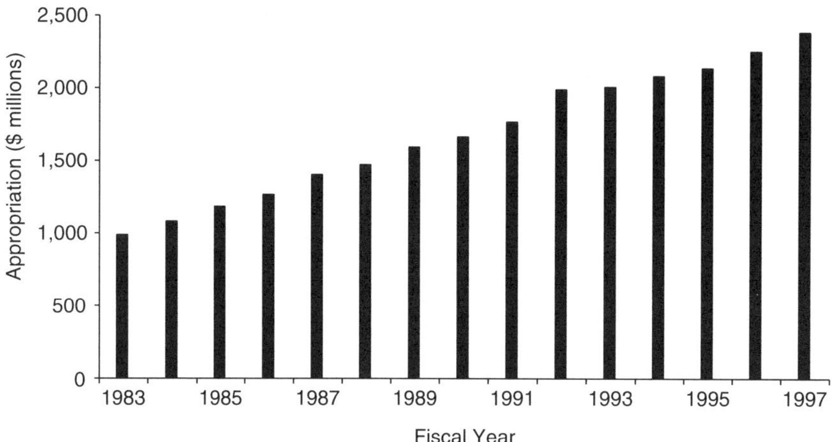

FIGURE 3-1 National Cancer Institute appropriations, 1983–1997. SOURCE: National Cancer Institute.

million was reserved for intramural research and $231 million was allocated for cancer prevention and control.

NCI has appeared to prioritize extramural spending on traditional R01 grants (increasing allocations for R01 grants from $356 million in FY 1986 to $377 million in FY 1989, even though the number of such grants declined from 2,508 to 2,239), outstanding investigator grants (increasing spending from $23.2 million in FY 1986 to nearly $53 million in FY 1989), cooperative agreements (doubling spending of $10 million in FY 1986 to $20 million by FY 1989), and intramural research (increasing spending from nearly $214 million in FY 1986 to $294 million by FY 1989; National Cancer Institute, 1998e). (See Box 3-1 for a description of common NIH research grant mechanisms.)

By FY 1993, NCI's budget topped $2 billion for the first time, allowing the Institute to increase funding for R01 grants to $430 million (although the number of grants awarded decreased again to 1,955), increasing MERIT awards from $32 million in FY 1989 to $51.6 million in FY 1993, increasing spending on cancer control contracts from $33 million in FY 1989 to more than $52 million in FY 1993, and nearly doubling the cancer career grant program over FY 1989 levels to $14 million (National Cancer Institute, 1998e).

Congressional appropriations for NCI topped $2.38 billion in FY 1997 and fueled increases in both funding and the number of R01 grants made by the institute (more than $577 million was applied to 2,194 awardees). The number and amount allocated for First Independent Research Sup-

Box 3-1
Common Research Grant Award Mechanisms at NIH

F31	Predoctoral Individual National Research Service Award
K01	Research Scientist Development Award—Research and Training
K08	Clinical Investigator Award
P20	Exploratory Grants
R01	Traditional Research Project Award
R03	Small Grant Award
R13	Conference Grant Award
R15	Academic Research Enhancement Awards
R21	Exploratory/Developmental Grants
R25	Education Projects
R43	Small Business Innovation Research Grants—Phase I
R55	James A. Shannon Director's Award
S06	Minority Biomedical Research Support
U01	Cooperative Agreement Research Support

port and Transition awards also increased ($47 million in awards to 446 grantees, an increase of more than $18 million from FY 1993 levels), as was the case for U01 cooperative agreements (more than $81 million in awards, up from $56 million in FY 1993) and the Clinical Cooperative Program (more than $86 million in awards, an increase of more than $12 million from FY 1993). Spending on cancer control grants and contracts more than doubled to more than $70 million and $110 million each, respectively (National Cancer Institute, 1998e).

CANCER RESEARCH AT OTHER ICDs

Although the increases outlined above do not represent the sum of spending on all cancer-related research at NIH, NCI has traditionally allocated the largest amount of any of NIH's ICDs on cancer research. Over the past several years, NCI's share of this budget has hovered at slightly greater than 85 percent of the total amount of NIH money spent on cancer-related research (National Institutes of Health, 1998). Many cancer-related grant programs sponsored by ICDs other than NCI enjoy joint sponsorship with NCI. In FY 1997, NIH spent approximately $2.76 billion on cancer research, more than 86 percent of which was funded directly by NCI. It is expected that by FY 1999 overall spending by NIH on cancer-related research will exceed $3.23 billion, fueled in large part by the Clinton Administration's request for NCI appropriations of $2.77 billion.

The National Institute of Environmental Health Sciences (NIEHS) holds the second largest portfolio of cancer-related research among the institutes at NIH, with allocations of $84.44 million in FY 1997, a figure that approached nearly $90 million in FY 1998. The National Heart, Lung, and Blood Institute (NHLBI) is third in cancer-related funding with funding, of $57.6 million in FY 1997, followed by the National Institute of Allergy and Infectious Diseases (NIAID) with funding of $43 million and the National Institute on Diabetes and Digestive and Kidney Diseases (NIDDKD) with funding of $33.4 million (see Table 3-1).

Examined by spending on specific cancer sites, cancer types, diseases related to cancer, and types of research mechanisms, NIH reports spending the greatest amount of money on cancer clinical trials (more than $400 million in FY 1997, an increase of more than $150 million from FY 1990), followed by funding for breast cancer (more than $330 million in FY 1997, a fourfold increase over FY 1990 levels of $81 million), cancer prevention and control activities (nearly $240 million in FY 1997, up from $80.5 million in FY 1990), AIDS-related cancers ($224 million spend in FY 1997, up from $149 million in FY 1990), and lung cancer ($132 million in FY 1997, up from $65 million in FY 1990). Among cancers that disproportionately affect ethnic minority and medically underserved communities (in addition to the cancer types described above), NIH spent $74 million across ICDs on prostate cancer-related research in FY 1997 (up from $13.2 million in FY 1990), $54 million on cervical cancer (an increase of $30 million from FY 1990 levels), approximately $100 million on colorectal cancer (nearly doubling spending from $51.2 million in FY 1990), and $39 million on ovarian cancer (nearly four times the $10.5 million spent in FY 1990). In contrast, other cancers that disproportionately affect minority and medically underserved groups, such as liver cancer ($33 million in FY 1997) and uterine cancer ($8.6 million in FY 1997), have not received substantial increases in funding, with increases of only about $5 million and $2 million, respectively, since FY 1990. It must be noted, however, that funding for these disease areas can and often does overlap. Basic research and clinical research that benefits more than one type of cancer site are included in estimates of total funding for each cancer (see Table 3-2; National Institutes of Health, 1998).

OFFICE OF RESEARCH ON MINORITY HEALTH

The NIH Office of Research on Minority Health (ORMH) was established in 1990 by then-director of NIH William Raub and was authorized by the U.S. Congress in the 1993 National Institutes of Health Revitaliza-

TABLE 3-1 National Institutes of Health Cancer Research Initiative

	Dollars (in thousands)			
Participating ICDS	FY 1997 Actual	FY 1998 Estimate	FY 1999 Estimate	% Change 1999/1998
NCI	$2,389,041	$2,547,314	$2,776,267	9.0
Cancer % to Total	**86.50%**	**86.6%**	**85.9%**	
NHLBI*	57,620	59,815	67,539	12.9
NIDR	16,448	17,313	19,811	14.4
NIDDK	33,430	36,450	39,350	8.0
NINDS	17,929	18,734	24,468	30.6
NIAID	43,085	44,377	47,927	8.0
NIGMS	22,574	24,421	30,421	24.6
NICHD	10,311	11,000	11,900	8.2
NEI	8,616	9,242	9,508	2.9
NIEHS	84,368	89,430	94,796	6.0
NIA	12,183	12,730	14,990	17.8
NIAMS	5,303	5,690	6,220	9.3
NIDCD	2,910	3,087	4,296	39.2
NIMH	4,287	3,823	4,116	7.7
NIAAA	2,700	2,000	2,500	25.0
NINR	3,570	4,250	4,570	7.5
NHGRI	17,084	22,158	30,151	36.1
NCRR	25,926	28,754	37,874	31.7
FIC	195	575	600	4.3
NLM	0	0	4,500	0.0
NIH	2,760,698	2,941,163	3,231,804	9.9

*All years adjusted to reflect Women's Health Initiative.
SOURCE: National Institutes of Health.

tion Act (P.L. 103-43). Its mission, as established by Congress, is to coordinate the development of NIH policies, goals, and objectives related to minority health research and research training programs and to expand the level of participation of minorities in all aspects of biomedical research (including training of minority scientists and participation of ethnic minority individuals in NIH-sponsored clinical trials). ORMH seeks to accomplish these goals largely by working in partnership with other NIH ICDs, as well as other governmental agencies.

ORMH holds no independent grant-making authority; its primary function in addressing minority health research needs is to leverage research support by creating partnerships with other NIH institutes. In effect, ORMH collaborates with NIH institutes and centers (ICs) to support research and training projects. Administrative and professional support

TABLE 3-2 Research Dollars (in millions) by Various Cancers

	1990 Actual	1991 Actual	1992 Actual	1993 Actual	1994 Actual	1995 Actual	1996 Actual	1997 Actual	President's Budget
Total NCI*	$1,644.3	$1,712.7	$1,947.6	$1,978.3	$2,076.2	$2,130.3	$2,254.9	$2,381.1	$2,441.7
AIDS	$149.2	$160.9	$165.7	$173.0	$213.0	$217.4	$225.4	$224.7	$224.3
Brain and central nervous system	29.8	31.5	32.5	40.5	41.7	43.0	41.6	44.2	46.3
Breast cancer	81.0	92.7	145.0	211.5	267.6	308.7	317.5	332.9	338.9
Cancer prevention and control	80.5	90.8	114.9	112.6	153.9	205.0	22.0	248.7	251.0
Cervical cancer	21.9	22.3	30.7	42.2	42.3	45.5	51.6	54.0	56.0
Clinical trials	246.0	254.4	314.5	326.8	339.0	384.8	393.8	403.9	412.6
Colorectal cancer	51.2	56.5	69.2	74.2	83.1	96.5	98.0	99.0	100.0
Hodgkins disease	7.5	7.8	6.7	6.8	6.7	7.8	8.0	8.4	8.8
Leukemia	50.4	60.1	64.6	74.2	77.7	77.5	79.3	83.0	86.0
Liver cancer	28.3	29.8	30.7	37.5	37.9	38.0	31.4	33.2	34.7
Lung cancer	65.1	68.7	76.3	92.9	106.4	113.9	119.4	123.3	128.2
Melanoma	21.2	26.2	24.8	29.8	33.4	31.8	36.0	37.3	38.3
Non Hodgkin's lymphoma*			33.4	40.1	38.7	39.7	49.9	51.5	52.7
Ovarian cancer	10.5	13.6	20.7	32.5	33.5	33.9	36.5	39.0	40.6
Prostate cancer	13.2	13.8	31.4	51.1	56.1	64.3	71.1	74.0	77.5
Uterine cancer	6.5	7.0	7.8	6.3	7.2	7.7	8.1	8.6	9.0

*Includes AIDS funding.
SOURCE: National Institutes of Health.

for these collaborations is conducted by IC staff following an interagency transfer of funds from ORMH to ICs.

The ORMH priority-setting and funding processes appear to be driven by the professional judgment and research priorities of an ad hoc panel, as well as those of other ICs. In response to an inquiry from the study committee, ORMH writes:

> ORMH begins its funding process by asking the ICs, "What is it that we should be doing that we are not doing?" In practice the ORMH sends out two communications to the ICs annually. The first call is for the confirmation of projects for which ORMH has committed out-year support. The second call is for the submission of new projects or programs that the ICs consider meritorious and which fill a gap in minority health research and/or research training. Because the level of support requested by the ICs usually exceed the budget for the Minority Health Initiative, an ad hoc review panel is convened to assist ORMH in prioritizing the projects to support (National Institutes of Health, Office of Research on Minority Health, 1998a).

Research initiatives proposed by other ICs for ORMH co-funding are evaluated by the Center for Scientific Review and individual IC advisory councils for appropriateness. Proposals are then forwarded to ORMH for evaluation and prioritization.

Although the ORMH proposal review process has been conducted by an ad hoc panel since the office's inception, as of recently the newly appointed Advisory Committee on Research on Minority Health will advise the ORMH director on prioritizing the projects that ORMH will support. This committee, which held its first meeting in April 1998, is composed of 12 individuals with expertise in minority health research or research training, or both. The committee will advise the ORMH director regarding appropriate research priorities and activities for the enhancement of minority health for the inclusion of minority groups as subjects in clinical research and for the enhancement of minority participation in research and training programs. The committee is expected to meet twice a year and to produce a biennial report summarizing its advice and recommendations regarding NIH programs. The establishment of the Advisory Committee appears to represent the first step toward a "formalized" process of internal review of ORMH activities (see Chapter 4 for a more detailed discussion of the ORMH priority-setting process).

Specifically, at the first meeting of the committee, ORMH Director John Ruffin and NIH Director Harold Varmus asked for the committee's assistance in several areas, including reviewing the current portfolio of research co-funded by ORMH to identify potential gaps, assessing whether critical minority health research issues are being appropriately addressed through the Minority Health Initiative, and advising NIH regarding optimal approaches for recruiting and training minorities for health research. Ruffin specifically asked for assistance in responding to new challenges, including developments in human genome research and changes to federal affirmative action policies that may affect minority scientist recruitment and training.

ORMH Research Funding

Funding for ORMH has increased significantly since the office was created in 1991, but its overall funding remains minuscule in comparison to the $14 billion overall budget of NIH. In FY 1991 the office initiated activities with a budget of $1.5 million. Funding increased sixfold in FY 1992, to more than $9.5 million. In FY 1993 ORMH's budget allocation increased to $48.4 million, coinciding with passage of the Minority Health Improvement Act of 1993. In FY 1994 and FY 1995 ORMH funding increased to $62.7 million and $67.8 million, respectively, but it saw its first budget decline in FY 1997, when the ORMH allocation dropped to $70.1 million from a high of $71.1 million in FY 1996.

In research relevant to the study of cancer among ethnic minority populations, ORMH reports that from 1992 to 1997, it provided nearly $20 million in funding to assist NCI minority initiatives. The bulk of this funding has been to support the Minority Adolescent HIV Prevention and Treatment Project (approximately $10 million from FY 1994 to FY 1997). Other significant expenditures include funding for grants to improve ethnic minority recruitment and retention in clinical trials, funds for training of minority investigators, and small research supplements. In FY 1997 ORMH allocated slightly less than $6 million to NCI (see Table 3-3), including $1.75 million to support the Minority Adolescent HIV Prevention and Treatment Project, $1 million to cancer centers to support minority recruitment to NCI-sponsored clinical trials, and nearly $750,000 to support other efforts to increase minority participation in clinical trials. These expenditures for cancer-related projects were approximately 9 percent of ORMH's total budget in FY 1997. ORMH reports that NCI did not provide additional funds beyond initial funding (e.g., for overall cancer center or clinical trial operations) to support these projects.

Estimated ORMH expenditures on cancer in FY 1998 reflect its twofold mission. The office allocated $6.22 million to assist NCI projects on cancer among minorities in FY 1998. The three largest NCI projects supported by ORMH are the Minority Adolescent HIV Prevention and Treatment Project ($1.75 million), funds to encourage minority participation in NCI-sponsored trials ($1 million), and training supplements for underrepresented minorities ($750,000; see Training of Minority Scientists below). Other expenditures include grants for regional workshops for mi-

TABLE 3-3 National Cancer Institute Minority Initiatives Supported by the NIH Office of Research on Minority Health (FY 1997)

Projects	ORMH $	Institute $
Minority Adolescent HIV and Treatment Project	1,750,000	0
Enrollment of Minorities in NCI Clinical Trials	59,535	0
Overcoming Impediments to Participation of Minorities and Special Populations in Clinical Trials	500,000	0
Minority Participation in NCI-Sponsored Clinical Trials	1,000,000	0
Barriers to Latino-American Participation in Cancer Clinical Trials	21,011	0
Procurement of Prostate Tumor Tissues from African-American Patients	52,326	0
Determination of Correlation Between Androgen Receptor CAG Trinucleotide Repeat Length and Prostate Cancer Risk	291,000	0
Small Grant for Women and Minority Recruitment	68,120	0
Cohort Study of African-American Men with Prostate Cancer	77,225	0
Caucus on Prostate Cancer and Minorities	45,528	0
Preventing Cancer in Hispanic Communities	249,954	0
Collaborative Clinical and Molecular Correlative Studies	350,000	0
Institute of Medicine Minority Cancer Study	600,000	0
Baylor College of Medicine—Biennial Symposium on Cancer and Minorities	30,000	0
NCI International Program Middle East Conference	250,000	0
Regional Grantsmanship Workshops for Minority Investigators	100,000	0
Minority Research Supplements	750,000	0
TOTAL	**6,179,171**	**0**

SOURCE: NIH Office of Research on Minority Health.

nority investigators, for grants conferences to stimulate ethnic minority participation in clinical trials, supplemental funding for basic research related to prostate cancer and ethnic minorities, and small supplements for minority cancer control and prevention programs.

ORMH's estimates of its expenditures on cancer-related research may overstate the amount of funding that directly addresses the cancer research needs of ethnic minority and medically underserved populations. As noted above, funding for the Minority Adolescent HIV and Treatment project represents a large proportion of ORMH's allocation for cancer research. The committee questions, however, the relevance of this project for cancer research. Although neoplasms are a significant health concern among patients suffering from AIDS and HIV-related complications, an overview of the Minority Adolescent HIV and Treatment Project supplied to the committee by ORMH does not mention the words "cancer," "neoplasms," or other related terms. Rather, this project's main focus appears to be the establishment of a community-based, comprehensive, and multidisciplinary health care center to monitor, treat, and enroll HIV-infected ethnic minority children and adolescents in HIV and AIDS Malignancy Branch clinical trials. It is unclear how many, if any, of the population enrolled in this program were treated for AIDS-related carcinomas. In addition, results of this research project may be limited; ORMH reports that the project was terminated in late FY 1998 "due to insurmountable contractual and legal issues" (National Institutes of Health, Office of Research on Minority Health, 1998a).

Assessment of ORMH Activities

ORMH serves as a focal point for the coordination of research on ethnic minority health at NIH. One of the office's major functions is to stimulate research on minority populations at relevant ICs of NIH by providing research supplements (including Minority Health Initiative funds) to "leverage" IC resources. ORMH has only recently, however, established a standing advisory panel to help guide the establishment of research priorities (this function had previously been assumed by an ad hoc panel) and does not participate in the Research Enhancement Awards Program with other specialty offices at NIH to coordinate funding proposals and priorities. Its criteria for program funding and research priorities have therefore been less open to public scrutiny. In addition, OMRH program funding appears to have supplanted, rather than leveraged, NCI resources for important research and program activities in many instances. The committee offers the following recommendation to strengthen ORMH's stated functions:

Recommendation 3-1: The Office of Research on Minority Health should more actively serve a coordinating, planning, and facilitative function regarding research relevant to cancer among ethnic minority and medically underserved populations across relevant institutes and centers of NIH. To further this goal, the Office of Research on Minority Health should:

- **make criteria for Minority Health Initiative project support explicit;**
- **coordinate with other specialty offices (e.g., the Office of Research on Women's Health) by participating in NIH-wide coordination efforts such as the Research Enhancement Awards Program; and**

- **ensure that Minority Health Initiative funding does not supplant funding from institutes and centers for research and programs relevant to ethnic minority and medically underserved populations.**

OVERVIEW OF SCIENTIFIC INFRASTRUCTURE AT NCI

Since 1996, NCI has undertaken several significant changes in its internal structure that affect both intramural and extramural scientific programs. Many of the these changes were initiated in response to a series of internal program reviews, including the 1995 Bishop-Calabresi report (Ad Hoc Working Group of the National Cancer Advisory Board, 1995), which recommended a complete organizational separation of intramural and extramural programs. Two new extramural divisions, the Division of Cancer Prevention (DCP) and the Division of Cancer Control and Population Sciences (DCCPS), were created. DCP was created to add "visibility, prominence, and strength to the NCI's prevention programs" (National Cancer Institute, 1998d, p. 11), whereas DCCPS was created from programs of the Division of Cancer Prevention and Control, which has been eliminated, as well as extramural portions of the Division of Cancer Epidemiology and Genetics.

Perhaps most significantly for ethnic minority and medically underserved groups, three new offices were created to develop partnerships with community-based groups that focus on cancer. The Office of Special Populations Research (OSPR) was formed to provide a focal point and coordinating center for research related to "special populations," defined by NCI as economically disadvantaged people, elderly people, and certain ethnic minority groups. OSPR works with other NCI offices to assist in defining scientific questions relating to special populations, as well as in evaluating the effectiveness of outreach efforts aimed at these populations. The Office of Liaison Activities links to national cancer advocacy organizations to facilitate communication between NCI and community-based groups. Similarly, the Office of Cancer Survivorship develops and coordinates research on cancer survivorship to address "the unique physical, social, psychological, and economic issues faced by these individuals" (National Cancer Institute, 1998d).

Intramural Research

Intramural research at NCI is conducted principally in the Divisions of Basic Sciences, Clinical Sciences, and Epidemiology and Genetics. This research encompasses basic, clinical, and population-based research. In addition, NCI intramural laboratories and clinics train cancer research specialists. The intramural research relevant to ethnic minority and medically underserved populations is described below.

Extramural Research

NCI's principal activity involves the funding of extramural research. Extramural research accounts for more than 75 percent of the institute's budget and includes both laboratory and clinical investigations (including individual or program project grants and cooperative agreements), epidemiologic studies and surveys, cancer control projects, cancer centers, construction and general medical infrastructure, and education. These extramural programs are categorized under cancer research activities, cancer control, and cancer resource development (National Cancer Institute, 1998f).

NCI's extramural research program is driven largely by investigator-initiated proposals for funding, consistent with the philosophy of its director, Richard Klausner. Proposals are evaluated on the basis of several criteria, principally, whether the research affords the greatest scientific opportunities to increase the level of knowledge about cancer. A second factor that guides funding is the degree of burden posed by specific cancers. All investigator-initiated research proposals are evaluated by any of more than 100 study sections or peer-review groups, which evaluate the importance of the research topic, the rigor of the proposed methodologies or techniques, and the investigator's ability to meet the aims of the study. NCI anticipates awarding more than $1.19 billion in extramural research awards in FY 1998 to support 3,700 research grants, more than 1,000 of which are new or competing renewal projects (National Cancer Institute, 1998d).

Much of the extramural research infrastructure is supported by other peer-reviewed mechanisms, including the network of cancer centers, community clinical oncology programs, clinical cooperative groups, tissue banks, some surveillance activities, and training programs. Other components are funded by contract with NCI, including major cancer registries (see the description of the Surveillance, Epidemiology, and End Result [SEER] program below).

Cancer Centers

NCI currently supports 57 cancer centers for the purposes of conducting interdisciplinary research, training, and education. The Cancer Centers Program is designed to create a flexible infrastructure for innovative research and clinical and community applications to promote collaboration between basic, clinical, and population research scientists. A key element of the cancer centers is to bring "the benefits of research more directly to local communities and regions of the country" (National Cancer Institute, 1998d, p. 34) by linking research and clinical application activities. Cancer center activities include the development of linkages with industry, state and local health agencies, and community organizations. However, no funding is provided for the development of such linkages.

Clinical Trials Infrastructure

Many of the NCI-supported cancer centers are involved in clinical trials. The largest source of support for clinical trials, however, is the NCI Community Clinical Oncology Program (CCOP) and Clinical Trials Cooperative Group program. NCI supports hundreds of clinical trials via these mechanisms. Fifty-two CCOPs are currently funded in 30 states, with an additional eight minority-based CCOPs (MBCCOPs) funded to increase the numbers of ethnic minority patients in clinical trials research. The Clinical Trials Cooperative Group program includes 12 groups that annually place approximately 20,000 new patients into cancer treatment protocols.

Training and Education

NCI's Cancer Training Program supports individual fellowship and career awards and education grants to support the cancer research infrastructure. The institute pursues four strategies to achieve this goal: (1) maintaining the numbers of basic scientists studying underlying genetic and biological mechanisms of disease; (2) encouraging a greater proportion of basic scientists to develop interests in model systems of human disease; (3) attracting more young physicians, public health specialists, and other health care professionals into cancer research, especially in biostatistical, epidemiologic, behavioral, and other prevention and control sciences; and (4) using education grants to improve the curricula for health care and public health students.

Cancer Control

NCI-supported cancer control activities attempt to disseminate and apply new medical knowledge to routine practice. This includes research on the behavioral, psychosocial, health services, communication, and cancer surveillance aspects of cancer control.

Dissemination

NCI conducts several dissemination activities through the Office of Cancer Information, Communication, and Education (OCICE). The Cancer Information Service (CIS) provides information to cancer patients and their families through a toll-free telephone information service and through community outreach efforts and educational campaigns. The International Cancer Information Center (ICIC) provides cancer information to scientists, health care professionals, and the public through PDQ, the NCI's cancer information database, and the bibliographic CANCERLIT database. NCI also disseminates information via its site on the World Wide Web.

NCI FY 1997 PROGRAMS AND RESOURCES ALLOCATED TO ADDRESSING ETHNIC MINORITY AND MEDICALLY UNDERSERVED POPULATIONS

NCI categorizes research and training programs relevant to special populations (including ethnic minority and medically underserved populations) into two subgroups. Category I programs are defined as "research or training targeted to, or for, a specific special population or populations," whereas Category II programs are "research on a problem affecting all populations (thus, not targeted to any specific group). This research is, however, of special significance to a specific special population or populations" (National Cancer Institute, 1998b, p. 4). Both program subtypes are reported here.

Cancer Surveillance Activities

NCI's cancer surveillance effort is aimed at identifying and reporting on the disease frequencies in the U.S. population that may be useful in identifying trends and generating causal hypotheses. At the core of this effort is the SEER program, which is described in greater detail in Chapter 2. SEER program data emanate from 11 population-based registries including registries in the states of Connecticut, Iowa, New Mexico, Utah, and Hawaii and the metropolitan areas of Detroit, San Francisco-Oakland and the San Jose area south of San Francisco, Los Angeles, Seattle-Puget Sound, and Atlanta and the 10 counties in Georgia surrounding Atlanta. According to NCI, the population in geographic areas in the SEER program represent approximately 14 percent of the U.S. population, including 25 percent of the Hispanic American population, 41 percent of the Asian/Pacific Islander population (including 43 percent of all Chinese Americans and 60 percent of all Japanese Americans), 27 percent of American Indian and Alaska Native populations, and 12 percent of the African-American population. More than half of the African-American population in SEER program coverage areas resides in either Los Angeles or Detroit, more than two-thirds of the SEER program Chinese-American population resides in either Los Angeles or San Francisco-Oakland, and 60 percent of the SEER program Hispanic population resides in Los Angeles.

The SEER program recently expanded its coverage explicitly to improve the coverage of minority populations (see Chapter 2). NCI allocated approximately $2.3 million in FY 1996 to expand the SEER program database to increase the coverage of the Hispanic population and $250,000 to increase the coverage of the Native American population.

To enhance SEER program data with regard to American Indian and Alaska Native populations, NCI is supporting and planning several Category I initiatives. The New Mexico SEER program registry receives NCI support to collect and report on data for American Indians in Arizona. NCI is also planning an operational system for the establishment of a cancer registry among the Cherokee population in Oklahoma. In addition, NCI has worked in collaboration with the Indian Health Service to support the Alaska Native Tumor Registry for cancer surveillance among Alaska Natives and previously supported a project to describe cancer incidence, mortality, and patterns of care, risk factors, and cultural obstacles to early detection and treatment of cancer among American Indians and Alaska Natives.

Among the products of the SEER program relevant to the study of ethnic minority and medically underserved populations is the program monograph entitled *Racial/Ethnic Patterns of Cancer in the United States 1988–1992* (Miller et al., 1996). This publication provides incidence and mortality data for 13 U.S. "racial" and ethnic groups (mortality data are compiled from National Center for Health Statistics [NCHS] data).

A summary of other cancer surveillance activities based on information provided to the study committee by request is provided below (National Cancer Institute, 1998b).

Data Resources

To address questions regarding the effects of cancer, the use of cancer-related services, costs of the disease, and patterns of care among special populations, NCI has supported a number of special initiatives, some in collaboration with other organizations and federal agencies.

Staff of the Division of Cancer Epidemiology and Genetics (DCEG) and the DCCPS recently published an atlas of cancer mortality maps for U.S. non-white populations, a Category I and II project that illuminates rates of mortality from cancer at a range of anatomic sites by geographic region. State economic areas experiencing variations in cancer risk among minority populations are also highlighted. Data from this study may provide leads about etiology and cancer risk that may be pursued by further epidemiologic research. The study has revealed noteworthy patterns, such as a higher rate of prostate cancer among African-American men in the south Atlantic states, increasing rates of stomach cancer among American Indians in the Southwest, and "limited declines" in cervical cancer among African-American women in the Southeast.

In addition, DCEG staff, in collaboration with the National Institute for Occupational Safety and Health and NCHS, have jointly sponsored a study of occupation and industry codes on death certificates for purposes of understanding cancer prevalence by occupational risk. This study now encompasses 24 states and includes more than 5 million records. NCI reports that data from this Category I and II study are available for whites, African Americans, and all minority populations combined.

NCI is also planning several case-control studies of specific cancers and cohort studies of non-cancerous conditions that are disproportionately prevalent among African-American men using data from the U.S. Department of Veterans Affairs (VA) inpatient and outpatient medical records. These data are available for more than 1 million African-American male veterans, as well as 4 million white male veterans, and can be used to examine the risk of various cancers associated with serious medical conditions and procedures.

NCI is also collaborating with the Health Care Financing Administration (HCFA) to link SEER program data with Medicare data to assess costs and the use of selected screening procedures, diagnostic procedures, and treatment patterns for older patients (ages 65 years and older). Health claims data will be examined by race, income, education, and related variables to understand how screening and treatment patterns may differ for subpopulations. In addition, the data will be analyzed by using census tract information to detect differences by the socioeconomic status of geographic areas for this Category I and II study.

In 1994, NCI established the Breast Cancer Surveillance Consortium to study mammography access and utilization among women in community-based settings and the impact of access and utilization on cancer outcomes. This Category II study is expected to yield data on mammography screening practices and mammography performance. It will also provide data on screening among ethnic minority women, as well as other factors that influence mammography access and utilization, such as education, income, and urban-rural location.

In addition, NCI has funded five grants specifically related to special populations to assess the utility of health claims data for cancer surveillance. These Category I and II projects will explore the completeness and accuracy of information reported in claims-based data systems to determine the utility of reimbursement claims for tracking cancer incidence and stage, the use of screening and diagnostic tests, long-term treatment, and cancer-related health care utilization.

Surveys

To address questions regarding health risk behaviors (e.g., diet, health habits, and use of cancer screening), NCI conducts or uses a number of surveys that may identify ethnic group differences related to cancer risk. As indicated above, many of these efforts are conducted in collaboration with other federal agencies or organizations.

NCI has collaborated with the U.S. Bureau of the Census to generate supplemental questions for the Current Population Survey, a monthly survey of approximately 50,000 households used to obtain information about the labor force. NCI questions provide surveillance information on tobacco use and tobacco control attitudes. These data have been used to provide estimates of tobacco use among minority and medically underserved populations and were published in the *Journal of the National Cancer Institute* in 1996.

NCI also periodically provides supplemental questions to the Centers for Disease Control and Prevention's (CDC's) annual National Health Interview Survey (NHIS), a nationally representative survey administered in person. NCI supplements to NHIS in 1987 and 1992 pertained to cancer risk factors, including tobacco use, diet and nutrition, knowledge and attitudes about cancer, use of cancer screening, and cancer survivorship. The survey has been translated into Spanish and has included a measure of "acculturation to the Hispanic population" (National Cancer Institute, 1998b, p. 12). NCI's supplemental questions to NHIS in the year 2000 will expand the acculturation section to include questions on health beliefs and health service use and will expand acculturation questions to Asian Americans, as well as Hispanics. NCI has also collaborated with CDC in the prospective National Health and Nutrition Examination Survey (NHANES), which investigated the health and nutrition status of the U.S. population with a particular focus on high-risk populations. Several cohorts have been followed prospectively since the 1970s to obtain data on diet and health. Both NHANES and NHIS are classified by NCI as Category II studies.

As part of the effort to understand dietary patterns and cancer risk, DCCPS staff have also studied data from the U.S. Department of Agriculture's Continuing Surveys of Food Intakes by Individuals to explore ethnic group differences in dietary intake and compliance with recommended daily nutritional guidelines.

Differences in breast cancer screening practices among elderly women in various ethnic groups have been examined in an NCI-supported study to measure the effect of legislation allowing Medicare reimbursement for breast cancer screening. Analyses comparing African-American and white women's usage patterns are ongoing. In addition, NCI has sponsored a national survey of mammography facilities to understand the characteristics of mammography services and providers and participation in price-subsidized programs for low-income women. NCI classifies these studies as Category I and II studies.

NCI is also supporting a Category I study to develop and validate needs assessment instruments to measure the effectiveness of cancer control methods among American Samoans. This project will develop a culturally sensitive survey instrument to assess knowledge and attitudes regarding cancer among a sample of American Samoans in Los Angeles, Hawaii, and American Samoa.

Studies That Use Databases

DCCPS sponsors several population-based studies relevant to ethnic minority populations. The Black/White Cancer Survival Study, begun in 1983, investigates the role of "social, behavioral, lifestyle, biological, treatment, and health care factors as contributors to the observed differences in survival" among African-American and white cancer patients (National Cancer Institute, 1998b, p. 18). NCI notes that several publications have developed from this study, which followed 3,400 individuals with breast, colon, corpus uteri, or urinary bladder cancers. In addition, SEER program and Medicare data have been used by DCCPS staff to examine patterns of care and costs of cancer treatment, in some studies according to clinical and sociodemographic factors. These studies are described by NCI as Category I and II studies.

Several SEER program special studies are ongoing. They report on data on patterns of care and treatment outcomes among white and nonwhite populations collected as part of the SEER program. One project reports on differences in treatment outcomes for African-American and white men with non-metastatic prostate cancer and has found differences related to race and socioeconomic status. Another study examines quality-of-life issues for Asian-American and Pacific Islander cancer survivors. Another series of studies examines trends in treatment for early-stage breast cancer by age, race, geographic region, and socioeconomic characteristics. Similarly, the Prostate Cancer Outcomes Study provides information about diagnostic and treatment practice patterns for prostate cancer and describes health-related quality of life according to geographic region, racial or ethnic subgroup, income, education, and health insurance status of patients. Of the more than 3,300 men participating in the study, approximately 500 African-American and 430 Hispanic men participated in the initial survey. Finally, feasibility studies are being conducted to examine patterns of care from several data sources, including the Indian Health Service, to provide more information on American Indian cancer patients, particularly those suffering from colon, lung, breast, prostate, and cervical cancers.

Epidemiologic and Etiologic Research

Nutrition Studies

To address questions about links between dietary patterns and cancer incidence and mortality, particularly among ethnic minority and medically underserved populations, NCI supports a number of nutrition studies.

The Women's Health Trial: Feasibility Study in Minority Populations was initiated to assess whether ethnic minority and low-income women could be recruited into a trial in sufficient numbers to evaluate a dietary intervention and test the intervention's effects on lowering fat consumption. More than 2,000 minority and low-income women were recruited for this randomized trial. Similarly, DCCPS supports a study assessing diet and breast cancer risk among a sample of 400 black women. This Category I study seeks to "yield statistical methods for enhancing the ability to assess diet-related breast cancer risks in Black women as well as provide relevant pilot data to support future studies" (National Cancer Institute, 1998b, p. 24).

DCEG staff are investigating the relationship between fatty acids and prostate cancer risk among African-American and white males. The levels of a variety of fatty acids are being measured in plasma collected from both African-American and white men in a large, multicenter, population-based case-control study to search for relationships between fatty acid profiles and prostate cancer risk. Ethnic-group differences in these profiles and their relationship to prostate cancer will be assessed, as will the relationship between diet and fatty acid profiles. NCI has classified this research as a Category I and II study.

The Multiethnic/Minority Cohort Study of Diet and Cancer prospectively examines the relationship of dietary and other lifestyle risk factors to cancer. Investigators at the University of Hawaii at Manoa are studying a total of 215,000 African-American, Japanese-American, Hispanic, and white subjects in the western United States to assess dietary patterns and group differences. Slightly more than $1 million was allocated to this Category I activity in FY 1997. In addition, NCI staff are collaborating on analyses of the contributions of dietary and nutritional patterns to the high incidence of esophageal, pancreatic, and prostate cancer and multiple myeloma in African Americans.

NCI lists three other ongoing, prospective studies (the Nurses' Health Study, the FELS Early Nutrition and Growth Study, and the Framingham Heart Study) that examine the relationship between nutritional and other risk factors and cancer in special populations. By NCI's own admission, however, these studies include very few ethnic minority participants and unknown numbers of lower-income or medically underserved participants. It is therefore unclear how research questions specific to these populations (e.g., "How is diet affected by acculturation?" or "Is poor childhood nutrition among African-American women linked to premenopausal breast cancer?") may be answered.

Environmental Risk Factor Research

Many ethnic minority populations are at greater risk for a range of environmental exposures (e.g., some forms of radiation or chemicals and pesticides) and infectious diseases (e.g., human immunodeficiency virus [HIV] and human papillomavirus [HPV] infections) that are known carcinogens or that may be linked with cancer. NCI supports a number of studies that investigate the physical, chemical, and viral causes of cancer and their disproportionate burdens on ethnic minority and medically underserved populations.

DCEG is supporting a study of breast cancer, benign breast disease, and pesticide exposure among a predominantly African-American population in Triana, Alabama, that has been exposed to high levels of the insecticide dichlorodiphenyltrichloroethane (DDT) in a tributary of the Tennessee River. Mammographic screenings, clinical examinations, and blood chemistries will be provided to the study participants. Other health and health education needs of participants will be identified and provided. The Category I study will evaluate the relationship between serum DDT levels and the risk for breast cancer and breast disease.

NCI, in collaboration with the Indian Health Service, CDC, and the Alaska Area Native Health Service, has funded pilot research exploring associations between breast cancer and elevated levels of organochlorines among Alaska Native women. These women are at increased risk due to diets high in protein and fat from marine sources established as having high concentrations of organochlorines. Components of this Category I study will involve the collection of serum, urine, and adipose tissue samples from Alaska Native women undergoing breast surgery and analysis of samples for organochlorines.

HIV infection now disproportionately affects ethnic minority individuals in the United States. NCI is investigating techniques that can be used to identify HIV-infected individuals who are at risk for rapid disease progression and who may benefit from early therapeutic intervention, thereby reducing associated cancer risks. In addition, NCI and the National Institute of Child Health and Human Development are sponsoring research to reduce the rate of mother-to-infant transmission of HIV.

Several studies are under way to understand adult T-cell leukemia (ATL) and human T-cell lymphotropic virus type I (HTLV-I) and type II (HTLV-II) infection. ATL and infection with its causal agent, HTLV-I, are more common among African Americans than among whites. NCI staff seek to define host susceptibility to infection and modes of transmission of HTLV-I and improve surveillance of ATL patients. Epidemiologic studies are also conducted to better understand the modes of transmission of HTLV-II. Similarly, Category I and II studies are being conducted to assess the roles of Epstein-Barr virus in Hodgkin's disease among Hispanic patients, Burkitt's lymphoma among Ghanaians, and gastric cancers among Japanese Americans. DCEG and DCP staff are also studying the relationship of HPV and the etiology of lymphoma, hepatocellular cancer, and cervical cancer in American Indians.

DCEG staff are also engaged in studies of occupational exposure to hazardous agents and cancer risk. These Category I studies examine links between exposure to chemical and other environmental agents across a range of occupations, racial and ethnic groups, and socioeconomic backgrounds, given that lower-income and ethnic minority workers are often exposed to carcinogens at higher levels. A number of studies assess cancer risks for farmers or individuals living in rural areas and have found excess incidence rates for several cancers. Another project assessed the feasibility of conducting studies on cancer risks among migrant workers of African, Hispanic, and Asian backgrounds. In addition, intramural staff are working in collaboration with investigators at the University of Minnesota to assess the linkages between occupational and environmental risk factors among women in Shanghai, China.

Access to Care and Cancer

NCI has attempted to stimulate research on patterns of health care, cancer, and variations by socioeconomic differences and racial and ethnic groups. This research also attempts to identify barriers to state-of-the-art diagnosis and care for patients in rural areas.

NCI sponsored two workshops, one in 1989 and another in 1992, on patterns of care and the economic and social burdens of cancer on families. In addition, NCI issued a program announcement to improve the understanding of the economics of cancer care. "Grants funded under this Program Announcement," according to an NCI report, "include studies of the cost-effectiveness of increasing breast cancer screening and effective follow-up among African American women, the effects of tobacco taxation on tobacco use, the cost effectiveness of alternative strategies of managing Pap smear results, patterns of care for breast cancer in [health maintenance organization] HMO and fee-for-service settings, and the application of econometric techniques to cost and outcomes studies using Medicare data" (National Cancer Institute, 1998b, p. 34). NCI has collaborated with other federal agencies, including the Agency for Health Care Policy and Research, HCFA, and the National Institute on Aging, in sponsoring this research. Finally, DCP recently released a request for applications (RFAs) to assess ways of improving cancer diagnosis and treatment in rural areas. The aim of the RFA is to "strengthen the application of state-of-the-art cancer diagnosis and management practices in rural areas by enhancing links between rural health care providers and regional cancer specialists" (National Cancer Institute, 1998b, p. 34).

Cancer Etiology

NCI intramural staff are investigating a range of possible and confirmed etiologic factors, including genetic susceptibility, environmental carcinogens, diet, behavior and lifestyle, and other risk factors, and their relationship with race and ethnicity in conferring a risk for cancer. For example, NCI scientists examined the relationship of rare variable nucleotide tandem repeat alleles of Ha-*ras*-1 in African Americans and whites as a possible predisposing factor in lung cancer and determined that differences in lung cancer rates between the two groups were due to differences in smoking patterns and not polymorphic gene variance.

Other studies on cancer etiology are summarized below by cancer site.

Prostate Cancer NCI scientists are studying the relationship between a variety of genetic, biochemical, behavioral, and environmental factors and prostate cancer in two large case-control investigations of African-American and white men in the United States and a sample of men in China at low risk for the disease. In that study vasectomy at a young age and family history are among the risk factors associated with prostate cancer, whereas researchers continue to examine the role of androgen metabolism and other biochemical markers in prostate cancer. DCEG and DCP staff are also studying these relationships in the NCI-sponsored Prostate, Lung, Colon, and Ovarian (PLCO) Cancer Screening Trial. These research efforts have been classified as Category I and II studies.

Breast Cancer DCEG supports a wide range of Category I and II research aimed at understanding the causes of breast cancer and whether etiology varies by racial or ethnic group. A population-based, case-control study in North Carolina focuses on the causes of breast cancer among African-American and white women who live in suburban and rural areas of eastern and central North Carolina. The study integrates epidemiology and molecular biology to explore risk factors and possible gene-environment interactions as causes of cancer. Other studies are aimed at understanding differences in breast cancer incidence among younger (under age 40) African-American and white women, diet and risk of breast cancer among Asian-American women, and whether racial or ethnic variations in breast cancer incidence and prognosis are attributable to various exogenous mutagens.

Cervical Cancer The incidence of cervical cancer is disproportionately high among African-American, Hispanic, and some Asian-American women. NCI supports case-control studies in Jamaica to understand the etiologic risks for cervical cancer associated with HPV, HIV, and HTLV, as well as a large study in Costa Rica that examines genetic susceptibility markers and nutrition to assess why common HPV infections sometimes persist and progress to cervical cancer. Both are Category I studies.

Nasopharyngeal Cancer NCI-supported scientists are studying the role of a range of environmental, lifestyle, and genetic factors in the development of nasopharyngeal cancer (NPC), the incidence of which is particularly high in Southeast Asia and among individuals of Chinese descent. A case-control study in the Philippines has revealed a strong link between occupational exposures to chemicals (e.g., formaldehyde), smoking, and other environmental risk factors and NPC. Scientists are also examining the role of oncogenes and tumor suppressor genes in the pathogenesis of NPC. The interplay of genetic factors and environmental exposures is also being assessed in a family-based study recently initiated in Taiwan. Finally, NCI is also supporting a study of 60,000 Chinese men in Singapore to investigate the relationship between diet, particularly ethnic foods such as salted fish, and NPC. These studies have been classified as Category I and II studies.

Oral and Pharyngeal Cancers DCEG staff are investigating the relationship between smoking and alcohol consumption and oral and pharyngeal cancers, the rates of which are 30 to 100 percent higher among African Americans than whites. When the rates for African-American and white nonsmokers and nondrinkers are compared, they are nearly equivalent. These relationships are being studied further in a case-control study in Puerto Rico, an area with high rates of oral and pharyngeal cancers. This study has revealed a greater risk for oral cancer with increasing alcohol consumption among persons with the *ADH 31-1* genotype. These studies have been classified as Category I and II studies.

Esophageal Cancer African Americans and Chinese Americans suffer from higher rates of esophageal cancer than whites. NCI-supported scientists are studying tumors that occur in excess among African Americans in a series of case-control studies. In addition, studies are in progress to collect DNA from samples of populations at high and low risk for esophageal cancer in Shanghai, China. In Linxian, China, NCI researchers are studying the impact of a nutritional intervention on late-stage progression of esophageal cancer among individuals in a high-risk population. These studies have been classified as Category I studies.

Stomach Cancer Asian Americans, African Americans, and farmers all suffer from higher rates of stomach cancers than other Americans. NCI is studying the effect of a nutritional intervention on the progression of precancerous gastric lesions among subjects in Shandong, China. A screening program in China is also sponsored by NCI to evaluate the role of diet on precancerous lesions of the stomach. Similarly, DCEG staff are evaluating the risk posed by agricultural hazards such as pesticides, fertilizers, and dust on stomach cancers in a case-control study in Nebraska. In addition, DCEG staff, working with the U.S. Environmental Protection Agency and NIEHS, are evaluating stomach cancer and agricultural exposures among African-American and white farmers in North Carolina and Iowa in the Agricultural Health Study. To encourage further research in this area, NCI, along with NIDDKD, NIAID, the NIH Office of Research on Minority Health, and the American Digestive Health Foundation, recently issued an RFA on *Helicobacter pylori* and its relationship to digestive diseases and cancer, with an emphasis on research related to minority populations. This research has been classified as Category I research by NCI.

Colorectal Cancer NCI supports several studies that are investigating a range of risk factors associated with colorectal cancer. In a case-control study being conducted in China and the United States, researchers found that Chinese-American men and white men have colorectal cancer rates seven times higher than those of men in China. High-fat diets and low levels of physical activity were among the identified risk factors. In addition, a new multicenter study is assessing the independent and combined effects of dietary factors, physical activity, body size, reproductive factors, and family history on the risk of colon cancer among African Americans and whites. Finally, staff of the Cancer Prevention Studies Branch of NCI are collaborating with VA to collect blood and tissue specimens from patients in VA medical centers to create a large specimen bank for a prospective study of nutritional and genetic hypotheses of colorectal neoplasia. Specimens will be obtained from patients with large adenomas, patients with small polyps, and asymptomatic individuals to assess their relationship with serum micronutrients and molecular genetic markers. These studies are classified as Category I and II research by NCI.

Pancreatic Cancer NCI-supported research on the etiology of pancreatic cancer includes a series of case-control studies among African Americans that examine the roles of smoking, diet, various medical conditions, and genetic factors. The role of hepatitis viruses in conjunction with other environmental and lifestyle risk factors in the development of pancreatic cancer is also being investigated in a case-control study in Senegal, West Africa. These studies are classified as Category I studies.

Multiple Myeloma NCI-supported case-control studies are comparing risk factors for multiple myeloma among African-American and white populations. Findings indicate that occupational exposures (especially for those residing on farms and reporting exposure to pesticides) increase the risk for this cancer. NCI also supported a workshop on the epidemiology of multiple myeloma, with special attention to factors that may contribute to the excess incidence among African Americans.

Cancer Prevention and Control

An NCI document notes that behavioral and environmental influences are responsible for the majority of cancers in the United States. Reducing the cancer burden therefore requires "a balanced partnership between the biomedical and behavioral/public health sectors" (National Cancer Institute, 1998b, p. 46). NCI's definition of cancer control research attempts to reflect this view: "cancer control research is now defined as basic and applied research in the behavioral, social, and population sciences to create or enhance interventions that, independently or in combination with biomedical approaches, reduce cancer risk, incidence, morbidity, and mortality" (National Cancer Institute, 1998b, p. 46). Much of this research is funded through the newly established DCCPS.

Primary Prevention and Intervention Studies

Tobacco Use and African Americans NCI has funded Category I research examining the effectiveness of culturally appropriate behavioral interventions to decrease the level of tobacco use among African Americans. In one study, the incremental benefits of "culturally sensitive" adjuvant behavioral therapy and use of the transdermal nicotine patch are assessed among a population of urban African Americans. In another study, gender and racial or ethnic variations in perceptions of cancer risk are assessed by using population-sensitive measures of risk perception. Improved cancer-risk communication in this study is expected to lead to reduced smoking rates and increased rates of use of screening mammography among African Americans. Finally, the Enhancing Cancer Control in a Community Health Center project assessed the effectiveness of patient-, physician-, and system-directed interventions aimed at promoting the early detection of breast and cervical cancers and smoking cessation in a predominantly African-American population. Ethnically appropriate patient education materials and telephone counseling were combined with physician education and other interventions in a community health center setting.

Tobacco Use and Hispanic Americans An NCI-funded Category I study is examining the effectiveness of a social influence model on cancer-risk behavior among migrant Hispanic adolescents. The intervention includes social skills development and enhancement of parental skills to reduce the rates of tobacco consumption and other cancer-risk behaviors. A total of 700 adolescents will be randomly assigned to intervention and control conditions, with 12- and 24-month follow-ups.

Tobacco Use and Native Americans Several Category I studies supported by NCI examine the use of culturally sensitive interventions to reduce the rates of tobacco use and improve diet. A study in California adapted a Quit for Life smoking cessation program for the needs of Indian health clinics and health care providers, followed by home visits to patients by Indian Community Health representatives. Another study examined the effects of culturally relevant community interventions with the family to augment a school-based health curriculum on health knowledge among southwestern Indian children. In the Northeast, NCI-supported investigators studied the effects of an integrated overall health curriculum on decision making among Native American youth related to diet and tobacco use. In the Northwest, a study examined the effects of a consultative process and the use of materials to assist tribal councils in developing and implementing more stringent tobacco-use policies.

Tobacco and Disadvantaged Youth NCI is funding a Category I study to develop and test community-based cancer prevention strategies among high-risk youth in New York whose families' incomes fall below the federal poverty line. Skills intervention techniques for youth and parental skills intervention techniques will be used and their effects will be assessed. In addition, NCI has reissued an RFA for studies relating to the control of tobacco use among youth, including the "identification and evaluation of factors influencing the decline of tobacco use among particular groups, for example, African American youth" (National Cancer Institute, 1998b, p. 51).

The American Stop Smoking Intervention Study The American Stop Smoking Intervention Study (ASSIST) is a community-based intervention directed by local voluntary coalitions that plan and support tobacco control activities with the support of NCI, the American Cancer Society (ACS), and state and local health departments. More than 6,000 community organizations are involved in the initiative in 17 states. The ASSIST intervention model is based on smoking prevention and control methods established by research supported by NCI, as well as other research. NCI reports that although this Category II initiative is aimed at all populations in the targeted states, those groups with elevated smoking rates relative to that for the majority population, as well as those groups "that have displayed slower rates of decline (e.g., women, youth, the medically underserved, the less educated, and several ethnic minority populations)," will receive special focus (National Cancer Institute, 1998b, p. 52).

Noticeably absent from this portfolio of research on smoking interventions among specific ethnic groups and disadvantaged populations are smoking cessation research programs targeted to Asian-American and Pacific Islander populations (especially Southeast Asian populations, among whom tobacco use is among the highest of all U.S. ethnic groups) and medically underserved individuals (who also suffer from a high incidence of tobacco use).

Reducing Dietary Risk Behavior in Adolescents The NCI-supported Category I and II study Reducing Cancer-Related Dietary Risk Behaviors in Adolescents targets a multiethnic population of lower-income students from two inner-city school districts in Minnesota to increase students' levels of consumption of fruits and vegetables and reduce their levels of intake of calories from total fat. Intervention components include a school curriculum addressing eating cues and the influence of advertising on food choices, a home intervention program to facilitate student-parent discussions of dietary choices, and a school environment component targeting food availability and incentives. Interventions will be implemented over a 2-year period, and evaluations will assess culturally appropriate strategies.

Risk Factor Prevention for Hispanic Youth NCI is supporting a Category I study evaluating a comprehensive cancer-risk prevention intervention targeting preadolescents in schools serving predominantly low-income Hispanic families. School-based and parent interventions are coupled with a school food service intervention in 14 schools in San Jose, California, to increase healthful eating practices and levels of physical activity among youth and provide instruction in weight regulation skills. A primary objective is to reduce the level of prevalence of obesity at the end of the 2-year intervention, whereas secondary objectives include increasing the level of consumption of low-fat foods (including fruits and vegetables and dietary fiber), increasing the level of physical activity, and decreasing the level of consumption of dietary fat.

5 A Day Behavioral Research and Evaluation NCI's 5 A Day program seeks to increase awareness of healthy dietary patterns and to increase levels of consumption of fruits and vegetables. These programs have been adapted to serve the needs of ethnic minority consumers. In North Carolina, an NCI-funded project mobilized community and religious organizations to tailor a 5 A Day program to the needs of an African-American community. Local businesses, churches, and media worked collaboratively with local health officials and cooperative extension staff to help implement the program. In Minnesota, an NCI-funded 5 A Day program targeted a multiethnic (45 percent minority) cohort of schoolchildren, including Asian-American, African-American, Hispanic, and American-Indian children, with a school-based intervention involving school curriculum, food service menu changes, and industry and media support. In Arizona, the 5 A Day-Healthier Eating for the Overlooked Worker project targeted a predominantly Hispanic population to compare the impacts of peer educational programs at work sites to those of traditional work-site wellness programs. The Treatwell 5 A Day Worksite Nutrition Intervention in Massachusetts serves a population that is approximately 33 percent African American and 33 percent Hispanic with a work-site intervention and family involvement component to assess their synergistic effects. The program is sponsored collaboratively by an NCI-supported comprehensive cancer center, the state health agency, cooperative extension, and industry. In Maryland, the effects of a program combining nutrition education, lay counseling, print materials, and community-based family involvement on levels of fruit and vegetable consumption among a low-income, primarily African-American population was assessed in the 5 A Day WIC Promotion Program (WIC is the Special Supplemental Food Program for Women, Infants, and Children). Finally, NCI has supported communications research, including focus groups with African-American men and women, to explore perceptions about food and to develop strategies to improve 5 A Day messages tailored to the African-American community. Results of this research are found in messages in radio segments, media newsletters, and other outreach activities.

Chemoprevention Trials

NCI is sponsoring more than 60 chemoprevention trials to test compounds that may block, suppress, or retard cancer. Although none appear to be focused on issues of chemoprevention among ethnic minority or medically underserved populations, NCI provided information on two such trials that are "of extreme importance to several special population groups" and are therefore classified by NCI as Category II studies (National Cancer Institute, 1998b, p. 61). The Breast Cancer Prevention Trial, initiated in April 1992, tested the effects of tamoxifen in the prevention of breast cancer among high-risk subjects. Similarly, the Prostate Cancer Prevention Trial is designed to test the effectiveness of finasteride in the prevention of prostate cancer. Both studies, however, suffer from disproportionately low ethnic minority enrollment (see Chapter 4).

Secondary Prevention (Early Detection)

Breast Cancer Screening The Breast Cancer Screening Consortium, funded through an NCI interactive grant mechanism, is a five-site study focused on identifying means of increasing the utilization of screening programs by women over age 50 who have not adhered to recommended screening guidelines. Telephone counseling and other interventions are examined in this study. NCI provided no information regarding the enrollment of ethnic minority or medically underserved women in this trial. A smaller study, the Increasing Breast Screening Among Nonadherent Women study, evaluated the effectiveness and cost effectiveness of tailored telephone counseling and other intervention strategies in five regions of the United States in increasing the rates of breast cancer screening among nonadherent women, including elderly ethnic minority women. NCI classifies this study as a Category I and II study.

PLCO Cancer Screening Trial The PLCO Cancer Screening Trial is a large-scale randomized study to determine whether screening tests will reduce the number of deaths related to prostate, lung, colorectal, and ovarian cancers. As of 1997, 89 percent of the participants in this Category II trial were white, 4.4 percent were African American, 1.4 percent were Hispanic, 4.3 percent were Asian American, and less than 0.5 percent were

Pacific Islanders, American Indians, or of other racial or ethnic backgrounds. To increase the levels of ethnic minority participation in the PLCO Cancer Screening Trial, NCI plans to cosponsor (with CDC) a new screening center to focus on the recruitment of African Americans and initiate another new center to focus on recruitment of Hispanics. A special study sponsored by CDC will assess psychosocial factors that influence older African Americans' decisions to undergo cancer screening. In addition, NCI is sponsoring a study to test literacy and develop culturally appropriate educational materials to encourage cancer screening among low-income African-American women.

Cervical Cancer Screening The ASCUS/LSIL Triage Study is a 6-year clinical trial designed to determine the proper means of evaluating and managing minor Pap smear abnormalities. Four clinical centers are funded by NCI to enroll approximately 7,200 women with a recent diagnosis of abnormal Pap smears, of which nearly 40 percent are African American or Hispanic. Participants will be randomly assigned to one of three management groups and monitored for 3 years to help determine which patients are likely to experience progression to cancerous conditions.

Colorectal Cancer Screening The South Carolina Colorectal Cancer Screening Study is an NCI-funded Category I study designed to develop new methods of recruiting low-income African-American women into colorectal cancer screening trials and to test literacy and develop culturally appropriate educational materials.

Other Screening Studies with Multiethnic Populations NCI funded a large grant for a multicenter project administered by the Northern California Cancer Center, Pathways to Screening in Four Ethnic Groups. This project developed and evaluated culturally targeted cancer control interventions on the basis of the Pathways to Screening framework, a model of early cancer detection that focuses on the continuum from basic knowledge and attitudes to the procedural and organizational aspects of the delivery process. Pathway models were developed and evaluated for the Hispanic, Vietnamese, African-American, and Chinese-American communities in the San Francisco Bay area. Evaluation will assist in the development of culturally tailored interventions appropriate for racial and ethnic groups in other regions of the United States.

Clinical Trials

NCI Intramural Clinical Research Trials

NCI's Division of Clinical Sciences (DCS) supports ongoing intramural clinical trials on the NIH campus in Bethesda, Maryland. These trials include studies of clinical treatment protocols for lung, breast, ovarian, prostate, and bladder cancers and lymphoma. DCS maintains a central referral office that prospective patients can contact and a toll-free telephone number that prospective patients can call to obtain information or help in finding appropriate studies. All care at the clinical center is free of charge. In addition, NCI contributes to the Special Ambulatory Care Program to supplement travel, housing, and guardian expenses for patients while they are at the clinical center and for transportation to and from NIH. In addition, NCI has contributed to the Patient Emergency Fund, which is available to provide financial assistance to patients participating in clinical trials.

NCI reports that "statistical and financial evaluations of the populations recruited to intramural trials at NIH indicate that the majority of [NCI's] patients, and particularly pediatric patients, represent indigent populations from rural or inner-city areas" (National Cancer Institute, 1998b, p. 10). In FY 1996, 2,798 patients were enrolled at the NCI clinical center. Of these, 83 percent were white, 10.8 percent were African American, 2.5 percent were Hispanic, 1.4 percent were Asian or Pacific Islander, 0.1 percent were Native American, and 2.1 percent were of unknown racial or ethnic backgrounds.

Extramural Clinical Trials

CCOP CCOP links patients and community-based physicians with researchers at clinical cooperative groups and cancer centers, thereby providing cancer patients, their physicians, and researchers with access to NCI-approved clinical trials and state-of-the-art care. NCI has funded nine clinical cooperative groups and three cancer centers to develop and manage clinical trials through CCOP. In addition, 51 community-based programs in 30 states were funded through CCOP and involved the participation of more than 300 hospitals and 3,300 physicians. NCI reports that nearly 20 percent of the more than 20,000 patients entering clinical treatment trials each year are ethnic minorities.

To increase the numbers of ethnic minority participants in CCOP, NCI initiated MBCCOPs in 1990. MBCCOPs are funded in seven states and Puerto Rico and have accounted for more than 50 percent of the accrual of new ethnic minority cancer patients. NCI reports that minority accrual in CCOPs is proportionate to their representation in the United States (see Chapter 4 for more detailed information on minority enrollment) but adds that recruitment of minority and underserved populations remains a "special focus" of recruitment efforts (National Cancer Institute, 1998b). Approximately $2.5 million was allocated to this activity in FY 1997.

In addition, NCI's Cancer Therapy Evaluation Program has provided $1.1 million in funding in FY 1997 to 5 of the 11 cooperative groups to enhance the accrual of minorities in trials. Funds have been used to support community outreach in institutions with large minority patient populations, focus groups and educational opportunities for minority professionals, and advertising to increase minority awareness of clinical trials. Within the past 2 years, NCI has also reached agreement with VA and the Department of Defense to include eligible veterans and active-duty military personnel in clinical trial programs, potentially increasing the pool of minority participants. Finally, as noted above, ORMH of NIH has supported specific minority accrual projects at the NCI cancer centers, including the development of outreach literature for people with low levels of literacy, hiring of bilingual patient liaisons and a minority recruitment data manager, and other projects.

Conferences to Increase Accrual of Minorities NCI has sponsored a series of conferences "to share current information and strategies that would aid cancer clinical investigators in recruiting and retaining minority participants in cancer clinical research" (National Cancer Institute, 1998b, p. 10). An RFA was issued to provide support for regional conferences; the RFA was preceded by a National Conference on the Recruitment and Retention of Minority Participants in Clinical Cancer Research. The national conference was cosponsored by NCI, ACS, the Oncology Nursing Society, NIH, and NIH's ORMH, and NIH's Office of Research on Women's Health. A monograph was published as a result of the national conference, and publication of the proceedings of each of the regional conferences is under way.

Basic Research

Basic research is the foundation of cancer research at NCI. This emphasis is reflected in the NCI FY 1999 budget request, which outlines four areas of "exceptional promise" for advancing knowledge of cancer: cancer genetics, including efforts to identify every human gene predisposing an individual to cancer; preclinical models of research, including the development of appropriate animal models of human cancers; imaging techniques to improve diagnosis; and defining the signature of cancer cells to improve detection and diagnosis (National Cancer Institute, 1998d).

New developments in basic research have led to groundbreaking cancer treatments and prevention methods that have provided benefits to all populations. In some cases, significant gains have been made in technologies for the detection and treatment of cancers that disproportionately affect ethnic minority and medically underserved populations. Few examples of basic research at NCI dedicated to examinations of potential differences in underlying biological or genetic mechanisms among population groups exist, however. In a document provided to the study committee, NCI reports that "where there are biological differences among populations, these can only be found through basic research," yet it goes on to state that its "basic science projects are rarely categorized as 'targeted' research" (National Cancer Institute, 1998b, p. 80).

NCI provided to the study committee examples of ongoing basic research that may provide benefits for the detection, prevention, and treatment of several cancers that disproportionately affect ethnic minority and elderly populations. Only in the area of breast cancer was it apparent that research questions were directed toward understanding population-group differences in cancer etiologies, disease courses, and treatment responses. For example, NCI has initiated a study to investigate the reasons for the possible increased aggressiveness of breast cancer in African-American women. Analyses of breast tissue samples from African-American and white patients matched by age, stage of disease at diagnosis, and other critical factors are under way to determine if differences in molecular characteristics may account for the poorer prognosis of breast cancer in African-American women. In addition, NCI has supported research on Mapping by Admixture Linkage Disequilibrium (MALD) to assist in gene mapping among patients with sporadic cases of breast cancer. Such patients have no family history of the disease, precluding traditional genetic linkage analysis. Tissue specimens from African-American patients are being analyzed by MALD analysis to explore possible genetic links behind sporadic cases of breast cancer.

NCI is also supporting two pilot studies involving basic research on breast cancer among diverse population groups. One examines the kinetics as the well as the phenotypic and genotypic properties of breast cancer as they relate to tumor aggressiveness among African-American, Hispanic, and white women in south Florida. Another plans a comparative molecular analysis of the primary DNA sequence of the estrogen receptor gene in breast cancer tissue removed from African-American, Hispanic, and white women to look for potential gene rearrangements and deletions.

Information for the Public and Outreach Activities

NCI staff are involved in a wide range of outreach and public information efforts, some of which are tailored specifically to the needs of ethnic minority communities.

Information and Education

International Cancer Information Center OCICE supports ICIC, which maintains the NCI web site CancerNet, as well as two comprehensive cancer databases, PDQ and CANCERLIT. CancerNet (located at http://cancernet.nci.nih.gov) provides information to the general public and physicians and features a special section entitled "Information for Racial/Ethnic Groups." ICIC staff are working with advocacy groups on an initiative to provide layperson-oriented information about cancer clinical trials on CancerNet. PDQ is a database that describes the latest advances in cancer treatment, care, screening, and prevention and features a technical version for health professionals and a nontechnical version for patients and the general public. Users can obtain information on clinical trials in directories of more than 23,000 physicians and more than 11,000 organizations active in cancer care. PDQ is available in both English and Spanish. CANCERLIT is a bibliographic database that contains citations from the cancer literature published from 1963 to the present and contains more than 1.2 million citations.

ICIC has also sought to provide tailored outreach to the Hispanic community by using market research conducted by the Office of Cancer Communications (OCC). Direct mail communication with 37,000 Hispanic-serving health professionals, including information about NCI resources and how to access them, a Spanish-language brochure for patients, public service announcements in major Hispanic markets, and outreach to the National Council of Catholic Bishops are among the strategies used to target this population. ICIC is also sponsoring a pilot project in seven Maryland public libraries to increase the awareness and use of CancerNet in these settings, especially among individuals who are less likely to have access to computer resources at home or work.

Cancer Information Service Branch The Cancer Information Service Branch oversees CIS, a national information and education network and toll-free telephone service that provides information to individuals and communities about recent developments in cancer research, prevention, and treatment. The CIS toll-free telephone service operates in both English and Spanish. To improve outreach to minority communities, CIS has engaged in collaborations with minority-based and minority-serving organizations. For example, CIS is or has been working with the National Black Leadership Initiative on Cancer (NBLIC), the Appalachian Leadership Initiative on Cancer (ALIC), and the National Hispanic Leadership Initiative on Cancer (NHLIC) to support the development of community-based coalitions focused on cancer prevention, to promote nutritional awareness, and to air bilingual public service announcements as part of cancer prevention efforts, respectively. CIS staff have also worked directly with community groups to develop culturally sensitive cancer screening messages for Hawaii Natives and American Indians.

Patient Education Branch The Patient Education Branch (PEB) of OCI-CE is involved in the development, implementation, and promotion of educational programs for persons living with cancer and their families, including culturally tailored education and outreach services for minority and medically underserved populations. PEB assists extramural scientists with outreach efforts to increase patient accrual to clinical trials, including promotional efforts targeted to minority health professional organizations and minority-serving media outlets. These efforts include the Cancer Clinical Trials Education Program, an information and education program geared to health professionals regarding clinical trials, including culturally tailored information for professionals serving ethnic minority patients and individuals with low levels of literacy. A cancer survivorship training program has also been developed for health professionals addressing the common concerns of cancer survivors, including components tailored to minority audiences. Similarly, an information booklet was developed for health professionals to address patients'concerns regarding genetic testing. PEB has also supported demonstration projects to develop new and innovative ways of disseminating the Patient Information File for the PDQ database, including one demonstration specifically targeted to African-American and Hispanic consumers. Finally, PEB also supports the Cancer Patient Education database, which provides information on hundreds of cancer patient education resources and publications, including non-English publications and publications directed toward individuals with low levels of literacy, and disseminates educational resources to cancer patients and their families.

Health Promotion Branch The NCI Health Promotion Branch (HPB) conducts research on health communication and develops materials for distribution through the CIS outreach program. For example, HPB staff have conducted focus group research to learn more about Hispanic consumers' attitudes, beliefs, and behaviors related to cancer prevention, early detection, and treatment and to learn more about African-American,

Hispanic, Native American, Asian-American, and white women's attitudes and knowledge regarding breast cancer and mammography. HPB has also conducted consumer research to determine how to better frame 5 A Day health messages to the African-American community. In addition, NCI staff have developed a geodemographic marketing database that links demographic, marketing, and health information to better tailor messages to the needs of specific communities.

HPB staff have also developed a number of publications and public service announcements for ethnic minority populations (see Appendix C for examples of titles). In addition, HPB supports media campaigns, such as the recent national media campaign on cervical cancer screening, that feature efforts to reach out to ethnic minority populations. The cervical cancer screening campaign included information on the incidence and rates of mortality from cervical cancer among older minority women in a media kit distributed to majority and minority media outlets.

Overall, OCC reports spending $7.4 million in FY 1997 targeting cancer information to minority and underserved populations, although this figure is derived by using "percent relevancy" calculations for monies allocated on the basis of the percentage of minority group individuals in the overall target pool. Among those programs in FY 1996 listed as "100 percent" relevant to minority populations, Hawaii's CIS received $393,000 for outreach activities targeted to Native Hawaiians, $250,000 each was allocated to the development of nutrition education materials targeted to African Americans with low levels of literacy and to community-based education projects directed at urban African-American residents, and $150,000 was allocated to the development and dissemination of culturally appropriate messages and materials for American Indians, Native Alaskans, and Native Hawaiians.

Outreach Activities and Community Education

NCI has placed a great deal of emphasis on three leadership initiatives to support minority outreach, research, and cancer control efforts.

NBLIC seeks to promote the participation of African-American community leaders in the mobilization and stimulation of community cancer prevention and control activities. NBLIC's objectives are to reduce cancer incidence and mortality rates and improve cancer survival rates among African Americans and to address barriers to cancer control services among other objectives. More than 60 community coalitions have been established through the work of NBLIC's four regional offices. NCI allocated approximately $1.7 million to this activity in FY 1997.

Through NHLIC, an initiative implementing community demonstration and health communications research projects, NCI is addressing the cancer prevention and control needs of the Hispanic community. NCI has established two cooperative agreements for NHLIC, one with the Baylor College of Medicine and another with the National Coalition of Hispanic Health and Human Services Organizations (COSSMHO). COSSMHO has established nine local project sites across the United States and in Puerto Rico to address cancer research questions with community-based organizations. NHLIC's: *En Acción*, an NCI cooperative agreement with the Baylor College of Medicine, is a theory-based, research-oriented program combining national and regional health expertise with grassroots community leadership to reach the major Hispanic populations in six cities across the country. The project initiated the first comprehensive epidemiologic assessment of cancer risk factors among these Hispanic and Latino population groups and has developed state-of-the-art cancer prevention and control strategies tailored to those diverse Hispanic populations. NCI allocated approximately $1.2 million for these activities in FY 1997.

ALIC serves to facilitate the development of a strong cancer network in Appalachia. As a research program, ALIC is testing the effectiveness of community coalitions and partnerships as an intervention strategy for social and organizational change in achieving cancer control objectives. The program involves four individual projects, with four research universities as the lead agencies, working with a variety of partners in 10 different states in the Appalachian region. All four projects have initially focused their coalition development activities on the following specific outcomes: an increase in early-stage diagnosis of breast and cervical cancer with a concomitant decrease in late-stage diagnosis of these diseases, an increase in cancer survivorship, and a decrease in breast and cervix cancer mortality over time. A great deal of information about the society and about the health—and cancer problems—in Appalachia, and about the individual ALIC projects, can be found in a publication, *Sowing Seeds in the Mountains*, an ALIC monograph published by NCI in 1994. Preliminary results suggest that the ALIC intervention has enhanced capacity (defined as a greater degree of interconnectedness among partnering organizations involved in planned action) in the Appalachian cancer control system and that this additional capacity will increase screening activities for breast and cervical cancer in the region. NCI allocated approximately $1.5 million for these activities in FY 1997.

Cancer Research Networks

NCI supports two networks to coordinate meetings and enhance the efforts of researchers working to address the needs of ethnic minority and underserved populations. The Network for Cancer Control Research Among American Indian and Alaska Native Populations (NCCR-AIANP) was established in 1990 to disseminate information regarding cancer control and prevention among American Indian populations, to increase collaboration with the Indian Health Service and CDC, to expand cancer surveillance among American Indian populations, and to promote new studies on patterns of care and cancer survivorship. NCCR-AIANP has convened three national conferences to discuss research and training issues relevant to American Indian populations and developed a National Strategic Plan for Cancer Prevention and Control Research in 1992. The Network also established in 1997 the Cancer Information Resource Center and Learning Exchange (CIRCLE) at the Mayo Comprehensive Cancer Center. This learning and resource center serves to link young American Indian cancer prevention and control researchers with experienced mentors. The Native Hawaiian and American Samoan Cancer Control Research Network focuses on the cancer control and prevention needs of Pacific Islander populations. The Network collaborates with a variety of public and private organizations, including Papa Ola Lokahi (the Native Hawaiian Board of Health), the Office of Hawaiian Affairs, the Cancer Center of Hawaii, Native Hawaiian Health organizations, traditional healers, scientific and lay community leaders, and others. In 1995 the two networks collaborated to sponsor a Native American Cancer Conference III in Seattle, Washington, to discuss their mutual problems.

It is not clear from the information provided by NCI how these networks differ from the leadership initiatives in purpose or mission. Similarly, it is unclear why no such network or leadership initiative exists for cancer control activities among Asian-American populations.

Training of Minority Scientists

Many ethnic minority groups are disproportionately underrepresented among cancer researchers in all relevant fields of study (e.g., oncology, psychology, epidemiology, molecular genetics). Increasing the pool of well-trained ethnic minority researchers can help to increase the quality and quantity of research on ethnic minority and medically underserved populations. For example, the small percentage of ethnic minority health care professionals and researchers has been identified as a significant barrier to the participation of ethnic minorities in clinical trials (Swanson and Ward, 1995). Further, such researchers are often able to address cultural and linguistic considerations in the conceptualization of research on ethnic minority populations and the interpretation of research findings.

NCI offers a number of training and career development programs designed to increase the number of minority scientists in biomedical fields, as well as to enhance the careers of those already in the field. NCI's Comprehensive Minority Biomedical Section (CMBS) in the Division of Extramural Activities (DEA) and OSPR have funded the majority of these graduate, postgraduate, and collegiate fellowships and scholarships to encourage minority students to pursue careers in oncology research. In addition, funds are allocated to increase mentoring and training opportunities at minority-serving institutions.

Eligibility for minority training funds is typically restricted to U.S. citizens or resident aliens and to members of ethnic or racial groups determined by the granting institution to be underrepresented in biomedical or behavioral research. For minority research supplements, this definition includes African Americans, Hispanic Americans, American Indians, Alaska Natives, and Pacific Islanders but excludes many Asian-American groups. Furthermore, NIH gives priority to projects involving African Americans, Hispanic Americans, American Indians, Alaska Natives, and Pacific Islanders. The exclusion of Asian-American groups from these programs appears to reflect NCI's belief that Asian-American scientists are well represented within the cancer research field. Asian-American researchers, however, are underrepresented in behavioral and population sciences, highlighting the dangers of assessing the representativeness of populations in research on the basis of aggregated data across all cancer fields. NCI did not cite an empirical basis for the policy of exclusion of Asian Americans from training programs.

Dissemination of information regarding training programs appears to occur largely through government publications, such as the *NIH Guide.* Announcements about the minority research supplement grants, for example, are provided to principal investigators via the guide. Dissemination also occurs through the efforts of program staff attending professional conferences and meetings (e.g., the annual meeting of the American Association for Cancer Research [AACR]). Beyond these efforts, NCI did not provide evidence of any formal or systematic information dissemination or outreach plan regarding training opportunities for minorities.

NCI Programs for Underrepresented Minorities

Minority training and enrichment programs include the following:

• *Science Enrichment Program.* The Science Enrichment Program (SEP) is a 4- to 6-week summer residential science education program to encourage promising high school students to pursue professional careers in scientific research. SEP is open to youth from underrepresented minority and underserved groups, as well as those from areas where science education opportunities are limited. Three universities (the University of Kentucky at Lexington, the University of Massachusetts at Amherst, and the University of Southern California) now participate in the program. Approximately 150 youth participate in the program, which received funding of slightly more than $1 million in FY 1997.

- *Minority Access to Research Careers Summer Research Training Program.* NCI, in collaboration with the Minority Access to Research Careers (MARC) program of the National Institute for General Medical Sciences (NIGMS), provides support to students from MARC institutions to participate in a summer research traineeship program at NCI's intramural laboratories. The program is designed to increase research training opportunities for minority MARC scholars interested in cancer-related research careers. Approximately $25,000 was allocated in FY 1997 to fund six students.
- *Travel Awards.* CMBS provides travel fellowships for minority students to attend annual meetings of AACR. The program is intended to increase the participation of minority pre- and postdoctoral scientists in the annual meeting. Thirty-three awardees were funded in 1997; $73,000 was allocated for this activity in 1998. Similarly, funds were made available for the first time to support the travel of faculty at historically black colleges and universities (HBCUs) to attend the AACR conference.
- *Mentored Career Development Award.* NCI has invited individuals who have been recipients of an NIH Research Supplement for Underrepresented Minority Individuals in Postdoctoral Training or a Minority Investigator Supplement to apply for the Mentored Career Development Award, which is intended to provide a means of gaining scientific expertise while bridging the transition from a mentored research environment to an independent research or academic career. Approximately $950,000 was allocated for this K01 award, initially announced in an RFA in 1997, with approximately $1.25 million allocated in FY 1998. Ten awards were made in 1997.

More than $400,000 was allocated in FY 1997 for the following four Minority Health Professional Training Initiative awards:

- *Minority Oncology Leadership Academic Award.* This award, available to faculty members at minority health professional schools, is offered to promote independent cancer research.
- *Clinical Investigator Award for Research on Special Populations.* This K08 award is targeted to newly trained clinicians interested in designing research protocols aimed at improving the health of groups with disproportionately high cancer morbidity and mortality rates. The award enables clinicians to pursue 3 to 5 years of special study and supervised research experience and covers the transition between postdoctoral research and an independent research career.
- *Mentored Research Scientist Development Award.* This award supports

the development of faculty members at minority-serving institutions in areas relevant to cancer. The awardee is provided with a mentored relationship with outstanding cancer researchers at major research institutions. The objective of the award is to "broaden the experience of faculty members at minority schools, to increase the pool of biomedical and behavioral investigators in cancer research, and have graduate and undergraduate students, most of whom will be minority individuals, become more cognizant of research opportunities in cancer research" (National Cancer Institute, 1998b, p. 23). Two such awards were made in 1994 and 1995.

• *Minorities in Medical Oncology*. This award, first announced in an RFA in 1996, was reissued as a program announcement in 1997 and provides funds to encourage recently trained minority clinicians to gain research experience in medical oncology. Three awards were made in 1996.

Other Training and Career Development Programs

In addition to the awards described above, a number of NIH-wide funding mechanisms related to career development and training are offered by NCI, the majority of which are open to all cancer researchers.

Research Supplements for Underrepresented Minorities Nearly $2.2 million was allocated for both the Minority Investigator Supplement to NCI's cancer centers for minority research and NCI grantees to support minority researchers involved in research projects. Minority Investigator Supplements were also available for promising high school students, undergraduate students, and graduate research assistants (nearly $1.2 million in FY 1997). In 1997, 128 awards were made; these grants were overwhelmingly made to African-American (61 awards) and Hispanic (60 awards) researchers, with 4 awards made to American Indian researchers and 1 award made to a Pacific Islander. In 1996, 112 awards were made; these were made exclusively to African-American and Hispanic scientists.

National Research Service Awards Three National Research Service Awards (NRSA) are offered. A predoctoral fellowship for oncology nurses, minority students, and students with disabilities (F31 award) was established to increase the numbers of each group in the cancer research enterprise, whereas a postdoctoral fellowship (F32 award) is open to all cancer researchers holding the Ph.D. degree or its equivalent. Both fellowships require the awardee to work with an identified mentor at a sponsoring institution to supervise research and training. The NRSA Senior Fellowship (F33 award) was established for experienced scientists who seek to acquire new research capabilities or change the direction of their research careers.

Other Awards Other individual research training and career awards include the Howard Temin Award (K01 award), to enhance the research careers of the most promising doctoral-level scientists while they consolidate and focus their research programs and obtain independent funding; the Preventive Oncology Academic Award (K07 award), to promote the career development of researchers in the fields of cancer prevention, cancer control, and cancer etiology; the Mentored Clinical Scientist Development Award (K08 award), for clinically trained physicians who are committed to careers in cancer research to undertake 3 to 5 years of specialized study; and the Mentored Clinical Scientist Development Program Award (K12 award), an award to educational institutions to support career development experiences for clinicians that will lead to research independence in areas such as translation of basic research results into new clinical procedures and AIDS-related malignancies.

Overall, NCI reports that it allocated $80.4 million to training and education programs in FY 1997, including $43.7 million to the NRSA program, $20.9 million to the Research Career Program, and $12.2 million to the Cancer Education Program. DEA reports that it allocated approximately $15 million to minority training, including the programs cited above.

Other Extramural Research Support

NCI reports that several programs, in addition to the ones reported above, have been designed specifically to expand opportunities for minority researchers or to address research questions critical to minority and medically underserved communities. These are described in the following sections.

Minority Biomedical Research Support

More than $2.5 million was allocated for the Minority Biomedical Research Support program, which is offered in conjunction with NIGMS to expand opportunities for ethnic minority faculty and students by supporting specific cancer-related projects at minority-serving institutions. Nineteen such awards were provided in FY 1997.

Small Research Grants for HBCU Faculty

To increase the research base at historically black institutions, NCI offers funding to new faculty members at HBCUs to conduct basic science research relevant to the goals of NCI.

Small Business Innovative Research Grants and Technology Transfer Research Grants

The Small Business Innovation Research Grant and the Small Business Technology Transfer Research Grants provide funds to small businesses that develop technological, innovative, and cost-effective solutions to translating basic scientific knowledge into clinical and preventive cancer services. NCI reports that it made 10 such awards for ethnic minority projects in FY 1997, including several projects that develop targeted cancer prevention and education messages for African-American, Hispanic, or Native American populations, and 2 awards for the development of cancer information materials for populations with low levels of literacy.

Small Grant Program

NCI has established an R03 award mechanism to fund projects solicited by RFAs or program announcements that are preliminary short-term research projects limited in time (typically 2 to 3 years) and amount of support ($50,000 annually). NCI provided examples of five projects related to special populations funded through this mechanism, which typically allows investigators to test new ideas or conduct pilot studies. In addition, NCI funded eight awards pertaining to underserved minority women in FY 1997. These awards were made following the release of an RFA pertaining to the recruitment and retention of ethnic minority women in clinical and prevention trials.

Funding for Extramural Research Relevant to Ethnic Minority and Medically Underserved Populations

NCI reports that 127 extramural awards were made in FY 1997 to address the needs of specific special populations, including some of the research projects summarized above. "Special populations" include ethnic minorities, medically underserved groups, elderly people, blue-collar workers, and people living in rural areas (see Chapter 2). Awards are included in this tabulation only if the grant primarily targets one or more special populations. Nearly $44 million in funding was allocated to special populations research in FY 1997, an increase of more than $30 million since FY 1990 (see Table 3-4 and Figure 3-2).

TABLE 3-4 Minority/Special Populations Awards (CRISP 1997; last update January 20, 1998)

Activity Code	No. of Awards	Award Amount
F31	2	$30,814
F32	1	28,600
K07	3	161,095
N01	9	14,408,361
P01	4	704,346
P30	8	1,307,744
P50	2	367,519
R01	59	17,514,524
R03	12	1,297,779
R13	1	50,000
R25	12	1,445,109
R29	1	132,937
R43	2	199,493
R44	3	1,022,700
U01	4	3,967,931
U10	5	1,175,872
Total	128	43,903,168

SOURCE: National Cancer Institute.

Among these awards, NCI reports that 59 R01 awards—the principal NIH research mechanism for investigator-initiated awards—totaling more than $17.5 million were provided. Nine N01 awards totaling $14.4 million were granted. The awards principally support the PLCO Cancer Screening Trial and the recruitment of minority individuals into these screening trials. Twelve R03 and R25 awards supported small grants for time- and scope-limited projects (these were primarily projects to stimulate recruitment and retention of minorities in clinical trials) (nearly $1.3 million) and educational projects to develop programs in areas of education, information, technical assistance, or evaluation ($1.44 million), respectively. Eight P30 center core grant awards totaling $1.3 million were made to consortiums, including the Charles R. Drew University of Medicine and Science in Los Angeles. Nearly $4 million in funding was provided to support four U01 cooperative agreements, including the minority-serving leadership initiatives. A total of $704,000 in four P01 awards was awarded to support broad-based, multidisciplinary research. Many other awards were provided in other categories (see Table 3-4 for details).

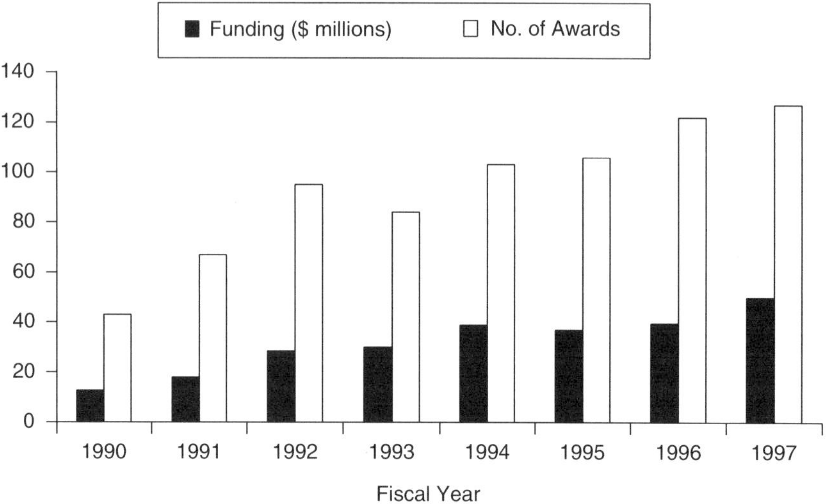

FIGURE 3-2 National Cancer Institute awards targetting special populations (total funding in millions of dollars). SOURCE: National Cancer Institute.

ALLOCATION OF NCI RESOURCES FOR RESEARCH ON ETHNIC MINORITY AND MEDICALLY UNDERSERVED GROUPS

The summaries of programs of research at NCI relevant to minority and underserved populations presented above include information regarding specific funding amounts, where available. Attempts to estimate the overall percentage of the NCI budget that has been allocated to the study of minority and medically underserved populations is difficult, in part because many basic and applied research programs that are geared to improving cancer prevention, treatment, and control among general populations may reap benefits for minority and medically underserved groups.

Another difficulty in accounting for funding allocated to the study of specific populations is posed by the accounting methods that NCI uses to estimate resource allocation. NCI, along with other agencies of the U.S. Department of Health and Human Services, is required to produce annual reports on the allocation of research funds for Minority Health and Assistance Programs (MHAPs). These include programs that are fully targeted to minority populations (100 percent relevant), in addition to those that are not specifically targeted to these populations but that have some bearing to minority populations by virtue of having minority groups among study samples, clinical trial groups, or the like. For the latter programs, NCI calculates the "percent relevancy" of the program on the basis of the percentage of minority individuals targeted in a research grant or contract. This percentage is then used to estimate the amount of funding from the project that can be added to the total funding for minority health programs. For example, if a clinical trial research grant is funded at a total of $1 million and if 30 percent of the patients in the trial are ethnic minorities, $300,000 is counted toward total institute expenditures on minority health. No such calculations or figures are reported for medically underserved populations.

Such accounting methods, however, obscure and perhaps overstate the benefits of research for minority populations. If research questions are not geared toward illuminating unique issues in cancer treatment, control, and prevention for minority populations, then the findings may be of limited value in addressing disparities in health outcomes between minority and nonminority populations. It is unclear from percent relevancy accounting methods whether such studies address unique issues for minority populations or whether subpopulation analyses are overlooked entirely. In addition, studies with very small percentages of minority populations may not provide the statistical power necessary to examine within- or between-group differences that are relevant for minority groups, yet these percentages are used in calculations of total resources allocated to minority programs.

Using "percent relevancy" accounting methods, NCI reports that $124,399,000 was allocated to MHAPs in FY 1997. Many of these research programs were summarized earlier in this chapter and include both intramural and extramural research, contract, and training programs. This figure represented approximately 5.25 percent of NCI's total budget in 1997. According to the committee's own calculations, however, inclusion of only those research programs listed as 100 percent relevant to minority populations would result in a total figure for FY 1997 of $24,234,000, or approximately 1 percent of the total NCI budget.

These projects almost certainly focus research hypotheses on issues for ethnic minority populations (i.e., that are *specific* to these groups), whereas NCI's report of $124.4 million may reflect both research targeted specifically to ethnic minority groups, as well as research that indirectly offers benefits to these populations (i.e., that are *relevant* to ethnic minority groups). Further, NCI's report of allocating $43.9 million in FY 1997 to research projects specific to "special populations" includes funding for projects targeted to elderly and blue-collar populations, groups that were not included in the committee's analysis.

The committee offers the following recommendations regarding resource allocation and accounting methods for programs of research and training relevant to ethnic minority and medically underserved populations:

Recommendation 3-2: Research and research funding relevant to cancer among ethnic minority and medically (as per Recommendation 3-3) underserved populations should be more adequately assessed and should be increased.

NCI reports that it allocated more than $124 million for research and training programs relevant to cancer among ethnic minority and medically underserved populations. This figure represents approximately 5.25 percent of the total NCI budget. The committee believes, however, that this is an overrepresentation of the amount of resources allocated to addressing the needs of ethnic minority and medically underserved groups (see Recommendation 3-3 below). When allocations are summed for projects exclusively directed to these populations, the figure is slightly more than $24 million, or approximately 1 percent of the total NCI budget. Other NIH ICs report on their allocations of money to minority health research and training programs, but these figures are small relative to the overall budgets of the respective ICs. The committee finds that these resources are insufficient relative to three criteria:

- the burden of disease in ethnic minority and medically underserved communities;
- the changing U.S. demographic picture (which indicates that the growth of many ethnic minority groups, such as Hispanics and Asians and Pacific Islanders, will significantly outpace that of other groups and that no ethnic group will constitute a "majority" by the year 2050); and
- scientific opportunities inherent in the study of diverse populations.

Recommendation 3-3: NIH should improve the accuracy of its assessment of research that is relevant to ethnic minority and medically underserved groups by replacing the current "percent relevancy" accounting method with one that identifies studies whose purpose is to address a priori research questions uniquely affecting ethnic minority and medically underserved groups.

NIH calculates the amount of money allocated to minority health research on the basis of the percentage of ethnic minority individuals in NIH study populations. Such percent relevancy accounting methods are inappropriate as an indicator of overall expenditures for studies that address minority health needs because they overstate the relevance of research for addressing ethnic minority health issues. Estimates of expenditures on minority-related health research should be determined by assessing whether research questions for specific programs are focused on illuminating the particular needs of ethnic minority and medically underserved communities.

The committee found no evidence that NIH calculates total expenditures for research on medically underserved groups, apart from calculations derived for ethnic minority populations. A consistent definition of medically underserved individuals is needed (as discussed above), and calculations of research expenditures for these groups should be based on whether research questions specifically address the unique needs of these populations.

RESEARCH ON CANCER AMONG ETHNIC MINORITY AND MEDICALLY UNDERSERVED GROUPS AT OTHER ICDS

As noted above, several ICDs are conducting research, either in collaboration with NCI or independently, on cancer among minority and medically underserved populations.

National Institute of Environmental Health Sciences

As noted above, NIEHS supports the second-largest portfolio of cancer-related research at NIH, with overall funding of more than $84 million in FY 1997. Of this amount, NIEHS reports that it allocated $26.7 million to fund 138 extramural projects, including investigator-initiated research, co-funded projects, and Superfund and center grants (described below). Of these, NIEHS reports that 71 awards are relevant to minority and medically underserved populations, in that the awards specifically target minority or low-income communities or the research topic disproportionately affects minority and medically underserved populations. Total expenditures on these awards fell slightly under $9.5 million; eight awards were cosponsored with NCI, with a total of $672,389 expended by NIEHS. Several relevant programs are described below.

Community Outreach and Education Program

NIEHS supports community outreach efforts through the Environmental Health Sciences Center Grants Program, a program of core center support that seeks to address specific regional or community needs through outreach and educational activities. Centers serve to define environmental health issues of greatest concern to communities, with a focus on populations that may be at greatest risk as a result of environmental insults, including children, elderly people, and low-income communities. Centers are encouraged to sponsor local efforts through community organizations and to collaborate with other existing outreach programs, especially those supported by other federal agencies (e.g., other NIH institutes, CDC, and the National Institute for Occupational Safety and Health).

Developmental centers, in particular, are encouraged to foster collaborations and develop outreach programs for ethnic minority and low-income communities. NIEHS currently supports three such centers. Columbia University's Harlem Center for Health Promotion and Disease Prevention, for example, has formed partnerships with community groups in Harlem and Washington Heights, New York, to promote public education, outreach, and environmental monitoring. Interdisciplinary and inter-institutional programs with Harlem Hospital, for example, have also provided a forum for sharing environmental health research findings across institutions. Community outreach forums have addressed a wide range of community concerns about environmental pollutants and public health problems. Similarly, the Tulane/Xavier Center for Bioenvironmental Research provides comprehensive environmental research and education for the City of New Orleans and the Gulf South region. This center combines the resources of a major research institution and historically black college to foster collaboration between local organizations; state, local and federal governments; industry; and students.

Community-Based Prevention/Intervention Research in Environmental Health Science

This initiative aims to implement culturally relevant prevention and intervention activities among economically disadvantaged and underserved populations that are adversely affected by an environmental contaminant. It is intended to foster refinement of scientifically valid intervention methods, whereas it also strengthens the participation of the affected communities in this effort. The long-range goal of this program is to reduce the incidence and mortality from environment-associated diseases among these populations. Five grants that concentrate on Native American, African-American, and Hispanic populations have been awarded. This program also serves as a model for other federal, state, and local agencies in designing their own environmental justice contaminant prevention programs.

Environmental Justice: Partnerships for Communication

The Partnerships for Communication program provides multiyear grants that foster collaboration between health providers and community residents to examine and assess environmental contamination specifically located in communities. The primary goal of the grants is to investigate the relationship between economic factors, social factors, and the health status of the community members exposed to environmental hazards. Currently, 12 grants have been awarded across the United States. The majority of these grantees are located in lower-income communities confronting the redevelopment of brownfields.

Minority Worker Training Program

NIEHS, working in collaboration with the Environmental Protection Agency, has developed the Minority Worker Training Program as a series of national pilot programs designed to test strategies for the recruitment and training of young people for future environmental careers. The people selected live near hazardous waste sites or in communities at risk of exposure to contaminated properties. This program seeks to provide sustainable job development and training for young adults who live in areas with hazardous exposure potential, such as brownfields sites in urban communities. Community groups and HBCUs are involved in this partnership to teach math, science, and life skills to assist in reinforcing worker knowledge and positive behavior on the job.

Environmental Health Science Centers: Agricultural Chemicals and Farm Workers

The NIEHS Environmental Health Science Centers are academic institutions throughout the country that bring together individuals from many scientific disciplines to focus on particular environmental health problems. Three of these centers (those at the University of Iowa, University of California at Davis, and Oregon State University) focus on the health concerns of agricultural workers, many of whom are migrant workers or disadvantaged minorities. The results of this research will help define the true risks to this occupational group so that better prevention and intervention strategies can be developed to protect their health.

Agricultural Health Study

NIEHS is assisting NCI in a prospective study of cancer risk in a cohort of 75,000 pesticide applicators and their spouses. NIEHS manages and evaluates the part of the study devoted to noncancer endpoints and has assisted in recruiting African Americans into the study population. This study examines, in part, the unique risks to rural African Americans and other minority populations exposed to pesticides. Minority populations may have increased susceptibility to the effects of pesticides. For example, there is increasing evidence of racial differences in the prevalence of gene polymorphisms that affect the metabolism of chemicals including pesticides and the organic solvents in which they are mixed. In addition, such groups may have enhanced vulnerability to pesticides due to underlying nutritional deficiencies or concomitant health problems often associated with poverty.

Brownfields National Partnership Action Agenda

NIEHS is participating to help support the Brownfields National Partnership Action Agenda, a public, private, and community initiative to redevelop brownfields into safer living areas. Brownfields are abandoned, idled, or underused industrial and commercial facilities where expansion or redevelopment is complicated by environmental contamination. These areas are not as toxic as Superfund sites but still face immense barriers to their redevelopment. Although brownfields are typically found in urban areas, they are prominent in rural areas as well. A large proportion of medically underserved and economically disadvantaged citizens reside near brownfields.

Mississippi Delta Project

The Mississippi Delta Project is a collaborative effort of government, academia, grassroots organizations in communities, and local and state health agencies to address environmental contamination in the Mississippi Delta Region, one of the poorest regions in the country and a region that is greatly affected by environmental pollution. NIEHS works with other federal agencies to identify key environmental hazards, promote environmental quality, and reduce and, where possible, prevent these hazards from affecting the health and environment of residents.

Working in collaboration with ORMH, NIEHS has initiated the Columbia Project, a community outreach program of the Mississippi Delta Project. This is a community-based effort to augment community participation and involvement in decisions concerning the environmental health of residents in the Delta Region. A Needs Assessment Workshop to identify demonstration projects in the Delta Region was held in February 1998 and included representatives from federal agencies, state and local health departments, HBCUs, grassroots organizations in communities, and health care professionals.

Institutional Capacity Building

NIEHS has supported several programs designed to enhance environmental health research and training capacity in underserved populations. NIEHS has initiated a series of planning activities organized through HB-

CUs and majority academic institutions to assess the needs and opportunities for building environmental health research and training capacity for underserved populations. In addition, a state-of-the-art Molecular Research and Training Center has been established at a local (Durham, North Carolina) high school that is attended by a large number of African-American students.

Training and Education Workshop

NIEHS sponsors several programs designed to increase the number of minority scientists involved in biomedical research, increase the levels of awareness and participation of minorities in NIEHS and NIH intramural and extramural activities, and facilitate cooperative research between minority and majority scientists on the health problems that may disproportionately affect minorities and lower-income populations. For example, the Minority Faculty Development program is designed to strengthen the ability of minority institutions to provide instruction of the environmental health discipline.

National Institute of Allergy and Infectious Diseases

NIAID supports a number of research projects relevant to cancer among minority and medically underserved populations. This research focuses largely on cancer associated with AIDS and neoplastic complications of HIV infection, notably Kaposi's sarcoma, but also includes basic studies of the abnormal proliferation of immune cells and immune responses to cell proliferation. Given that HIV infection disproportionately affects ethnic minority populations, particularly African-American and Hispanic communities, NIAID's portfolio of research in this area is highly relevant to the overall NIH effort to address cancer among minority and medically underserved populations.

As noted above, NIAID supports the fourth-largest portfolio of cancer research among NIH ICDs, with $43 million in funding for 177 cancer-related research projects in FY 1997. Of these, NIAID reports that 63 projects, with funding totaling $4.49 million, are relevant to minority and medically underserved populations.

Clinical Trials

Through a range of intramural and extramural programs, NIAID directs a large national clinical trials network that tests and provides therapies for the treatment and prevention of HIV infection and its complications. These programs have enjoyed, on the whole, significant success in the recruitment of minority candidates into clinical trials. NIAID works with these networks to identify and help develop culturally sensitive educational materials and to identify and overcome barriers to recruitment and retention of minority patients. Among the patients enrolled in the Adult AIDS Clinical Trials Group in 1996, for example, 35 percent were African American and 25 percent were Hispanic. Three institutions serving predominantly minority communities were originally funded in 1993 to assist in minority accrual to these trials. Similarly, the Terry Beirn Community Programs for Clinical Research on AIDS (CPCRA) enrolled 31 percent African-American patients and 12 percent Hispanic patients among new enrollees in 1996. CPCRA is a community-based trials network located in community settings such as health care clinics and centers, making these trials much more accessible to women and ethnic minorities.

NIAID supports epidemiologic research, clinical research, and research on the natural history and transmission of HIV infection in a variety of populations. Urban women and children are the focus of the Women and Infants Transmission Study, which evaluates issues of perinatal HIV transmission and disease progression in women and children. In 1996, 86 percent of the women enrolled in this program were ethnic minorities. Similarly, the Women's Interagency HIV Study examines the spectrum and clinical course of HIV infection in women and has enrolled 56 percent African-American and 24 percent Hispanic women. In contrast, NIAID's Multicenter AIDS Cohort Study, which examines the mechanisms by which HIV damages the immune system and how the immune system combats HIV infection among homosexual and bisexual men, has enrolled only 15 percent ethnic minority participants.

Training and Infrastructure Development

NIAID has provided support for a number of programs designed to increase the numbers of minority biomedical researchers and support the development of the biomedical research infrastructure at minority-serving institutions.

The Research Supplements for Underrepresented Minorities program served to increase the number of minorities in biomedical research by providing supplemental training funds for research grants currently being funded by NIH. In 1996, NIAID funded 40 such supplements at $3.6 million for minority investigators at the junior faculty, postdoctoral, predoctoral, undergraduate, and high school levels. Similarly, the Research Centers in Minority Institutions (RCMI) program assists predominantly minority institutions that offer doctoral degrees via grant support for laboratory and infrastructure development, faculty expansion, and other areas to assist these institutions in becoming more competitive in seeking research funding. NIAID co-funds the AIDS Infrastructure Initiative of RCMI and supported 15 RCMI projects at eight institutions in FY 1996. To further enhance these efforts, NIAID offered its own AIDS Infrastructure for Minority Institutions RFA in FY 1990 and FY 1993 to provide funding for RCMI projects at three additional institutions.

NIAID has also collaborated with the National Institute of Mental Health to support an initiative pairing NIAID's 12 Centers for AIDS Research investigators with RCMI investigators to increase collaborations between ethnic minority and majority institutions. Eleven projects at seven schools were ultimately funded. In 1995, NIAID established its own Enhancement Awards for Underrepresented Minority Researchers to enable these individuals to establish clinical or basic AIDS research programs. Nine individuals were funded. Furthermore, NIAID's Office of Research on Minority and Women's Health has developed a number of outreach programs, including one for Washington, D.C., area high school science students and teachers, and other collaborations with the Interamerican College of Physicians and Scientists to increase awareness of NIAID programs and resources among Hispanic investigators.

Ethnic Minority Issues at NIAID

In 1994, the NIAID director established the Minority Scientists Advisory Committee (MINSAC) as a standing committee to advise the director on issues and concerns of the minority scientific community and provide suggestions on ways that the Institute can attract highly qualified minority scientists to its intramural and extramural programs. In particular, MINSAC has conveyed concerns regarding the underrepresentation of minorities in tenure, tenure-track, and postdoctoral positions within NIAID's intramural research program, resulting in the creation of additional lines to attract minority scientists. In addition, MINSAC has initiated the development of a minority constituency catalog, including minority scientists, institutions, and organizations, to assist in the identification of qualified minorities to participate in the NIH peer-review system.

National Institute of Diabetes and Digestive and Kidney Diseases

NIDDKD directs approximately 70 percent of its budget to investigator-initiated grants. These awards are largely focused on basic research to understand underlying mechanisms of disease and pathogenesis. Like other ICDs, NIDDKD uses RFAs or program announcements sparingly and largely in response to congressional directives or the need to stimulate research in small program areas.

Priority setting at NIDDKD is determined by a planning process that establishes a framework for program activities. This program plan is submitted to the NIDDKD Advisory Council for discussion. Of the six sections in the current program plan, one references "minority activities" and highlights minority initiatives, research projects, center activities, and training and career development programs.

NIDDKD's cancer-related research is coordinated with NCI via a formalized memorandum of understanding that establishes NCI's primary responsibility for research on carcinoma of the prostate and NIDDKD's primary responsibility for research on noncancerous conditions, including research on the growth, development, and maturation of the prostate.

NIDDKD reports that it allocated a total of $33.4 million for research related to cancer among minority and medically underserved groups. This funding supports 142 programs or research grants. Nearly $1.5 million of this funding was allocated to the minority emphasis within the NIDDKD clinical trial on Medical Treatment of Prostatic Symptoms (MTOPS); this money represents 20 percent of the total funding for MTOPS. NIDDKD supported a workshop to identify barriers to the successful recruitment and retention of minority participants in this study and provided funding for 11 of 17 participating clinical centers to develop minority recruitment plans specific to their locales.

In collaboration with NCI and NIAID, NIDDKD has sought to stimulate research on *Helicobacter pylori* and its relationship to digestive diseases and cancer, particularly in minority populations, by establishing an RFA in January 1997. The RFA calls for studies on the epidemiology of *Helicobacter* in minority populations, genetic susceptibility to *Helicobacter* infection, and the clinical course of infection. The RFA notes that 10 to 12 awards are anticipated, with $2.5 million in funding available for awards. Before FY 1997, NIDDKD offered RFAs for studies of the regulation of prostate growth, the molecular epidemiology of prostate carcinogenesis, clinical trials of medical therapy in benign prostatis hyperplasia, hormonal regulation of breast-specific growth factors, and other studies of cancers that disproportionately affect ethnic minority populations.

National Heart, Lung, and Blood Institute

NHLBI reported a dramatic increase in cancer-related research expenditures from FY 1985 to FY 1997. In 1985, NHLBI allocated $3.87 million to cancer-related research; this figure increased to $50.7 million in FY 1993 and $57.6 million in FY 1997, spurred in large part by the cancer portion of the Women's Health Initiative (WHI; see below), of which $16.7 million is included in the FY 1993 total and $19.5 million is included in the FY 1997 total. The bulk of NHLBI's cancer-related research funding is for basic scientific projects that are not targeted to specific populations.

NHLBI reports that before FY 1997 it did not support any cancer research relevant to minority and medically underserved populations. According to NHLBI Director Claude Lenfant, "The NHLBI does not have any processes for establishing priorities for cancer-related research among minority and medically underserved populations. Research on cancer and research on cancer in minorities are not part of the mission of the NHLBI, except for the WHI which NHLBI administers as part of a NIH consortium with the National Cancer Institute (NCI), the National Institute of Arthritis and Musculoskeletal and Skin Diseases (NIAMS), and the National Institute on Aging (NIA)" (Lenfant, 1998, p. 1).

In FY 1997, NHLBI supported aspects of WHI that included research on cancer (approximately 40 percent of the total WHI contract). NHLBI estimates that the minority population of these study trials is approximately 20 percent. WHI is a cross-institute collaboration that examines the effects of promising interventions, such as hormone replacement therapy and dietary modification, in preventing a number of common diseases among women, including coronary heart disease, osteoporosis, and cancer (specifically, breast and colorectal cancers). In addition, WHI attempts to identify risk factors for these diseases and assess the feasibility of various community-based programs of preventive care.

National Human Genome Research Institute

The National Human Genome Research Institute (NHGRI) was established in 1989 first as a center, then as an Institute in 1997 to lead NIH's efforts in the Human Genome Project, including chromosome mapping, DNA sequencing, DNA-based diagnostics and gene therapy development, database development, technology development for genome research, and studies of the ethical, legal, and social implications of genetics research. Cancer-related research represents a significant proportion of NHGRI's portfolio, including work conducted in the Laboratory of Cancer Genetics, where researchers are seeking to understand genetic changes in somatic cells that lead to cancer, inherited mutations that predispose individuals to cancer, and genes involved in the development of malignant characteristics in cancer cells, such as drug resistance and metastasis.

Of note in NHGRI's cancer research portfolio is a collaborative effort between NHGRI and NIH's ORMH to establish an intramural research project, the Center for Collaborative Research on Genomic Analyses of Diseases that Disproportionately Affect African Americans, at Howard University in Washington, D.C., an historically black university. NHGRI and ORMH have identified four principal objectives of this collaboration:

- to increase the competitiveness of minority researchers and minority institutions by developing a center that will become a self-sustaining entity through competitive grants and contracts;
- to promote collaborative research between majority and minority institutions (NHGRI and Howard University scientists will be involved in an exchange between the two campuses to foster cross-fertilization and training);
- to increase the inclusion of minorities in study populations; and
- to promote the study of diseases that disproportionately affect African Americans, such as diabetes and hereditary prostate cancer, which will be a focus of the Center.

In a summary of this initiative, NHGRI notes that there is a paucity of standardized, population-based data on the genetic and epidemiologic factors underlying the diseases that disproportionately affect African Americans. To address this need, the help of African-American physicians, research scientists, and institutions is needed to increase the participation of African Americans in research. The Center's initial objectives include the recruitment of African-American families for genomic research; the development of standardized protocols for the collection of genetic, clinical, and epidemiologic data; and the establishment of core facilities for the isolation, characterization, and storage of cells and DNA for study. Specific projects emerging from this collaboration include a study of sibling pairs with non-insulin-dependent diabetes mellitus in West Africa, genetic linkage studies of hereditary prostate cancer among African Americans (which has also received research support from NCI), and studies of the ethical, social, and legal aspects of genetic research and testing, such as the informed-consent process and the psychosocial impact of a genetic diagnosis on African-American patients and their families.

The training and education of young African-American scientists is also a major goal of the collaboration with Howard University. With funding from ORMH, several African Americans at the doctorate level have been recruited for these projects, and additional training for pre- and postdoctoral scientists will occur at NHGRI's laboratories in the Division of Intramural Research.

NHGRI proposes that the Center be supported for 5 years, with assistance from ORMH.

SUMMARY AND RECOMMENDATIONS

NIH, and particularly NCI, has funded an impressive array of research projects and training initiatives that may have a demonstrable impact in addressing the disproportionate burden of cancer incidence and mortality among minority and medically underserved populations. The committee finds, however, that no "blueprint" or strategic plan exists to direct or coordinate this research activity (see discussion of priority setting in Chapter 4). As a result, model programs in one or more institutes are not replicated by other ICDs where indicated, some areas of research emphasis receive greater attention than others, and overall funding to address the needs of minority and medically underserved populations is inadequate. Several recommendations are therefore indicated:

Recommendation 3-1: The Office of Research on Minority Health should more actively serve a coordinating, planning, and facilitative function regarding research relevant to cancer among ethnic minority and medically underserved populations across relevant institutes and centers of NIH. To further this goal, the Office of Research on Minority Health should:

- **make criteria for Minority Health Initiative project support explicit;**
- **coordinate with other specialty offices (e.g., the Office of Research on Women's Health) by participating in NIH-wide coordination efforts such as the Research Enhancement Awards Program; and**
- **ensure that Minority Health Initiative funding does not supplant funding from institutes and centers for research and programs relevant to ethnic minority and medically underserved populations.**

Recommendation 3-2: Research and research funding relevant to cancer among ethnic minority and medically underserved populations should be more adequately assessed (as per Recommendation 3-3) and should be increased.

Recommendation 3-3: NIH should improve the accuracy of its assessment of research that is relevant to ethnic minority and medically underserved groups by replacing the current "percent relevancy" accounting method with one that identifies studies whose purpose is to address a priori research questions uniquely affecting ethnic minority and medically underserved groups.

Although the committee found evidence that NCI sponsors significant behavioral and social science research aimed at examining the range of behavioral, psychosocial, dietary, and other factors that enhance the risk for cancer or poor cancer outcomes among ethnic minority and medically underserved groups, behavioral and social science research should be expanded, particularly with respect to prevention and outreach efforts. Lerman et al. (1997) note that approximately 65 percent of cancer deaths are attributable to behaviors such as smoking, sexual risk behavior, and to factors such as diet. For example, over the past half-century, more than 300,000 women have died from cervical cancer, including a disproportionate number of women from ethnic minority and medically underserved backgrounds, even though the technological tools have been available since the 1940s to vastly decrease mortality due to cervical cancer. Similarly, greater research is needed to illuminate barriers to cancer care (Chapter 5) and strategies to overcome them.

Although the committee does not seek to imply that NCI's research resources should be allocated entirely on the basis of likely etiologic factors, it is noteworthy that the NCI division with primary responsibility for funding behavioral and population-based research, DCCPS, allocated approximately $21 million to "minority health and assistance programs" in FY 1997 (as noted above, this figure is based on a percent relevancy calculation, which suggests that many projects were not specifically targeted to ethnic minority and medically underserved populations). This figure represents approximately 17 percent of the total NCI funding for MHAPs and is likely an inflated estimate of funding for behavioral and social science research, given that a large percentage of DCCPS's resources are allocated to important programs such as the SEER program and other nonbehavioral research.

The agenda for such research should be based on an analysis of the prevalence of particular cancers in these population and their preventability (Chen, 1994). Particularly for ethnic minority populations, this research should include investigations of ethnically appropriate interventions, including culturally competent and linguistically appropriate approaches. In addition, more research is needed on barriers to cancer care among these populations, and strategies to overcome them.

Recommendation 3-4: The newly established program of behavioral and social science research at NCI addresses an area of research that has been neglected in the past. The committee urges that this program of research identify as one of its highest priorities a focus on the cancer prevention, control, and treatment needs of ethnic minority and medically underserved groups.

Such focused research will require collaboration and coordination between DCCPS and the NCI Divisions of Cancer Prevention and Cancer Treatment. As will be discussed in Chapter 4, coordination of this research activity is appropriately led by OSPR, provided that sufficient resources and authority are granted to OSPR to carry out this agenda.

The NHGRI-Howard University collaboration stands as an outstanding, but unfortunately rare, example of a partnership between the federal scientific research infrastructure and an historically black institution that meets multiple goals. Not only will this partnership result in improved recruitment of ethnic minority patients as research subjects but it will also improve opportunities for the training of minority scientists and allow focused investigation of genetic risk as it applies to some segments of the African-American population.

Recommendation 3-5: Collaborations between NIH and research and medical institutions that serve ethnic minority and medically underserved populations should be increased to improve the study of cancers that affect these groups and to increase the involvement of such entities and populations in scientific research.

Although the committee found evidence that NCI sponsors a significant portfolio of training programs designed to increase the numbers of ethnic minority investigators in cancer-related research fields, there is little evidence that NCI or NIH has undertaken a thorough assessment of training programs to determine whether these programs are producing adequate numbers of ethnic minority researchers in all appropriate cancer research fields (e.g., behavioral and social sciences, epidemiology, genetics, and cell biology) and to determine whether training programs have resulted in the increased representation of ethnic minorities in cancer research fields. Furthermore, there is little evidence that guidelines or other training criteria have been established by NCI or NIH to ensure that all trainees can receive high-quality instruction and mentoring. Such efforts would improve the planning and implementation of future training programs.

Recommendation 3-6: NIH should increase its efforts to expand the number of ethnic minority investigators in the broad spectrum of cancer research to improve minority health research. These efforts should (1) assess relevant areas of research needs and ensure that trainees are representative of these disciplines and areas of inquiry, (2) determine guidelines for the quality and expected outcomes of training experiences, and (3) maintain funding for a sufficient period of time to assess the impact of training programs on the goal of increasing minority representation in cancer research fields.

4
Evaluation of Priority Setting and Programs of Research on Ethnic Minority and Medically Underserved Populations at the National Institutes of Health

As noted in Chapter 3, the National Institutes of Health (NIH) and the National Cancer Institute (NCI) sponsor a wide range of research and training programs relevant to cancer among ethnic minority and medically underserved populations. In addition to evaluating this research and program portfolio, the committee was asked to evaluate NIH's mechanisms for prioritizing research on cancer among ethnic minority and medically underserved groups, as stated in the committee's charge: "review . . . NIH's ability to prioritize its cancer research agenda for minorities and the role of minority scientists in decision making on research priorities."

This chapter summarizes the committee's assessment and includes an evaluation of opportunities for minority scientists and members of lay and community groups to provide input into the priority-setting process, the rationale by which policy decisions are made with regard to research priorities, and the adequacy of mechanisms for their implementation.

To understand the context for NIH's priority-setting processes and mechanisms for receiving input, it is necessary to understand how these processes are perceived by the scientific and lay communities. The first section of this chapter summarizes data that the committee collected with regard to these perceptions, including data from a survey of researchers interested in cancer among minority and medically underserved populations and a panel of individuals representing the perspectives of members of cancer survivor groups in ethnic minority and medically underserved communities. A review of NIH mechanisms for community and researcher input follows. Finally, an analysis of the NIH priority-setting process for addressing cancer among minority and medically underserved communities is presented.

SURVEY OF RESEARCH STAKEHOLDERS

The committee sought input both from ethnic minority researchers in the field of cancer research and from minority and nonminority investigators interested in cancer among minority and medically underserved populations. It sought this input as part of its attempt to understand the experiences of investigators across a broad range of disciplines who either have applied for NIH funding or have been involved in proposal review. These include individuals who either have some familiarity with the NIH portfolio of research on cancer among ethnic minority and medically underserved populations or may have benefited from NIH training programs designed to increase the level of representation of minority investigators in the field of cancer research.

It must be noted that the committee did not seek to identify a representative sample of the populations described above. Rather, the purpose of this survey was to identify some of the range of experiences and perceptions, both positive and negative, that minority investigators and those investigators interested in cancer among minority and medically underserved populations may have had with regard to NIH's priority-setting process and current program of research in this area. The survey results should therefore be interpreted with caution—they are likely not representative of any particular population of researchers, clinicians, or health policy analysts. They do, however, provide some insight into the kinds of perceptions that the extramural scientific community holds with regard to research on minority and medically underserved populations.

Sample

The pool of potential survey respondents was selected by obtaining the names and mailing addresses of 839 individuals who hold membership or who are otherwise affiliated with one of several organizations or cancer-related research programs. Specifically, names were obtained from the American Association of Cancer Research (minority research section), the Society for the Advancement of Chicanos and Native Americans in Science (members in cancer research-related fields), the Intercultural Cancer Council membership database, the Hispanic Cancer Control Network, the National Institute of General Medical Sciences (recent recipients of NIH minority training funds in cancer-related fields), and the Appalachian Leadership Initiative on Cancer (principal investigators). Whenever possible, membership overlap was identified and duplication of survey solicitation was avoided. Data on the racial and ethnic distributions of the potential respondents are not available.

The committee received 220 completed responses to the survey. Among these, 33 identified their ethnicity as "white or Caucasian," 65 identified themselves as "African American," 90 identified themselves as "Hispanic," 12 identified themselves as "American Indian or Alaska Native," and 10 each identified themselves as "Asian American or Pacific Islander" and "other." Respondents were primarily doctoral degree holders; 92 reported their highest education level as the Ph.D. or other doctorate, and 74 reported holding M.D. degrees (several reported holding both the M.D. and the Ph.D.). The majority reported working in research or teaching settings, often in combination with clinical work. Forty percent of the respondents listed laboratory, clinical, or field-based research as their primary occupation, although many were also involved in clinical practice or teaching. Only 14 percent of respondents listed teaching alone as their primary activity, and only 16 percent listed clinical practice alone as their primary work. The majority (52 percent) reported working for a nonprofit educational or research institution.

Survey Questions

An example of the survey is provided in Appendix D. Survey respondents were asked to provide demographic and educational information about themselves (race or ethnicity and highest degree obtained), as well as information about the nature of their current work (primarily research, teaching, clinical practice, or other) and employer (federal, state, or local government; nonprofit educational or research institution; health care service delivery; or other). In addition, respondents were asked whether they had submitted a research proposal to NIH for funding, whether they had responded to an NIH Request for Applications (RFA) or Program Announcements (PA), and whether they had received funding in the form of either a research or program grant or a training grant. Individuals who applied for funding were asked to rate and comment on their experience with the process.

In addition, respondents were asked how familiar they are with the NIH research priority-setting process and whether they had provided input into this process, either formally (via service on an NIH advisory body) or informally (e.g., ad hoc feedback to NIH staff).

Respondents were asked to rate and provide their perception of the receptivity of NIH to research proposals focusing on the health needs of minority and medically underserved populations, of the value that NIH places on research relevant to these groups, and of the value that NIH places on the training of minority scientists. Subsequent questions asked respondents to provide examples of NIH programs that they feel have worked well in addressing the health needs of minority and medically underserved groups and to provide specific recommendations on how NIH might improve its approach to addressing research among these populations. Finally, respondents were asked to provide any additional comments in areas of the study charge.

Results

The majority of respondents (74 percent) reported having submitted a research proposal to NIH or its institutes at some point in their careers. Nearly two-thirds (66 percent) reported having responded to an RFA or a PA from an NIH institute. More than half (58 percent) reported that they had received some form of research support from NIH. Only 16 percent reported having received research training funding from NIH or its institutes.

The survey questions tended to elicit widely varying responses. In some cases, responses appeared to be based upon a lack of information about NIH programs and resources, suggesting that outreach programs to targeted groups, such as underrepresented minority investigators, had failed to reach many of them. For example, several respondents expressed frustration that no research funds were available for minority investigators, especially young researchers transitioning from graduate or postdoctoral work to faculty positions. In fact, NCI sponsors several programs geared to young investigators and new faculty (see Chapter 3). For these survey respondents, however, the absence of such programs was viewed as detrimental to the development of ethnic minority cancer researchers, as noted in the comments of one respondent: "NIH seeks to train minority scientists yet fails to ensure adequate support once scientists reach a faculty position. A transition period of three years could make a big difference."

Peer Review and Priority Setting

With regard to the experiences of investigators applying for NIH research funds, many comments appeared to be critical of the process generally, irrespective of whether the proposal was specific to minority and medically underserved populations. "Deadlines are (after PAs) not realistic. Redundant paperwork," wrote one respondent, whereas another respondent noted, "The criticisms by and large focused on trivial details and often reflect ignorance of the reviewer in a particular field." Others found NIH staff to be unresponsive in the process. "Study section administrations generally [are] not helpful," wrote one respondent. This sentiment was echoed by others: "The peer review process is increasingly idiosyncratic, with the review being conducted by junior investigators who have little experience in research," and "No real helpful input as to how to make the proposal fundable, and a very impersonal experience. No direct communication or discussion." Another respondent described proposal review as a "triage process" whereby staff make decisions regarding whether proposals fit RFAs, thereby limiting the number of proposals that advance.

Many others, however, offered praise for the peer-review process. "Excellent program directors," wrote one respondent, who continued: "Weakness of numerous staff changes over [the past] six years but quality of support is excellent." "Comments were helpful," wrote another and the, "Executive Secretary was helpful."

Significantly, several respondents pointed to aspects of peer review and the priority-setting process that are particularly problematic for minority researchers or those studying issues relevant to minority and medically underserved populations. Among the comments that reflected this point: "I believe in the peer review process for the most part. In times of budget constraints, funding decisions are sometimes skewed toward the more established scientists. This is not good for budding investigators." "[The] process [is] not supportive of community-based and community-driven research." "Big drawback [of the peer review process] is focus on researchers who have already done this—NIH reinforces success, [making it] very hard to get started." "Program staff and contracting staff were helpful. . . . However, few at the top understand the need to fund research adequately or address the resource issues that (minority) researchers face in conducting cancer research in minority and medically underserved communities." "Good in general. Sometimes [there exists] a perception that connections and old school ties are more important than science." Several others felt that it was particularly difficult for investigators at historically black colleges and universities (HBCUs) to successfully compete for funding.

Few respondents reported attempting to provide input into the NIH research priority-setting process, but several commented on the process. Some comments reflected a theme similar to that described above: that minority investigators feel "shut out" of the process. "This is an 'old boys' network [and] it is difficult for a minority woman to . . . approach," wrote one respondent. "Have more of the review[ers] coming from HBCUs and breaking 'good-old-boy networks' among large white institutions," wrote another. Still others advocated that the level of representation of researchers from minority and medically underserved communities on NIH advisory and policy boards should be increased. "Appoint more minority investigators and administrators to key advisory committees and review committees or study sections," "Include more qualified minorities in goal setting and identification of priority areas as they pertain to minorities," and "Include more minorities on review panels" were among the comments supporting this concern.

NIH Receptivity to Special Populations Research

Few respondents felt that NIH was receptive to research proposals focusing on the needs of minority and medically underserved populations. One respondent noted that "they [NIH] seem not to understand minority health issues" and added that there exists a critical need for researchers to work in partnership with community groups. The following comments reflect this sentiment: "NIH appears to be receptive, but funding priorities often place these [minority- and underserved-oriented] proposals at the end of the funding chain. . . . [T]he funding is often inadequate. Programs are funded at a level to fail." Research on minority and medically underserved populations "appear[s] to be a low priority or not a primary concern of many institutes." "Depending on politics—sometimes the need [for minority and underserved research] is not well received. [The lack of research in this area] is rationalized through issues of 'no earmarks' or [poor] quality of proposals submitted." A minority of respondents, however, were more positive about NIH's receptivity to special populations research: "I think it is improving thanks to a center [sic] overseeing minority research," wrote one respondent, whereas another respondent noted that NIH is "flexible enough to be reactive [to minority health research needs] within constraints of research-based programs."

Similarly, many respondents felt that research on minority and medically underserved communities was not a high priority for NIH. Priorities are "biased toward academic institutions," wrote one respondent from a community-based group. Among the comments of other respondents: "NIH recognizes the need for research relevant to minority and medically underserved communities, but does not invest in building the appropriate mechanisms to fund such research. Investment must be in the development of research training programs for minority researchers and . . . in the area of community-driven research." "Some specific programs [relevant to minority and medically underserved populations] have been terrific but then are ended." Special populations research is "a very recent concern [and] not a priority of Dr. Varmus."

Training Programs

Respondents were more positive regarding NIH training programs for minority scientists, and the value that NIH places on these. "I believe NIH has made special efforts to provide training for minority graduate students and scientists," commented one respondent. Many were critical, however, of perceived gaps in funding and programs at two critical ends of the training "pipeline": outreach programs for promising high school students from minority and medically underserved communities and support for young researchers transitioning to faculty positions. Among the comments supporting this position: "Excellent options for training. Nothing specific for junior faculty." "NCI could improve the support of minority clinical scientists, especially during the transition period to independent investigation." "NIH seeks to train minority scientists yet fails to ensure adequate support once scientists reach a faculty position. A transition period of three years would make a big difference." Still others believe the problem of encouraging more individuals from underrepresented groups into the sciences is a problem beyond NIH's resources. Among the comments reflecting this view: "There is a framework for training minority scientists; however, there is an insufficient critical mass of either applicants or mentors to make the process work," and "There is a great deal of effort going on into recruiting and training minorities and scientists [sic]. There is, however, a scarcity of candidates that hinders the best NIH efforts."

Effective Programs

Many respondents listed minority training programs, however, as among the NIH programs that have worked well to address the research needs of minority and medically underserved communities. Several respondents pointed to NCI's Minority Supplement and Minority Access to Research Careers and Minority Biomedical Research Support training programs as highly effective in preparing well-trained minority scientists for work in cancer research fields. NCI programs that offer funds to assist young scholars—criticized by some in this survey as nonexistent—were praised by others. "The NCI program to support the transition from postdoctoral positions to faculty positions is excellent. It should be supported and extended to other NIH institutes," wrote one respondent. Many other respondents stated that the quantity and quality of cancer research among minority and medically underserved populations would increase as the number of scientists from these groups increased, suggesting that training programs are viewed as a critical link to improving research.

Other respondents pointed to NCI's Leadership Initiatives—the National Black Leadership Initiative on Cancer, the National Hispanic Leadership Initiative on Cancer, and the Appalachian Leadership Initiative on Cancer—as very effective in addressing the cancer control and research needs of these populations. Finally, other respondents pointed to specific programs as having worked well to address the needs of special populations, including NCI-sponsored smoking cessation programs.

Recommendations

The respondents made recommendations in several general categories. These are summarized below. Representative comments related to each of the recommendations are presented in Appendix D.

1. Involve community members and community-based researchers as partners in the research process.

Many respondents felt strongly that community leaders and grassroots community health organizations offer invaluable expertise in assisting researchers who are planning community-based research. Community members are an underused resource who can assist in the design and implementation of research strategies, but only if they are involved as full partners in the process. NIH should encourage community collaboration, in the view of many respondents.

2. Improvements should be made in training and grant programs to increase the capacity for scientific research among minority and medically underserved populations.

Many respondents felt that the quality and quantity of proposals for health research among minority and medically underserved populations will improve only when the numbers of minority scientists are increased. Although most respondents praised NIH's minority scientist training programs, many urged greater attention to the needs of minority scientists at early career stages (i.e., at the postdoctoral and junior faculty stages of their careers). Others advocated for more outreach efforts to inform minority scientists of research funding opportunities and mentoring for successful grant competition.

3. Scientists from minority and medically underserved communities should be involved in the NIH priority-setting process and in staffing of NIH positions.

Several respondents pointed to a lack of cultural sensitivity and awareness of the needs of ethnic minority and medically underserved communities on the part of NIH scientific review groups and staff as a key impediment to increasing the number of programs targeted to these populations and funding research targeted to these populations.

4. Involve community members and community-based researchers as partners in research priority-setting.

As in Recommendation 1 above, some respondents felt that the knowledge of community leaders and grassroots health advocates could be better used by NIH if these individuals were consulted in the research priority-setting process. Community members' knowledge of the health problems, resources, and needs of their communities would not only help to better inform NIH of the most pressing issues faced by minority and medically underserved communities, but such consultation and involvement in the priority-setting process would foster greater collaboration and community participation in research.

5. Research issues for minority and underserved populations must be integrated into a national cancer research agenda.

Some respondents questioned whether research on minority and medically underserved populations was a significant component of a national cancer plan. These respondents stressed that research among minority and medically underserved populations should not be an "afterthought" or compartmentalized within limited areas of NIH's research portfolio but should be integrated into areas of key focus.

6. Define special populations research more adequately.

Several respondents were critical of how "special populations" are defined at NIH, arguing that a better assessment of "underserved" groups is needed. Some argued that use of the term *minority* is pejorative and should be replaced in favor of terminology that more accurately describes cancer risk.

7. Involve institutions serving ethnic minority and medically underserved communities in cancer research.

Several respondents argued that institutes serving minority and medically underserved communities, such as HBCUs and institutions that serve the Hispanic populations, have the greatest ability to perform culturally appropriate research with minority and medically underserved populations. In addition, these institutions would have greater access to minority and medically underserved study populations and have greater opportunities to train ethnic minority scientists and researchers. Respondents urged NIH to make greater investments in these opportunities.

WHAT ARE THE NEEDS OF CANCER SURVIVORS IN ETHNIC MINORITY AND MEDICALLY UNDERSERVED COMMUNITIES?

To understand the needs of cancer survivors in ethnic minority and medically underserved communities, the committee received testimony from representatives of several community-based cancer prevention and health promotion organizations, as well as testimony from an individual at an academic center who has spearheaded several community-based health efforts, primarily in low-income, rural communities. These individuals were asked to comment on how well the NIH research results are communicated and applied to cancer treatment and prevention programs for minority and medically underserved communities.

Many of these individuals spoke from personal experiences as cancer survivors who sought information for themselves and their communities and who would address the specific needs that they faced. Zora Kramer Brown is founder and chair of the Breast Cancer Resource Committee, which addresses the prevention and treatment needs of African American women at risk of or living with breast cancer. The organization plans future initiatives to address cancer among African American men. Venus Gines is a 6-year survivor of breast cancer, a community activist from Atlanta, Georgia, and a member of the NCI Director's Consumer Liaison Group. Lucy Young is a 10-year survivor of breast cancer. After recovery, she founded the Chinese American Cancer Association (CACA) in Flushing, New York, to support and meet the needs of immigrant cancer patients, especially those with language difficulties.

Finally, Barbara Clinton, director of the Center for Health Services at Vanderbilt University, spoke from the perspective of her 17 years of work with community-based health initiatives in Tennessee, Kentucky, Virginia, West Virginia, Florida, Louisiana, and Arkansas. Much of her work involves mobilization and linkage of community resources to address health needs, including the promotion of lay health advisers, the provision of technical assistance to communities, and other efforts to assist low-income and medically underserved populations. Two other individuals with expertise in the survivorship needs of ethnic minority and medically underserved communities, James Williams (executive director of US-TOO, International, an organization focused on the needs of prostate cancer survivors) and Yvette Joseph Fox (executive director of the National Indian Health Board), were invited to discuss their perspectives and work with the committee but were unable to attend.

Zora Kramer Brown noted that African Americans have a greater vulnerability to cancer than the general population. African Americans contract cancer at earlier ages than the majority population and suffer from higher cancer mortality rates. Data are needed, she stated, to understand why these disparities exist: "Is it genetically based? Is it environmentally based? Is it dietarily based? Is it the result of cultural values or belief systems, or is it economically based?" she asked.

Brown stated that "by and large, the National Institutes of Health and other federal agencies have been most supportive of these [community and advocacy] groups. The Breast Cancer Resource Committee, in fact, has enjoyed a productive collaboration with NIH regarding breast cancer education and survival issues among African-American women . . . [F]ederal agencies, generally, have been particularly supportive in helping to communicate research data to minority communities, in supporting education and early detection in underserved populations, and in addressing to some extent other overall survival needs of cancer victims."

She added, however, that NIH must improve its record with regard to the accrual of minority populations in clinical trials, in establishing collaborations between comprehensive cancer centers and historically black medical schools, and in increasing the participation of minorities in cancer review panels (see below).

Venus Gines noted that in the Latino culture, feelings of fatalism regarding cancer are high: cancer is viewed as a "death sentence." This fatalism prompted Gines to seek more information regarding her breast cancer diagnosis of 6 years ago. She found very little information in Spanish, her native language. Much of the information was merely translated from English and contained little information about cancer in Latinos. "In order for me to get the important data that are necessary for scientists to find out about Latinos and breast cancer, we need people who are of the culture who can help."

Gines developed Mi Nueva Esperanza (My New Hope), which provides education regarding breast cancer to Latina women in the form of a picture book with writing in clear, simple Spanish. More than 3,000 copies have been distributed nationwide, including in migrant worker camps. This effort was supported in collaboration with the American Cancer Society.

Gines also organized a health fair in the Atlanta, Georgia, area, in collaboration with Hispanic community organizations. This health fair offered clinical breast examinations and mobile units to provide mammograms and Pap smears. Child care was provided, and other barriers to participation were addressed.

Lucy Young founded CACA after finding little information in her native language as she battled breast cancer. In addition to helping Chinese-American cancer survivors to develop support networks, the group sponsors educational fora and develops and translates educational materials. CACA also offers free home care and free transportation services to low-income cancer patients. CACA was the first of the 3,500 local units sponsored by the American Cancer Society to focus on the needs of Asian American populations.

"Through my experience, I realized one thing," she stated, "that in suffering, one can sometimes discover one's life potential, as well as how to develop it. Ten years ago when I learned I had breast cancer, I asked God, 'Why? Why me? Why now?' But today, I know the answer."

Barbara Clinton has worked to develop and support community-based health initiatives ranging from maternal and infant health promotion to cancer prevention and screening. She has been extensively involved in the development of models in which lay health advisers are used for health intervention purposes. Much of this work takes place in rural communities in Appalachia. Clinton noted the link between cancer and environmental carcinogens, noting that "the South is the nation's biggest hazardous waste dump," especially in low-income communities in the South. She also addressed the need for greater provision of information from NIH to managed care organization, and for research on the use of lay health advisers.

The panel highlighted several themes and recommendations, as summarized below.

1. Inclusion of minorities in clinical trial research must be a high priority at NIH.

Zora Kramer Brown provided an example of how a lack of inclusion of minority women in breast cancer screening trials led to recommendations from an NIH Consensus Panel that may be appropriate for many women but not minority women. The Panel concluded that evidence was lacking to recommend breast cancer screening among women ages 40 to 49, but Brown stated that these data ignored the fact that the greatest increase in breast cancer is among African American women under the age of 40. The Panel's recommendation was later reversed, but the initial recommendation was based on studies from Sweden, Canada, and England that did not include African-American women.

"We have not done a good job of convincing the African-American community that clinical trial research actually does benefit them," said Brown. "And in order to do that there has to be education that is coupled with it. And I do believe that education is research." Brown added that minority patients and their providers need to better understand how to gain access to clinical trials.

Brown draws a distinction between poverty, illiteracy, and cultural beliefs. Poverty and illiteracy may pose barriers to clinical trial accrual, but these are not cultural factors, she indicated. NIH needs to attend to poverty and illiteracy, but it should not ignore cultural factors that may pose barriers to accrual in clinical trials.

2. Collaboration between comprehensive medical centers and historically black medical schools should be fostered.

Most clinical research is conducted in large research hospitals that do not serve African Americans, according to Brown. African Americans do, however, frequent hospitals associated with historically black colleges and medical schools. This limits NIH's ability to access black populations and incorporate findings from African-American researchers and institutions. "A teaming of representatives from our majority comprehensive medical centers with representatives from our HBCU institutions and facilities has the potential to greatly advance our understanding of cancer incidence and mortality among African Americans," she stated.

Brown pointed to the success of National Human Genome Research Institute-Howard University collaboration on genetically based risk among African Americans as an example of such a collaboration.

3. Greater participation of minorities in cancer review panels is needed.

Brown noted that NCI has simple nondiscrimination provisions in its requirements for the selection of cancer review panels. The U.S. Department of Defense, in contrast, actively recruits minorities for scientific review panels, with minority population representation on some panels being up to one-third or more of the total. Inclusion of minorities on panels can increase NIH's sensitivity to proposals from scientists, particularly minority scientists, who study minority populations, she noted.

4. The portfolio of "special populations" research at NIH must adequately address the range of possible etiologic factors for cancer among racial and ethnic groups.

Brown criticized the NIH portfolio of research on cancer etiology among racial and ethnic groups as too narrow and failing to examine possible biological or genetic differences. "The argument that the results of basic research can be extrapolated to all populations simply does not apply," she stated. "In fact, it is entirely inconceivable that the results of studies [with] African Americans, upon expanded scrutiny, might be legitimately extrapolated to one or more other ethnic groups."

"I have a concern that, in the absence of definitive results from other factors," she continued, "the standard explanation for cancer discrepancies in African Americans might become too comfortably and conveniently couched in terms of culture and economics. . . . [W]e owe it to the African-American population and to the nation to either rule out or to identify definitively the other factors to which I have alluded."

5. NIH staff must reflect the diversity of the U.S. population.

Brown stated that staff at NIH need to include minorities so that staff are representative of the populations that they study.

6. NIH must improve educational and outreach efforts to minority communities.

Venus Gines criticized NIH outreach efforts as inadequate. "I think what we need is more visibility of NCI people," she stated, "because in Atlanta, for instance, you mention NCI, nobody knows the National Cancer Institute [in] our community. They're up there in an ivory tower maybe, but they really don't know what the National Cancer Institute does. They hear [of] the American Cancer Society because of all the [information about] Relay for Life, and all this has been in the news. But NCI needs to be a little more visible in the communities, I think, for one thing."

Zora Kramer Brown added that health providers in minority communities are often overburdened. She also stated that NIH needs to be sensitive to the special circumstances and outreach needs faced by health providers and health educators in these communities.

Barbara Clinton stated that issues of understanding and addressing a diagnosis of cancer for many ethnic minority and medically underserved individuals are complex and require the patient to negotiate culturally and institutionally imposed barriers to the retrieval of information. Information should therefore be tailored to these needs, she indicated.

7. Greater sensitivity to culturally appropriate outreach efforts is needed.

Venus Gines noted that cancer prevention and control messages must be tailored to ethnic minority communities, a task that is often more complicated than it appears. "We should try to stay away from just straight translating from English to Spanish. We need to really focus on the culture, and I think that's very important."

Both Venus Gines and Lucy Young also noted the need for cancer prevention and outreach messages to address potential cancer stigma and "taboo" issues among minority communities. In the absence of having cancer survivors from these communities as visible role models, they stated, many ethnic minorities with cancer may not want to be publicly identified. Young added that many Chinese Americans living with cancer may not want others in the community to know of their condition.

8. Follow-up services should be made available for individuals after cancer screening.

The need to provide follow-up services, especially for ethnic minority patients for whom late diagnosis is a problem, is very important. Venus Gines described her frustration in trying to find appropriate follow-up services for women screened at the Atlanta community health fair with abnormal Pap smear results.

9. A strategic plan to address the survivorship needs of ethnic minority communities should be developed.

Lucy Young recommended that NCI form a diversity team to develop ongoing task force committees to develop strategic plans for different ethnic groups. "These committees should collect and gather information on cancer-related grassroots organizations to identify their needs," Young said. "Then, submit a proposal of suggestions to NIH or NCI to better serve the different ethnic groups." Population groups such as "Asians" should not be lumped together, because Chinese, Korean, Japanese, and other groups are culturally different.

10. Community-based groups need assistance in grant writing to be competitive for NIH grants.

Lucy Young, Barbara Clinton, and others agreed that community-based organizations with innovative cancer control or research proposals should be encouraged to submit proposals but that they often lack the time, resources, or skills to do so. NIH should provide technical assistance to these groups to improve their ability to compete for grants.

11. Environmental risk factors disproportionately affect ethnic minority and medically underserved groups, and therefore should be prominent in the NIH portfolio.

"At the community level, cancer prevention is inextricably linked to environmental degradation," noted Barbara Clinton. Scientists should move "beyond the notion that personal health behavior alone explains the increased mortality in low-income populations." NCI should "investigate the relationship between environmental exposures that occur early in life and the development of adult diseases as well as transgenerational effects that occur in the child of the person who was exposed to the environmental toxin."

Clinton also recommended that NIH "support leadership exchanges between staff of the NCI and national and local environmental organizations." Finally, she noted, cancer control research should support existing community-based efforts to address environmental issues.

12. NCI should expand investigations of lay community health workers, who may be especially effective in addressing the needs of cancer survivors in minority and medically underserved communities.

Lay community health workers, according to Barbara Clinton, provide locally tailored and culturally sensitive information to patients on subjects that are confusing and sometimes taboo. "These workers help people access available resources in cost-effective ways," she noted. NCI should also expand research on health navigators, who help patients understand treatment options, providers, and other choices. Research questions should investigate how and under what conditions these providers work best.

13. NCI should provide information to managed care organizations

to provide them with up-to-date information regarding best practice outcomes and cost data.

Clinton noted that "HMO [health maintenance organization] decision guidelines often deny payment for any treatment that is not approved by the FDA [Food and Drug Administration] on the grounds that the treatment is experimental, even though trial treatment may be a better and even more cost effective option for the patient." HMO coverage of clinical trial treatment may improve the accrual of minority patients.

MECHANISMS FOR ETHNIC MINORITY COMMUNITY AND RESEARCHER INPUT INTO THE CANCER AGENDA

The perceptions and experiences of community representatives and grassroots leaders, as well as those of researchers interested in cancer among minority and medically underserved groups, are important in helping to provide an understanding of NCI's mechanisms for the involvement of these constituencies in research priority setting. NCI's response to minority community and researcher input is led by the recently established Director's Consumer Liaison Group (DCLG) and the Office of Special Populations Research (OSPR). At the NIH level, the effort is led by the Office of Research on Minority Health (ORMH).

Office of Research on Minority Health, NIH

As noted in Chapter 3, ORMH, established by the director of NIH in 1990, was authorized by the U.S. Congress in 1993 (P.L. 103-43). Its mission is to improve the health status of minority Americans through biomedical research and to expand the participation of minorities in all aspects of biomedical and behavioral research. Part of its responsibilities includes an ongoing consultative process with outside organizations, a process that ORMH initiated in 1991 with the establishment of a 53-member fact-finding team. More recently, Congress has mandated that an Advisory Committee on Research on Minority Health be established to advise ORMH and NIH (this Advisory Committee is described in Chapter 3). ORMH reports that of the 9 members currently impaneled on the Advisory Committee, 6 are ethnic minorities (12 members are ultimately expected to be appointed).

Prior to passage of the congressional mandate for the establishment of an ORMH advisory panel, however, ORMH's research priority-setting processes appeared to be based largely on the research agendas of collaborating NIH institutes and centers (ICs) and the views of an ad hoc review panel, as noted in Chapter 3. Although a broad framework of 13 minority health research priorities was established by the advisory fact-finding team and was published in 1992 (National Institutes of Health, Office of Research on Minority Health, 1992), and six "priority areas" for funding minority health and training initiatives were established on the basis of "continuing consultation with the minority community and experts within the ICs" (Ruffin, 1996), criteria for the prioritization and funding of research on specific diseases such as cancer are not explicit. Further, it is apparent that ORMH and its newly established advisory body will be able to more effectively leverage NCI's resources to support minority cancer research programs if its NCI analogue, OSPR, is afforded greater authority and responsibility in establishing and implementing a minority cancer research agenda, as will be discussed below.

Office of Special Populations Research, NCI

OSPR grew out of a report of an NCI Special Action Committee, an internal group of program, planning, and management staff from all NCI divisions formed to ensure that the cancer research needs of special populations were being adequately addressed (National Cancer Institute, 1996a). Reports were presented in 1990, 1992, 1994, and 1996, with the last report recommending the abolishment of the committee and the establishment of a focal point within NCI's Office of Program Operations and Planning to provide leadership and to coordinate activities addressing the cancer research needs of special populations, including a multiethnic advisory committee made up of NCI staff that would replace the Special Action Committee. OSPR is also establishing an external liaison committee consisting of scientists, medical professionals, civil rights advocates, and others involved in minority health issues (O. Brawley, National Cancer Institute, personal communication, May 29, 1998). OSPR also collaborates with ORMH to establish research priorities, but OSPR lacks the appropriate funding mechanisms or program authority to exert influence over research priorities at NCI. OSPR and its advisory body therefore provides guidance within NCI, but without program funding or authority, it is relatively powerless in working with ORMH or acting independently to effect meaningful changes in the research agenda at NCI.

Director's Consumer Liaison Group, NCI

In 1997, the NCI director established DCLG to provide advice and make recommendations to the Advisory Committee to the Director of NCI. (The Advisory Committee is chaired by the NCI director and includes the chair of the National Cancer Advisory Board and the chairs and cochairs of the NCI Board of Scientific Counselors and Board of Scientific Advisors.) NCI's Office of Liaison Activities (OLA) coordinates and supports the activities of DCLG. OLA's goals are to create and maintain ongoing communications and information exchange between the national cancer advocacy organizations and NCI and to cooperate and collaborate with these groups in areas of mutual interest (National Cancer Institute, 1998f).

The purposes of DCLG are (1) to help develop and establish processes, mechanisms, and criteria for identifying appropriate consumer advocates to serve on a variety of program and policy advisory committees responsible for advancing the mission of NCI; (2) to serve as a primary forum for discussing issues and concerns and exchanging viewpoints that are important to the broad development of NCI programmatic and research priorities; and (3) to establish and maintain strong collaborations between NCI and the cancer advocacy community to reach common goals (National Cancer Institute, 1998f). DCLG is also described in greater detail in Chapter 5.

The Planning Group that led to the implementation of DCLG specifically addressed the means of achieving appropriate diversity within DCLG and wanted to ensure multicultural representation among DCLG's 15 members, along with other important characteristics among its members, such as individuals of both genders and of various ages, individuals with cancer at different sites, and individuals from various types of organizations. The Planning Group would have stipulated that at least one-third of DCLG members belong to a racial and ethnic minority but was precluded from doing so by a federal law prohibiting the selection of individuals on the basis of race. Thus, the Planning Group's final recommendation was that DCLG's membership: (1) be culturally diverse, (2) include individuals with cancer at different sites, (3) include medically underserved individuals, (4) include men and women, (5) include individuals from a range of organizations (local, regional, and national), (6) include individuals of various ages, and (7) include individuals from diverse geographic locations (including individuals from rural and urban areas). The initial DCLG includes African-American, Asian-American/Pacific Islander, Hispanic, Native American, and non-Hispanic white members (National Cancer Institute, 1998f).

One of the express purposes of DCLG was "to help NCI *widen the pool* of qualified consumer advocates who can be called upon to serve on NCI advisory committees and other groups" (emphasis added; National Cancer Institute, 1998f). Thus, at least the stage is set for participation of a more diverse and expansive array of minority community representatives in NCI's policy-making and priority-setting processes.

Other NCI Advisory Panels

No strategy for increasing the pool of qualified minority scientists to serve on NCI's advisory committees and other groups comparable to that established for consumers through DCLG currently exists. NCI's senior management turns to seven different advisory groups for advice and counsel: (1) the President's Cancer Panel, (2) the National Cancer Advisory Board, (3) the Board of Scientific Counselors, (4) the Board of Scientific Advisors, (5) the Intramural Advisory Board, (6) the Extramural Advisory Board, and (7) the DCLG. Currently, 19 percent (21 of 113) of the people serving on these groups are members of minority groups—9 Asian Americans/Pacific Islanders, 7 African Americans, 4 Hispanics, and 1 American Indian/Alaska Native—whereas that proportion was 14 percent (19 of 134) in 1992. There is wide variability, however, in ethnic minority representation among the various advisory groups. More than one-third (35 percent) of the National Cancer Advisory Board members (6 of 17) were ethnic minorities as of December 1997, yet among NCI's two most powerful advisory bodies, the Board of Scientific Advisors and the Board of Scientific Counselors, only 11 percent (3 of 26) and 17 percent (7 of 42) are ethnic minorities, respectively. NCI reports that consumers are represented on the majority of NCI advisory panels, but the numbers of these individuals on each panel were not specified.

It therefore appears that significant representation on advisory panels by members of ethnic minorities takes place primarily when NCI embraces a conscious plan for diversity: witness the original intent of the Planning Group for DCLG to have one third of its 15 members be ethnic minorities and the final makeup of the group, which includes representatives from five different minority groups.

Concern regarding ethnic minority representation on NCI advisory panels was also salient in the input to the committee from ethnic minority researchers in the field of cancer research, as well as from minority and nonminority investigators interested in cancer among minority and medically underserved populations. As indicated above, opinions about the ways of increasing the level of representation included (1) increased participation by researchers from minority and medically underserved communities in goal setting and identification of priority areas pertaining to minorities, (2) appointment of more minority investigators and administrators to key advisory committees and review committees or study sections, and (3) development of an advisory board to address the research needs of minority and medically underserved communities. Thus, a comparable strategy for widening the pool of minority investigators (and administrators) who serve on policy-making and priority-setting groups within NCI, as has been developed for consumers through DCLG, is an apparent need.

Recommendation 4-1: NCI should develop a process to increase the representation of ethnically diverse researchers and public rep-

resentatives serving on all advisory and program review committees so that the makeup of these committees reflects the changing diversity of the U.S. population. NCI should develop an evaluation plan to assess the effect of increased and more diversified ethnic minority community and researcher input on changes in NCI policies and priorities toward ethnic minority cancer issues.

Such increased and more widely based minority community and researcher input is not the desired end result but is one of many means of marshaling the considerable resources of NCI in reducing the burden of cancer among minorities and medically underserved individuals in terms of fewer deaths, fewer new cases, increased lengths of survival, and increased quality of life among cancer survivors. Such input at least ensures that ethnic minority and medically underserved populations will have a (substantial) voice at all levels of discussion in NCI's agenda. The committee believes that the impact of such a policy shift should be assessed to determine whether it will ultimately have a significant effect on NCI's policies and priorities.

Recommendation 4-2: The research needs of ethnic minority and medically underserved groups should be identified on the basis of the burden of cancer in these populations, with an assessment of the most appropriate areas of research (i.e., behavioral and social sciences, biology, epidemiology and genetics, prevention and control, treatment, etc.).

Another aspect of the potential influence of minority community and researcher input into NCI is the environment within which such input operates. NIH and NCI operate within a primary milieu of "greatest scientific opportunity." In the words of NCI's director: "The NCI's cancer research funding strategy is to assure that there is sufficient funding to enable scientists to pursue those research areas with the greatest scientific opportunity—that is, the greatest opportunity to increase our knowledge of cancer" (National Cancer Institute, 1998d, p. 26).

However, the director also acknowledges that "a second critical factor that guides program direction, in addition to scientific opportunity, is the burden of specific cancers" (National Cancer Institute, 1998d, p. 26). This "second critical factor" is essential for addressing the cancer problems of minority and medically underserved populations because NCI has acknowledged that "while we have seen a decline in overall cancer prevalence and mortality rates in the last five years, the decline did not occur in all American populations. Overall rates do reflect a story of success based on statistical averages, but when we examine specific ethnic and racial groups, and those in underserved situations, we find that declines in cancer incidence and death have not occurred for all populations" (National Cancer Institute, 1998b, p. 1).

Acknowledgment of the role of "burden of disease" in guiding NCI program direction and the acknowledgment that declines in cancer incidence and death have not occurred for many minorities are significant in view of a recommendation of the NCI Special Action Committee's 1996 report, which led to the creation of OSPR. In that report, the committee also recommended that "the NCI research portfolio needs to be [data driven and] reviewed with a focus on the cancers noted as significant in the minority cancer statistics monograph. Cancers that disproportionately affect special populations should be carefully examined to identify research opportunities. . . . [T]he results of such a review should be discussed in the broader context of NCI's mission under the auspices of the National Cancer Advisory Board and the Boards of Scientific Advisors/Counselors" (National Cancer Institute, 1996a, p. 11). The committee concurs with this recommendation, as will be discussed below in greater detail in a review of NCI and NIH mechanisms for research priority setting.

Recommendation 4-3: For NCI to address the needs of ethnically diverse and medically underserved populations effectively, the Office of Special Populations Research (or some other designated entity or entities) must possess the authority to coordinate and leverage programs and resources across the divisions and branches of NCI to stimulate research on ethnic minority and medically underserved populations. This authority can be established by providing such an office with:

- **a leadership role in major NCI-wide priority-setting bodies and**
- **special resources to fund programs specifically targeted to these populations, or**
- **accountability for the institution-wide allocation of program resources.**

SPECIAL POPULATIONS AND PRIORITY SETTING AT NCI

The evaluation of priority setting for research on cancer among special populations must be undertaken against the backdrop of three basic considerations. First, the fundamental missions of NCI and NIH frame the larger public policy context within which issues such as the types of research and levels of funding commitment for special populations should be judged. Second, a clear and persuasive rationale for any special research focus on specific subpopulations must be articulated, and the efforts to address the needs of special populations should conform to that rationale. Third, the criteria and procedures used to set research priorities for the general population must be examined with an eye to their adequacy to priority setting for special populations. This section discusses these three issues.

Mission

The mission statement of NIH states that its primary aim is research designed "to uncover new knowledge that will lead to better health for everyone." The mission statement of NCI embodies similar institutional goals tailored to its specific disease focus. The ultimate aim of NCI, according to a 1998 NCI report, *Priority Setting at the National Cancer Institute* (National Cancer Institute, 1998g) is "to prevent or cure cancer." Given the quite general language of the NIH and NCI mandates, a wide array of policy options and research priorities is compatible with fulfillment of their missions. Accordingly, the NCI report emphasizes that priority setting is necessary "because there are more mission-related things that could and should be done than there are resources available to do them" (National Cancer Institute, 1998g, p. 7).

A three-pronged approach is outlined in NCI's fiscal year 1999 bypass budget:

1. Sustain at full measure the proven research programs that have enabled NCI to come this far.
2. Seize extraordinary opportunities to further progress made possible by previous research discoveries.
3. Create and sustain mechanisms that will enable NCI to rapidly translate findings from the laboratory to practical applications that will benefit everyone.

NCI's approach reveals three especially noteworthy principles relevant to this committee's charge. As indicated in more detail below, these principles themselves offer no definitive guide to priority setting, but they do point the way toward reducing some common misunderstandings that sometimes color the public debates about the relation between NCI's mission and its choice among the many policy options in service of its mission.

First, the central aim of NIH and its institutes, including NCI, is the production of new knowledge about the causes, prevention, and cure of cancer. Both NCI and NIH emphasized the acute need to focus on the production of knowledge that might not otherwise be generated without the support of public agencies. This rationale is often articulated as the basis of a preponderance of emphasis on funding basic research that would not find sufficient support in the marketplace when no immediate financial rewards are expected. However, this principle has particular importance for setting research priorities for special populations as well.

For example, if knowledge about the etiology of cancer among low-income populations with greater than average exposures to suspected environmental contributors to an increased cancer incidence or increased mortality from cancer is known but studies are unlikely to be conducted within the private sector, then there is at least an initial rationale for giving research of this type the same careful consideration in the priority-setting process as other research that lacks commercial incentives. Indeed, not only may such research lack commercial incentives but there may also be commercial disincentives such that without sufficient commitment by public agencies, many scientific opportunities to learn about the fundamental causes and etiology of cancer may be missed.

Second, because the ultimate aim of publicly supported research is the improvement of the public's health, any and all types of research—whether it falls within traditional contrasting categories, such as basic or applied research, behavioral or molecular research, or fundamental or translational research—are appropriate candidates for consideration in the priority-setting process. From the perspective of a purely public health approach (again, this is not included as the general perspective that NCI should adopt), all types of research that may ultimately contribute to improved health outcomes are consistent with NCI's mission. In addition, if scientific opportunities in those areas are identified, fulfillment of NCI's mission dictates their careful consideration.

If, for example, as Richard Klausner, the director of NCI, has testified, more than 50 percent of the burden of cancer is due to behavioral and lifestyle factors; and if these differences frequently appear to be positively associated with differences in socioeconomic, educational, cultural, or other discernible characteristics of identifiable subpopulations, then their consideration within the priority-setting process is warranted. Moreover, if some portion of the increased burden of cancer appears to be attributable to the failure of some subpopulations to adopt proven behavioral modifications that would reduce their cancer burden, then research into effective mechanisms of communication is itself a scientific opportunity that merits thoughtful consideration within the priority-setting process.

Third, as the language of NCI and NIH mandates make clear, the obligations of the public agencies extend to all segments of the public. In the language of the NCI mandate, the aim is to develop "practical applications that will benefit everyone." A consequence of this commitment is an institutional obligation to monitor and revise the research portfolio on an ongoing basis with an eye to those populations whose health needs are underserved, especially when the differential health burden is attributable, at least in part, to a differential in the advancement of scientific knowledge regarding the causes and prevention of cancer among those subpopulations.

Alternative interpretations of the responsibilities and obligations of publicly supported research agencies exist, however. A narrowly construed focus on public health would dictate priority setting such that the aggregate public health is maximized, even if such policies do not allow some subpopulations to receive the expected benefits of such research. However, the committee rejects this interpretation of NCI's mission for several reasons. First, it is contrary to the plain language of NCI's own mission statement and incompatible with its institutional history and long-standing commitment to using data regarding differential health burdens as one factor among others pertinent to the priority-setting process.

Second, such an interpretation is incongruous with recent expressions of congressional policy with respect to the NIH priority-setting process. For example, the NIH Revitalization Act of 1993 (P.L. 103-43) mandated that women and minorities and their subpopulations be included in all human subject research, and federal regulations implementing this mandate for all NIH-supported research became effective in September 1994. The rationale for greater inclusion in clinical trials is the aspiration that "the manner in which scientific knowledge is acquired be generalizable to the entire population of the United States" (National Institutes of Health, 1994).

Rationale for Focus on Subpopulations

A proponent of crosscutting research as the sole means of addressing the needs of special populations might reject the use of targeted or special population-based approaches on the basis of the assumption that all issues of fairness and comprehensiveness of research policy can be accommodated by a combination of research strategies that are expected to yield information about causes and treatment of cancer within the general population and compliance with existing mandates for inclusion of members of those populations within ongoing clinical studies. Thus, it might be argued that the goal of obtaining broad generalizable knowledge is best met by inclusionary crosscutting studies. However, the committee rejects the adequacy of this approach.

Behind the desire for research that yields broad generalizable scientific knowledge is the more fundamental aspiration to interrupt a chain of research policy decisions that can result in some segments of the overall population receiving demonstrably fewer of the fruits of publicly supported research than others. The crux of the rationale for modification of clinical research guidelines is articulated with great clarity in a 1993 Institute of Medicine (IOM) report discussing issues of inclusion of women in clinical trials (Institute of Medicine, 1993). The report expressed its concern that steps be taken to avoid situations in which subpopulations bear differential health burdens as a partial consequence of disparities in clinical benefit, which are in turn due to disparities in scientific research applicable to conditions affecting them. Although the IOM report did not attempt to resolve the issue of whether or how much of the differential health burden experienced by women could be attributable to exclusionary policies toward women in research, the IOM committee that wrote the report opposed institutional policies that magnify the potential for leaving subpopulations systematically disfavored. In addition to inclusionary policies, the IOM report on the inclusion of women in federally funded research made clear that its underlying rationale supported the consideration of additional, targeted research into conditions that uniquely or differentially affect women.

The present IOM committee endorses the reasoning of the earlier IOM committee and finds that it is applicable to the need for vigilance in identifying and responding to the cancer burden disparities experienced by subpopulations as a fundamental requirement of fairness in the administration of publicly supported programs meant to benefit all segments of U.S. society. The message of the earlier report is one that the present committee reiterates: NIH should be on the lookout for differential health burdens among subpopulations, and when there are scientific opportunities to study the causes of such differential burdens or to reduce their magnitude, such research focused on these subpopulations is a legitimate option for consideration by a publicly accountable agency. In instances in which the differential health burdens are considerable, such options should be given the highest level of consideration within the NCI priority-setting process.

One important difference between the rationale for targeted research among women and the rationale for targeted research among groups defined as special populations in this report should be emphasized. That is, an additional rationale offered as partial support for targeted research among women is the assumption that some diseases are physiologically, hormonally, or genetically mediated by biologically based gender differences. As stated in Chapter 2, however, the committee rejects the view of race as a biologically based concept. Thus, no part of the committee's support for the appropriateness of cancer research targeted to subpopulations rests upon assumptions about the basis of group differences in disease expression similar to those for research targeted to women. Indeed, no analogous biologically based assumption is necessary. As documented in Chapter 2, the existence of differences in the occurrence of disease among subpopulations may be attributable to numerous causes including environmental exposures, and cultural and behavioral differences, among other factors. Instead, the reasons for such differences are open research questions rather than guiding assumptions meant to support targeted research.

Criteria and Priority-Setting Procedures

Thus far, the committee has argued that the statements of mission of NIH and NCI support and in some instances necessitate an important role for consideration of differential health status among subpopulations in the priority-setting process. Moreover, the committee has articulated a more fundamental rationale for the need for special vigilance and attention to the needs of those subpopulations. This rationale rejects the adequacy of approaches that merely seek to address the needs of those subpopulations in the routine portfolio of research initiatives in favor of supplementary strategies that focus directly on subpopulations. This section considers further whether the criteria and procedures used for priority setting are generally compatible with and sufficient for priority setting for the study of cancer among special populations.

The most detailed official discussion of criteria for priority setting used across the 21 institutes that make up NIH are elaborated in its recent pamphlet, *Setting Research Priorities at the National Institutes of Health* (National Institutes of Health, 1997). In defending what might be called an organic view of scientific discovery, the document states that "science is by nature structured and self-correcting" and that "science itself sets its own priorities" (p. 6). NIH thereby rejects the view that the growth of scientific knowledge can be managed with precision through the use of some top-down planning model or that any simple algorithm can be used to rank those areas of inquiry most requiring funding. Many factors must be taken into account in the priority-setting process, according to the NIH pamphlet; chief among them are the public health needs of the nation and the scientific opportunities or most promising avenues of research available given the state of scientific knowledge developed thus far. Thus, the ultimate choice of which among the many avenues should be explored is a complex one requiring a global appreciation of the current status of scientific research across all major areas of inquiry, the most promising theoretical approaches with crosscutting potential, and an awareness of the many conditions that impose large health burdens in the form of premature mortality, excess morbidity, loss or restriction of functioning, and pain.

The priority-setting policy of NCI (National Cancer Institute, 1998g) tracks that of NIH, often relying on language identical to that used in the

NIH pamphlet. NCI maintains that the decision as to what to study rests primarily on two guiding principles:

1. Scientific opportunity. What research areas and projects have the greatest potential to expand knowledge? The answer to this question comes primarily from the scientists themselves, working in hundreds of academic, medical, public, and private research institutions around the country.

2. The burden of cancer. Research funding is likewise guided by the degree to which specific cancers affect Americans. For example, lung and colon cancer, which account for high numbers of cancer deaths each year, are among NCI's priorities.

Although both the NCI and the NIH statements reject any simple algorithm for priority setting, both place great weight on the need for priority setting to be driven largely by scientific opportunities. The aim is to generate new knowledge along a broad frontier, and an underlying assumption behind the desire for a broad and diverse portfolio is the claim that the growth of scientific knowledge is unpredictable. Thus, the ability of science policy experts to develop a systematic plan is inevitably limited and is subject to frequent revision. Incorporating language borrowed from the NIH pamphlet (National Institutes of Health, 1997, p. 6), NCI argues that "the precision with which investigators and administrators describe the targets and outcomes of research . . . cannot alter the inescapable truth that many of the results of research are unpredictable . . .Thus, science has the ability to refresh its own priorities in order to seek opportunities that are ripe for pursuit and capture" (National Cancer Institute, 1998g, p. 7).

A cautionary observation contained in the NIH pamphlet points to the difficulty of relying too heavily on disease burden. One worry is that there are many incompatible but equally relevant ways of measuring disease burden. They include the number of people with the disease, the number of deaths caused by a disease, the economic and social costs of a disease, the number of premature deaths caused by a disease, or the extent of pain, disability, or suffering caused by a disease. No single agreed-upon measure of disease burden exists, nor should one exist when research priorities are being set. All measures of disease burden have some moral claim, and the adoption of none is plausible if it means the exclusion of the others.

Moreover, a recent IOM report on research priority setting at NIH cautions against using cost data as a proxy for ranking funding decisions (Institute of Medicine, 1998). The fact that funding for research on one disease is several times greater than funding for research on another disease on a per capita or per death basis may seem to disease-specific advocates or their friends in the U.S. Congress to involve some unfairness or unjustifiable inequality. However, the disease receiving greater research funding may differ from the less richly funded disease receiving less research funding in a number of relevant aspects. One disease may be more painful and debilitating, may result in more premature deaths, or may be a communicable disease that threatens the community as a whole; or given the current state of scientific understanding about a particular disease, investments in research on that disease may offer greater prospects for cure or prevention than a similar investment is likely to yield if it were devoted to research on another disease. Thus, such disparities in health outcomes, whether they track groups defined by disease or other criteria (e.g., ethnicity, geography, or occupation), provide the initial reasons for greater attentiveness to issues of health differentials within the research priority-setting process. Such differences alone, however, do not provide decisive reasons for altering funding priorities.

The inherent difficulties of assessing the relative health needs and the ineffectiveness of setting priorities on the basis of any of the available measures of disease burden tend to elevate the importance of scientific opportunities. Without an assessment of scientific opportunities, public funds are likely to be squandered with little or no demonstrable health benefits, and the obligation to pursue the well-being of the community as a whole will not be met. As a consequence of treating scientific opportunity as a necessary but not sufficient condition for according high priority to those areas in which advances are most likely, the primary emphasis of NCI and the other institutes within NIH is placed on individual investigator-initiated research proposals that are peer reviewed for scientific merit (National Institutes of Health, 1997).

The heavy emphasis on scientific opportunity has been endorsed by NCI Director Richard Klausner in his congressional testimony regarding priority setting at NCI. In addition, Klausner's testimony in hearings conducted by the present IOM committee further reflect a general preference for addressing the health needs of special populations through crosscutting research designed to lead to discoveries benefiting everyone. The value of the crosscutting approach is additionally supported by the claim of unpredictability in the growth of scientific knowledge. The pursuit of promising scientific leads in one area often reveals unexpected knowledge about the cause, prevention, or treatment of other medical conditions. Thus, the confidence in policies that concentrate efforts wherever the most promising leads emerge is reinforced by the reasonable expectation that approaches believed to yield the greatest anticipated gains in knowledge may be expected to yield the greatest serendipitous gains in knowledge.

Neither the importance of scientific opportunity nor the difficulties in assessing and weighing relative need, however, obviate the importance of taking account of differential health burdens in the priority-setting process. Nor does the expectation of serendipitous gains in knowledge undermine the justification for allocating some portion of the diversified research portfolio to the study of those conditions or populations differentially burdened by cancer. For several reasons, on the basis of considerations of both fairness and good science, such targeted approaches may be useful complements to the mainstream approach.

First, just as there are reasonable limits to the ability to plan science, there are similar limits to how much one can rely on the organic model of the growth of scientific knowledge. The maxim that "science is self-correcting" is true only within limits. Although parallel and subsequent inquiry can confirm, refute, or modify the state of knowledge gleaned from one avenue of inquiry, there is no guarantee that the organic growth of knowledge will be uniform and free of lumps and gaps. Indeed, the organic model assumes that its trajectory will be unpredictable, and just as its unpredictability can yield serendipitous benefits, it can also result in large gaps differentially affecting some portions of the population.

In fact, a substantial body of evidence in the history of science supports the claim that developments in scientific knowledge have been instigated and aided by exogenous forces that redirect scientists' attention toward the unexpected and away from the linear, highly focused approach that concentrates on well-defined problems with ready hypotheses to be tested. Thus, the fact that a large measure of unpredictability exists in science does not uniquely favor building exclusively on what is known but favors as well some attention to questions not readily answerable from within the conventional scientific consensus. For example, research devoted to a better understanding of medical conditions among those most burdened by a disease may yield insights into causes and prevention not readily obtainable through study of the overall population, and this in turn may yield a better understanding of the etiology and nature of disease in others as well. Such principles of focused, targeted research are mainstream operational assumptions guiding much of current genetic research, in which it is hypothesized that understanding of causal mechanisms in smaller populations at greater than average risk will lead to improved understanding of similar conditions in others who are not the direct focus of inquiry.

In short, if uncertainty is a persistent feature of the growth of scientific knowledge, then it would be unreasonable to sacrifice all targeted research for the sake of deliberate crosscutting research, and the serendipitous character of science ensures that pursuit of the most promising leads from the current baseline of knowledge in heavily studied areas can be expected to produce unanticipated gaps no less than unanticipated gains in knowledge. The prospect of the existence of such gaps in which substantial differential health burdens exist therefore warrants vigilant monitoring of differentials within subpopulations and attention to the need for research on the causes and mitigation of those differences as a supplement to the other parts of the research portfolio.

Moreover, a predictable consequence of the heavy reliance on researcher-initiated proposals is the increased likelihood that important questions regarding disease among those most heavily burdened will go unasked, especially if environmental and behavioral factors play an important mediating role and the incentives of the marketplace make their study less likely. Accordingly, various strategies designed to direct, motivate, and focus researcher imagination may be necessary as a supplement to the investigator-initiated approach if gaps in scientific knowledge contributing to differential health burdens are to be taken seriously.

Although NCI has provided the committee with many additional documents outlining its past and ongoing initiatives for special populations and its plans for the expansion of its Division of Cancer Control and Population Sciences, some unanswered questions remain. In oral testimony before the committee, Director Klausner emphasized the importance of crosscutting research and the fact that the differential cancer burdens experienced by some subpopulations will derive benefits from the knowledge gained from research on cancer generally. According to Klausner, much of the research not attributed to budgetary codes specific to research on cancer among special populations also produces secondary benefits for special populations, and thus, data regarding special initiatives alone fail to provide a full accounting of the level of NCI's commitment to meeting the health needs of those populations. The committee acknowledges the importance of these ancillary contributions that some critics may fail to appreciate.

However, the committee believes that Klausner's remarks emphasizing the secondary benefits derived from crosscutting research leave the status of NCI's commitment to special population research initiatives somewhat uncertain. In supplementary written testimony provided to the committee by Barbara Rimer in response to committee questioning (Rimer, communication with the study committee, 1998), NCI indicated that it intends to pursue both the traditional investigator-initiated approaches and RFAs targeted to special populations. In addition, Rimer shared budget proposals for future initiatives affecting many of the groups that NCI defines as special populations.

The committee applauds Rimer's statement of commitment to the continuation and expansion of such initiatives. However, important unresolved issues of both the process and the criteria used for priority setting for research among special populations remain. For example, the future role of the Director of Special Populations remains unclear. Klausner has indicated that he views the role of the Director of Special Populations as "the eyes and ears" on these matters. The committee believes that the director also needs to have a strong voice in priority-setting activities affecting special populations, as well as clear institutional guidance for identifying high-priority objectives for research on such populations.

Moreover, the Office of Special Populations Research currently lacks many of the institutional advantages that would ensure that an NCI commitment to research among special populations has a chance to be successful. It has no independent resources to fund a separate portfolio of initiatives for special populations research, has no clear criteria for recommending the priorities for such initiatives that are dependent upon the resources of other parts of NCI or means of guiding such initiatives, and holds no official position on any of the NCI advisory committees responsible for setting major intramural or extramural priorities.

In response to committee questions regarding the appropriateness of focusing research on special populations on the basis of burden of disease, Klausner indicated that the recommendations of the Special Action Committee on Minority/Special Populations did not represent current NCI policy. Although no specific recommendation of the Special Action Committee was repudiated in Klausner's testimony, the committee believes that many of the recommendations merit careful consideration. Among its useful recommendations were proposals to improve the input of staff and other persons knowledgeable about the needs of special populations, an acknowledgment of the importance of better incidence and mortality data among these groups, and the need for support for a data driven research agenda taking into account the top five cancers affecting each minority population (National Cancer Institute, 1996a).

The committee generally agrees, however, with the conclusion of the NIH priority-setting pamphlet (National Institutes of Health, 1997) regarding the difficulty and multiple ambiguities of the concept of burden of disease and how it is measured. The recommendations of the Special Action Committee Reports of 1992 and 1996 were silent on the issue of how those top five most burdensome cancers should be conceptualized, but this omission need not be fatal to NCI efforts to focus on neglected areas of research on cancers affecting each of the special populations. An increased burden can be detected in many ways, ranging from increased mortality to an increased incidence of particular cancers. No one-size-fits-all approach should be applied to each population. A more fruitful strategy will require the assessment of the unmet research needs of each population with whatever data are available regarding the type of burden specific to that subpopulation, in combination with an appraisal of the scientific opportunities. In short, no simple formula for addressing each group's top five most burdensome cancers will be adequate, and no uniform measure of burden across all subpopulations will be feasible.

The committee agrees with many of the conclusions of the recent IOM Committee on Priority Setting at NIH (Institute of Medicine, 1998), especially its general endorsement of the peer-review process and the central importance of scientific opportunity as a necessary condition for the allocation of scarce resources. However, lying beyond the scope of its charge are issues that this committee was asked to evaluate, and the committee concludes that in setting priorities for research among special populations, additional weight must be given to burden of disease. This does not mean that the demand for scientific opportunity should be sacrificed, however; it means only that unless NCI takes steps to initiate and stimulate research among special populations, the scientific opportunities from research within those communities will continue to lag behind those from research in areas where more effort has been expended in the past. Moreover, the committee concludes that as a supplement to the regular mechanisms for investigator-initiated research, additional steps are necessary to ensure that research questions for all of the subpopulations that NCI serves are adequately addressed. The committee concludes this chapter with the following recommendations.

Recommendation 4-4: Investigator-initiated research must be supplemented to ensure that the cancer research needs of ethnic minority and medically underserved populations are addressed.

SUMMARY

The committee finds that the research priority-setting process at NCI and NIH fails to serve the needs of minority and medically underserved populations. Although the processes for receiving input from interested scientists (e.g., ethnic minority scientists and those interested in research among ethnic minority and medically underserved populations), community groups, and consumers are improving (e.g., with the conception of DCLG), the level of representation of these groups on key NCI advisory panels should be improved. In addition, their impact on the priority-setting process should be evaluated to ensure that policy changes follow from increased representation. Assessment of the burden of cancer among minority and medically underserved populations and consideration of the burden of cancer within the large framework of scientific opportunity should be key aspects of the research priority-setting process. To stimulate research on cancer among minority and medically underserved populations, NCI must expand RFAs and other mechanisms, especially in areas where critical research gaps exist. The committee's specific recommendations are as follows:

Recommendation 4-1: NCI should develop a process to increase the representation of ethnically diverse researchers and public representatives serving on all advisory and program review committees so that the makeup of these committees reflects the changing diversity of the U.S. population. NCI should develop an evaluation plan assess the effect of increased and more diversified ethnic minority community and researcher input on changes in NCI policies and priorities toward ethnic minority cancer issues.

Recommendation 4-2: The research needs of ethnic minority and medically underserved groups should be identified on the basis of the burden of cancer in these populations, with an assessment of the most appropriate areas of research (i.e., behavioral and social sciences, biology, epidemiology and genetics, prevention and control, treatment, etc.).

Recommendation 4-3: For NCI to address needs of ethnically diverse and medically underserved populations effectively, the Office of Special Populations Research (or some other designated entity or entities) must possess the authority to coordinate and leverage programs and resources across divisions and branches of NCI to stimulate research on ethnic minority and medically underserved populations. This authority can be established by providing such an office with

- **a leadership role in major NCI-wide priority-setting bodies, and**
- **special resources to fund programs specifically targeted to these populations, or**
- **accountability for the institution-wide allocation of program resources.**

Recommendation 4-4: Investigator-initiated research must be supplemented to ensure that the cancer research needs of ethnic minority and medically underserved populations are addressed.

5

Advancing State-of-the-Art Treatment and Prevention

In the previous chapters, the committee has reviewed in detail the National Institutes of Health's (NIH) portfolio of research on cancer among ethnic minority and medically underserved populations and, pursuant to the study charge, has commented on the adequacy and comprehensiveness of this portfolio in addressing the cancer research needs of these populations. The committee has reviewed the priority-setting processes at NIH that underlie decisions regarding resource allocation and the areas of scientific inquiry that are emphasized. Ultimately, however, the utility of this research in reducing cancer incidence and mortality and increasing rates of survivorship among ethnic minority and medically underserved populations is dependent upon NIH's ability to bring the fruits of such research to affected communities. This includes the application and testing of new knowledge in field-based clinical and prevention trials and the dissemination of research findings to community-based health care providers, to organizations engaged in cancer prevention, and to members of affected communities. Accordingly, this chapter addresses two aspects of the study charge:

- It conducts "an examination of how well research results are communicated and applied to cancer prevention and treatment programs for minority and medically underserved communities"; and
- It assesses "the adequacy of NIH procedures for equitable recruitment and retention of minority and medically underserved populations in clinical trials."

This chapter begins with an assessment of NIH's efforts to include ethnic minority and medically underserved populations in NIH-sponsored cancer treatment and prevention trials. Particular attention is paid to the unique issues involved in recruiting these populations and retaining them in clinical trials, given the high quality of care generally afforded to patients enrolled in clinical trials and the importance of testing hypotheses with diverse populations to ensure the generalizability of findings. Next, the chapter reviews the strategies that NIH uses to disseminate information regarding cancer research to ethnic minority and medically underserved populations, their providers, and community-based health organizations.

RECRUITMENT AND RETENTION OF ETHNIC MINORITY AND MEDICALLY UNDERSERVED PARTICIPANTS IN CLINICAL CANCER RESEARCH

Clinical research forms the backbone of scientific advancements in medicine. New medications, preventive and rehabilitative interventions, and other innovations must be tested under the rigorous conditions of clinical trial research to understand whether these applications will work effectively, under what conditions they will work, and whether patients will be exposed to unintended harmful effects. Because patients are monitored closely under most clinical trial protocols, they often receive a higher quality of medical care and follow-up than patients who are not enrolled in clinical trials. This holds true even among patients in clinical trials assigned to "no-treatment" or "placebo" control groups in randomized trials.

Ethnic minority and medically underserved populations, however, have historically not participated in clinical trial research at rates proportional to participation rates among middle- and upper-income whites. Many factors may underlie this disparity. Examples of historical abuse of ethnic minorities in research abound; most researchers, and in particular, many in African-American communities, point to the Tuskegee syphilis experiment as a significant source of minority mistrust of the scientific establishment. In that study, federal researchers followed approximately 400 lower-income African-American men in rural Macon County, Alabama, who were infected with syphilis to study the natural history of the disease. Left untreated, syphilis can cause a host of life-threatening medical and cognitive complications. Yet, despite the availability of treatments such as penicillin, these men were denied treatment and were not informed of their infection. When news of the study became public in 1972, the study was abruptly halted, and the federal government and other public and private research entities began developing a series of procedures designed to protect the rights of human subjects participating in research.

Efforts to obtain informed consent and protect participants in clinical trials, however, may have resulted in the exclusion of ethnic minority and medically underserved populations from some clinical trial settings. Many researchers found recruitment of these populations into clinical trials to be challenging; some researchers who were unaccustomed to working with ethnic minorities as potential research subjects encountered difficulties in obtaining their informed consent for participation in trials, whereas other researchers may have been too cautious in attempting to protect research subjects from unethical behaviors (Durso, 1997). Such attitudes may have furthered the gap of mistrust between the scientific community and ethnic minority communities. Some researchers dismissed the possibility of recruiting research subjects from ethnic minority communities altogether, citing difficulties in recruitment.

Mistrust of the scientific community among ethnic minority populations is also heightened by well-publicized claims concluding that African Americans and other minority groups are genetically inferior to whites, despite the repudiation of such work by large segments of the scientific community. Publications such as Richard Hernnstein and R.J. Murray's, *The Bell Curve,* which argues that African Americans are intellectually inferior to whites and Asians as a result of genetic differences between these groups, may reinforce the perception of many ethnic minorities that the "scientific establishment" views them as inferior and less deserving of high-quality medical care (Durso, 1997). Similarly, a large body of evidence indicates that African Americans and other minorities receive a lower intensity of medical and surgical care (Sullivan, 1991), reinforcing this viewpoint.

Structural issues within the health care research industry also pose challenges to the recruitment of ethnic minority and medically underserved individuals. Many urban, low-income, uninsured, underinsured, or ethnic minority individuals receive treatment in large public hospitals, as opposed to private hospitals or university-affiliated research hospitals. The latter often capture a larger share of federal research dollars. Increasingly, time and financial constraints prevent many physicians working in public hospital settings from participating in research projects and enrolling their patients as subjects.

Researchers working with lower-income and minority communities may also face greater costs in conducting research as a result of the need to address financial barriers to participation in clinical trials. Recruitment often requires more than placing ads in newspapers; researchers must expend resources to build relationships with community groups and hire outreach personnel. Clinical trial participants often must visit a doctor's office or clinic regularly, which for some entails transportation and child-care costs, which typically are not covered by federal research grants. Some research programs have offered meals as a means of assisting low-income patients' participation.

Thus, the combination of historical experience and unequal access to health care has created a dynamic of mistrust on the part of ethnic minority and medically underserved communities and, in many quarters, resignation to low levels of minority participation in clinical research among investigators and health practitioners.

From a scientific perspective, however, it is critical to include diverse populations in clinical trials to ensure that research findings are generalizable to the entire population. (As discussed in Chapter 4, Zora Kramer Brown provides an example of the dangers involved when scientists and public health officials attempt to generalize research findings from relatively homogeneous study populations to broad, more diverse populations.) From a social justice perspective, it is important that research supported by taxpayer dollars be inclusive of and applicable to the diverse populations of the United States.

To address these needs, NIH and the U.S. Congress worked to develop standards in the late 1980s and early 1990s that mandated the participation of women and ethnic minorities in federally supported human subjects research. In 1993, as part of the NIH Revitalization Act (P.L. 103-43), Congress passed legislation that called for (1) the inclusion of women, ethnic minorities, and subpopulations into clinical trials; (2) the inclusion of adequate numbers of women and ethnic minorities for performance of valid analyses; (3) preventing cost from being an applicable reason for the exclusion of these groups; (4) a determination of the circumstances under which inclusion of these groups may be inappropriate; and (5) clinical trials and outreach programs to be designed and executed in ways that encourage recruitment and retention of women and ethnic minorities (Penn, 1996). This legislation was designed to ensure that biomedical and behavioral research results are applicable to all affected populations and include detailed information about the effects of gender, racial, and socioeconomic factors that might influence the development and outcomes of cancer.

In response to the law, guidelines for inclusion were developed and published (U.S. Department of Health and Human Services, 1994), and a 1-year comment period was provided. The policy states that women and ethnic minorities and their subpopulations must be included in all NIH-supported biomedical and behavioral research projects involving human subjects unless there is a clear and compelling justification that the inclusion of these groups is inappropriate with respect to the health of the subjects or the purpose of the research. NIH policy also demands that studies be designed to allow valid analyses to be performed (i.e., to detect a significant difference that is of clinical or public health importance on the basis of scientific data). Investigators are required to report on actual accrual and inclusion of women and minorities in progress reports and for supplementary grant applications. In the future, reporting on intent to recruit will also be mandated. A computerized tracking system that enables NIH institutes to report on the actual number of ethnic minorities and women included in NIH-sponsored research studies has been developed.

The NIH Revitalization Act did not, however, address the many practical and ethical concerns that affect recruitment of ethnic minorities into clinical trials. As noted above, the cost of research may vary, with some populations being more costly to recruit into clinical trials. Balancing cost considerations with the need for fair recruitment into clinical trials can be challenging and can involve trade-offs that constrain researchers. Another concern is the applicability of results of studies with the general population to each of the relevant subpopulations. If certain groups of individuals are not included in clinical trials, then the principle of justice would support the need for a remedy to this situation. This leads to a separate concern: whether it is ethical to target the recruitment of ethnic minorities into clinical trials. Targeted studies are based on the conceptual framework that individuals differ on the basis of gender, "race" or ethnicity, culture, age, and other factors. However, these studies also raise the concern that the researchers who are involved in these studies believe that there are biological differences among the "races," a concept that is controversial (see Chapter 2). In certain cases, such assumptions that individuals differ are reasonable, such as in the evaluation of biological differences in the context of genetic conditions or in behavioral studies, especially if the behavioral studies address institutional racism that is associated with outcome differences between ethnic minorities and nonminorities. Finally, trust is an important consideration in recruitment efforts. Much existing evidence indicates that African Americans are less trusting of clinical research efforts than whites. No data are available indicating whether low-income whites share this mistrust. These concerns are not unreasonable, given the large degree of evidence indicating the lower intensities of medical and surgical care for African Americans.

NIH Efforts to Increase Participation of Minority and Medically Underserved Groups in Clinical Trials

The National Cancer Institute (NCI) has reported on several initiatives that have been used to increase the participation of ethnic minority populations and groups with low levels of literacy in clinical trials.

Outreach efforts to inform ethnic minority groups and populations with low literacy levels about clinical trials include versions of the NCI publication *What Are Clinical Trials all About?* in Spanish and in a version for people with low literacy levels, and a Spanish-language version of the videotape *Patient to Patient: Cancer Clinical Trials and You.* Fact sheets on cancer prevention and treatment studies have been developed in both English and Spanish. Similarly, a new training program for health professionals that addresses common patient concerns about the trial process, from initial decision making to trial participation and follow-up, was developed in English and Spanish.

To address the increasing complexity of the informed-consent process, representatives from NCI, the Office of Protection from Research Risks, and the Food and Drug Administration have organized a working group charged with developing recommendations to make the informed-consent process more understandable. Informed-consent documents are lengthy, complex, and often difficult to understand, thereby hindering the process of providing accurate information to potential subjects. The working group developed recommendations for an informed-consent template and sample consent documents that are undergoing field testing.

NCI's Cancer Therapy Evaluation Program provided supplemental funding in fiscal year (FY) 1997 for 5 of the 11 Clinical Trials Cooperative Groups (see below for description) as part of an initiative to increase the accrual of ethnic minority populations. Funds were used to support focus groups and educational opportunities for ethnic minority health professionals, to advertise and support outreach efforts in ethnic minority communities, to hire translators, and to conduct other community-based education efforts.

To increase the number of ethnic minority patients enrolled in Community Clinical Oncology Programs (CCOPs), NCI developed the Minority-Based Community Clinical Oncology Programs (MBCCOPs) in 1990. The MBCCOP involve more than 300 physicians and eight program sites located in areas with large minority populations, such as San Juan, Puerto Rico; Mobile, Alabama; Honolulu, Hawaii; and San Antonio, Texas.

The NIH Office of Research on Minority Health (ORMH; see Chapter 3) has provided funding to the NCI Cancer Center Program to support programs and personnel to increase the accrual of ethnic minorities in cancer center trials. These funds have supported the hiring of personnel involved in minority recruitment efforts, such as translators, data managers, bilingual patient liaisons, and others and have supported activities such as the development of recruitment brochures specifically targeted to ethnic minority patients.

Finally, NCI has sponsored several conferences to promote strategies for the development and sharing of information among investigators to increase ethnic minority accrual. NCI released a request for applications in 1996 to support regional conferences on the recruitment and retention of ethnic minorities in clinical trials. Eleven such conferences were funded to address particular issues for investigators and patient populations at each locality. These regional conferences followed a national conference entitled Recruitment and Retention of Minority Participants Clinical Cancer Research, held in Washington, D.C., that was cosponsored by the American Cancer Society (ACS), the Oncology Nursing Society, the NIH Office of Research on Women's Health, and ORMH, among others. A monograph of the conference proceedings outlining specific needs and strategies for recruitment and retention of ethnic minority and underserved populations was published by NCI (see Box 5-1).

ETHNIC MINORITY ACCRUAL IN NIH-SPONSORED TRIALS

As noted in Chapter 3, NCI sponsors approximately 500 clinical trials, including those of the Clinical Trials Cooperative Groups and CCOP, intramural clinical trials, and trials conducted at NCI-funded cancer centers. The Clinical Trials Cooperative Group Program performs more than half of the NCI-sponsored trials, conducting approximately 900 of the 1,500 trials. Thirteen cooperative groups that included participants from 194 universities and 1,839 hospitals and more than 23,700 physicians were funded in 1977. CCOP links community-based physicians with Clinical Trials Cooperative Groups and cancer centers for cancer prevention and treatment trials. More than 50 community-based programs in 30 states, nine cooperative groups, and three cancer centers were funded in 1997 and involved more than 300 hospitals and 3,300 physicians. Finally, NCI sponsors four large cancer prevention trials, described in greater detail below and in Chapter 3: the atypical squamous cells of undetermined significance (ASCUS) or low-grade squamous intra-epithelial lesions (LSIL) Triage Study (ALTS) of cervical cancer screening, evaluation, and management; the Prostate, Lung, Colorectal, and Ovarian Cancer (PLCO) Screening Trial; the Prostate Cancer Prevention Trial (PCPT); and the Breast Cancer Prevention Trial (BCPT). The levels of ethnic minority accrual in these trial groups are summarized below. Except in a few instances as noted below, NCI and the trial groups did not report on accrual by socioeconomic status or other indicators of medically underserved populations.

Determinations of whether the level of accrual of ethnic minorities into trials is proportionate to cancer burden can typically be accomplished by comparing the percentage of cancer diagnoses among racial and ethnic groups in the U.S. population within a given time frame and the percentage of minority enrollment within trials for each cancer studied. Such

BOX 5-1
Factors Affecting Ethnic Accrual and Inclusion of Minorities in Research

In January 1996, the National Cancer Institute (NCI), in conjunction with the National Cancer Advisory Board, the American Cancer Society, the Oncology Nursing Society, and the National Institutes of Health (NIH) Office of Research on Women's Health and Office of Research on Minority Health, organized a conference entitled "Recruitment and Retention of Minority Participants in Clinical Cancer Research." The 2-day conference brought together national experts on minority health and clinical trials research to share perspectives and strategies to improve the rate of inclusion of ethnic minorities in research. The proceedings of the conference were published by NCI (National Cancer Institute, 1996d). In the Executive Summary, conference participants concluded that the achievement of equity in clinical trials will require that four goals be met:

- there must be professional and institutional commitment to increasing minority participation;
- data on the cancer burden in subpopulations must be collected and made available;
- there must be more research on the accrual and retention process in a whole range of clinical trials, with specific attention paid to accessibility, education, communication, and attitudes of participants, physicians, and communities; and
- there must be minority participation not only in clinical trials, but also in the conduct of clinical trials (National Cancer Institute, 1996d).

The committee supports the findings and recommendations of the five conference panels, some of which are summarized below with respect to specific issues and populations.

ETHICAL ISSUES IN RECRUITMENT OF MINORITY PARTICIPANTS

Three ethical principles should guide the behavior of individuals who conduct clinical research, particularly with respect to oversight by institutional review boards (IRBs), according to Nancy Kass of Johns Hopkins University. These ethical principles are respect for autonomy, beneficence, and justice. Occasionally, these principles conflict with each other, which requires priorities to be considered.

CULTURAL ADAPTATIONS FOR OVERCOMING BARRIERS

Native Americans

Cultural factors significantly affect the recruitment of Native Americans into clinical trials, according to Linda Burhansstipanov, Director of the Native American Cancer Research Program in Denver, Colorado. Relevant considerations include insurance, poverty, racial identification, and distrust of science and research, especially by underserved and underrepresented populations. IRB processes are very different for Native Americans, especially with respect to considerations of the protection of individuals and sovereignty. Although the Native American health care system provides excellent access to care, the rate of survival from cancer for this group is the poorest among all ethnic groups. Informed-consent forms and procedures may serve as a barrier to recruitment, as the language commonly used in such forms and procedures may be considered offensive by some Native Americans. In many cases, the informed-consent process is poorly understood by Native Americans. In addition, body language and styles of interaction between researchers and potential research subjects may affect recruitment. Other factors including intonation are important. Among this population, fear of research is real and telephone recruitment is generally unhelpful.

Involvement of the community elders is important in studies among Native Americans. Face-to-face recruitment is likely to be the most successful strategy. Incentives, such as food for research subjects' children or grandchildren, and other rewards are being tested, but they have yet to show results. Although programs such as the Native Sisters (a social and emotional support system) have been implemented, their success is limited. Tribal beliefs are difficult to change, and protocols are often inflexible. The result is that it may take three times as long to recruit Native Americans into clinical trials.

African Americans

As described by Carolyn Harvey, cultural variations in communication styles also affect the recruitment of African Americans to clinical trials. Linear models of information are preferred among whites, with an emphasis on written messages. In contrast, among African Americans, a cyclical model of consent and information is important, with information being disseminated through real-life situations rather than statistics or written messages. African Americans are more likely to communicate via a church or an interactive educational session and often need the freedom to respond and interrupt during a teaching session. African Americans may also require flexibility and are responsive to nonverbal aspects of communication, accounting for the importance of tone, inflection, and body language. A model for this approach has been developed in East Texas (the Visible Messenger Model), where people who are known, trusted, and accountable in the community are recruited to provide cancer awareness messages.

Continued

BOX 5-1 *Continued*

Asians/Pacific Islanders

As outlined by Marjorie Kagawa-Singer, among Asians/Pacific Islanders many factors are barriers to recruitment, including structural concerns (such as a wide range of fluencies in English), cultural considerations (e.g., different conceptions of health and fear of preventive interventions), and cultural differences (decisions are made by family conference and often take a long time). Confidentiality is also a concern because these individuals often require the town elder to participate in the consent process, representing a breach of confidentiality. Written consent forms are off-putting to the patients. Successful strategies include the use of research team members familiar with Asian and Pacific Island cultures. Allocation of adequate lead times with focus groups is also required, because additional services are often needed.

Hispanics

As outlined by Edward Trapido, Hispanics consist of individuals of diverse races and ethnicities, with many subpopulations. Differences exist within subpopulations according to culture, language, religion, race, age, gender, family role, education, and length of time in the United States. Focus groups consisting of individuals from Miami revealed several important beliefs of the Hispanic participants: physicians did not communicate well with patients; the medical staff was insensitive to their culture and language; they had not been well informed about their cancer; many felt that physicians had financial interests in prescribing surgery or advising enrollment in surgical trials; chemotherapy would bring on certain death; physicians were concerned that patients would not follow up with care; communication difficulties were common when physicians preferred to speak English, even if the patient understood the language (even if the patient's native language was Spanish); patients were often not asked to participate in the trials; and the participants had a high level of concern over Medicare fraud, inconsistent public health policies, the commercialization of medicine, and the need to involve pharmacists and nurses in the process. Other cultural considerations include a sense of fatalism. Patients are often not told their diagnosis to spare them from pain.

General recommendations of this panel included the following:

- recognize variability and diversity within and among ethnic groups;
- include provisions for transportation and family coverage;
- train more community members to work in clinical research;
- stress the importance of enrollment in trials to the family;

- promote the balance of spirituality, faith, medicine, and science; and
- adapt the language in written and oral communications to the patient.

PUBLIC AND PROVIDER EDUCATION

Approaching Community Physicians

Worta McKaskill-Stevens points out that community physician involvement in cooperative trials is needed. The National Medical Association (22,000 minority physicians, two-thirds of whom are primary care providers) is working closely with the Eastern Cooperative Oncology Group to develop a protocol-specific patient brochure. The text includes sections on IRBs and who the participants are, and a layperson is on the IRB. It provides general information for clinical trials.

Recruiting Asian Americans for Smoking Cessation Research

Moon Chen, Jr., points out that researchers are challenged to recruit Asian Americans if they overlook the tremendous diversity within Asian-American populations. The majority of Asian Americans are foreign born (especially true with regard to the Southeast Asian populations in the United States), thereby posing linguistic barriers to recruitment. There is a relative dearth of research information on these populations, which is especially alarming given the high rate of health risk behaviors such as smoking (for example, 57 percent of Southeast Asian males in the San Francisco Bay area smoke). A research project in Ohio solicited community support and hired workers from Asian ethnic groups to find study samples via the telephone book and home visits, in part to establish rapport for a long-term relationship instead of simply collecting data. Similarly, educational outreach efforts in California proved successful when antismoking messages were tailored to particular groups and were presented by use of outdoor billboards and educational classes in settings where community members gather.

Successful Recruitment of African-American Men: The DEED Program

Isaac Powell describes the Detroit Education and Early Detection (DEED) program, which studied prostate-specific antigen changes among African-American men enrolled in a prostate cancer screening program. Researchers assessed these men's attitudes toward the health care system and found that fear of a positive diagnosis was a significant barrier to participation (many men held fatalistic attitudes toward a diag-

Continued

BOX 5-1 *Continued*

nosis of cancer). Concern about the loss of sexual function and other quality-of-life issues was also a significant barrier. Another significant impediment was distrust: many African-American men sampled believed that they might be abused as medical subjects in large health care institutions. After identifying potential barriers, the DEED program recruited subjects via African-American churches and related networks. Researchers found that when the church minister and other leaders were recruited for testing, participation among church members increased two- to threefold. In addition, a group of prostate cancer survivors assisted in recruitment by discussing their experiences. DEED program researchers reported high levels of success in recruiting and retaining African-American men in the in the longitudinal project.

Working with Communities: A Key to Success

Noel Chavez described several efforts that are needed for health education and research outreach in medically underserved communities. Chavez stressed the need for assessment of community norms and beliefs, to find out who in the community is entrusted with leadership positions, and how the community relates to the larger social environment. In addition, researchers need to find ways to help communities gain "ownership" of research programs, including involvement in project planning and development, recruitment, and protocol design. Finally, researchers need to be prepared to assist communities in solving problems rather than assuming that work that can be done for or with a community. The development of trust and support within the community requires time, effort, flexibility, and resources, but the relationships built in this process will improve the likelihood of success.

General recommendations of this panel included the following:

- There is a need for active involvement of minority physicians in the community as well as community members.
- Researchers should factor in the time and cost of recruitment of minority and underserved populations in research budgets.

IMPLEMENTATION STRATEGIES

Alternative strategies for recruitment of ethnic minorities into clinical trials have not been evaluated in most settings. Roshan Bastani describes the experience of the University of California at Los Angeles (UCLA) in improving recruitment of ethnic minorities into clinical trials. An important consideration in this effort is the difficulty that some individuals have with the written informed-consent process. An appeal was made to the UCLA IRB to allow verbal consent in place of written consent, because in one study of low-income women (many of whom had low levels of literacy, were recent immigrants, or were illegal aliens), the written informed-consent process was too intimidating. The IRB allowed the use of verbal consent in conjunction with mailing of explanatory information on the study to all participants. Use of verbal consent dramatically increased the level of recruitment of members of this population.

Tom Welty described logistical considerations related to the recruitment of American Indians into cancer research. The Indian Health Service (IHS) acts like a health maintenance organization and is faced with the rationing of health care services because of budget constraints. IRB concerns are very lengthy, involving the IHS or tribal facility, a second level of federal approval, and tribal approval. Publication of trial results requires approval of the tribe, the Area Publication Committee, and the IHS Publication Committee. Strategies to improve the IRB process in the IHS setting are needed. However, the safeguards have been adopted for good reasons, because much of the previous work provided little benefit to the Indian population and was intrusive and offensive to many.

Recommendations from this panel included the following:

- Retrospective assessment may be useful in communities where recruitment into clinical trials has been unsuccessful, including an assessment of physicians' knowledge of the trials and eligibility criteria.
- Researchers must perform recruitment activities in institutions that serve as focal points of community life for many minority groups, such as churches and Head Start programs.

analyses, however, are sometimes complicated by several statistical and data limitations (J. Unger, Southwest Oncology Group, personal communications, 1998). For example, information regarding incidence is typically derived from Surveillance, Epidemiology, and End Result (SEER) program data, which are less reliable for some populations (e.g., American Indians) and nonexistent for others (e.g., rural medically underserved populations), as discussed in Chapter 2. Furthermore, as Tejeda et al. (1996) state:

> [T]rue determination of proportional representation [of minorities] in trials is difficult because the United States does not have a national, population-based cancer registry from which the racial/ethnic composition of the population with cancer can be counted. Such a registry would make the determination of racial/ethnic composition of the newly diagnosed population with cancer a simple arithmetic exercise (p. 815).

Calculation of the percentages of members of ethnic groups with cancer diagnoses is also dependent on the quality of the overall population data from the U.S. Bureau of the Census (i.e., the "denominator"), which are less reliable for some populations (especially many ethnic minority groups) within SEER program coverage areas. Finally, for many rare cancers and for cancers among smaller ethnic groups, incidence data are unreliable, therefore limiting the kinds of analyses that can be performed (Tejeda et al., 1996). Only a few published studies account for these limitations, and these are cited below. The committee therefore interprets the proportionality of ethnic minority participation in clinical trials with caution.

Sufficient data are not available from NCI to evaluate clinical trial accrual for medically underserved populations.

Cancer Cooperative Group Trials

Of the 13 cooperative groups funded in 1997, 4 are focused on pediatric cancers (the Children's Cancer Group [CCG], the National Wilms' Tumor Study [NWTS], the Intergroup Rhabdomyosarcoma Study Group [IRS], and the Pediatric Oncology Group [POG]), 5 are focused on specific cancers (the Brain Tumor Cancer Group, the Gynecologic Oncology Group [GOG], IRS, the National Surgical Adjuvant Breast and Bowel Project [NSABP], and NWTS), and 2 are small or regional groups (the M.D. Anderson Cancer Center [MDA] and the North Central Cancer Treatment Group [NCCTG]). These groups all face special circumstances that may affect the accrual of minorities in clinical trials. The groups focused on pediatric cancers, for example, enroll the majority of pediatric cancer patients in the United States (approximately 70 percent), making proportionate accrual of minority patients more likely (Bleyer, 1977; Tejeda et al., 1996). The remainder, however, are large nonspecialty trial groups that recruit subjects from broad adult patient populations.

NCI Clinical Trials Cooperative Group statistics indicate that the overall level of participation of U.S. cancer patients in Clinical Trials Cooperative Group is about 2.5 percent. In an examination of accrual patterns by ethnicity and age for all cooperative group trials during the period between January 1991 and June 1994, Tejeda et al. (1996) found that overall, ethnic minority representation is proportional in comparison to the incidence of cancer among ethnic minorities in the U.S. population. Specifically, the level of enrollment of African Americans was found to be 9.6 percent, that of Hispanics was 5.6 percent, and that of whites was 84.8 percent. These figures are very close to the estimated proportions of individuals with cancer in these groups in the United States (9.4 percent among African Americans, 3.4 percent among Hispanics, and 87.2 percent among whites).

Among the various age groups, Tejeda et al. (1996) found that overall, younger patients tend to be heavily represented in Clinical Trials Cooperative Groups, because slightly less than half of trial participants are under age 50 years, even though more than 85 percent of cancer diagnoses occur among people 50 years of age or older. Within age groups, the level of accrual of African-American and Hispanic patients appeared in most instances to be proportional to the incidence or slightly below the incidence of cancer in these populations. Among African-American and Hispanic patients ages 0 to 19 years, the level of enrollment (11.0 and 12.0 percent respectively) was very close to rates of incidence (12.4 and 11.9 percent, respectively); the same held true within the 20- to 49-year-old age group (10.6 and 4.8 percent enrollments for African Americans and Hispanics, respectively, compared to incidence rates of 11.4 and 6.0 percent, respectively) and the group consisting of those 50 years of age and older (8.5 and 2.5 percent enrollment for African Americans and Hispanics, respectively, compared to incidence rates of 9.1 and 2.9 percent, respectively).

When accrual was examined by specific cancer sites (leukemia and breast, colorectal, lung, and prostate cancer), Tejeda et al. (1996) found that, with a few exceptions, the level of ethnic minority enrollment in Clinical Trials Cooperative Groups generally was proportional to or greater than the expected incidences. Enrollment of African Americans in trials involving colorectal cancer (8.4 percent enrollment) and prostate cancer (9.8 percent enrollment) lagged slightly behind the incidence rate among this group (9.4 percent of cases of colorectal cancer and 11.1 percent of cases of prostate cancer among African Americans). Similarly, the level of enrollment of Hispanics in trials involving lung cancer (1.4 percent enrollment) also lagged slightly behind the incidence (2.2 percent). The greatest disparities in accrual were observed among African Americans ages 20 to 49 years with leukemia (9.4 percent enrollment compared with 12.4 percent incidence), colorectal cancer (10.2 percent enrollment compared with 15.7 percent incidence), and lung cancer (17.2 percent enrollment compared with 20.4 percent incidence) and among Hispanics ages 20 to 49 years with lung cancer (1.8 percent enrollment compared with 3.2 percent incidence).

The analysis of Tejeda et al. (1996), however, did not examine cancer incidence among Asian-American, Alaska Native, and American Indian populations in determining the proportionality of accrual patterns because of the small number of cases of cancer among these groups in the SEER program database. Similarly, the study does not report on the proportionality of accrual of low-income, low-literacy-level, rural, or otherwise medically underserved populations, presumably because these data are not reported in the SEER program registry (see Chapter 2).

NCI provided to the committee raw data and percentages of total enrollment for the Clinical Trials Cooperative Groups in 1997. Although the proportions of cases of cancer among ethnic minority patients during the period of trial enrollment were not provided by NCI, enrollment data are presented here for purposes of comparison across trial groups. Where data on expected incidences are available, these are reported, but the committee urges caution in their interpretation. Percent accrual of ethnic minorities in each trial group in 1997 is depicted in Figures 5-1 and 5-2.

Among the pediatric clinical trial groups, both CCG and POG appear to have high levels of representation of ethnic minority patients on the basis of 1997 enrollment data. Among the 2,300 children enrolled in CCG,

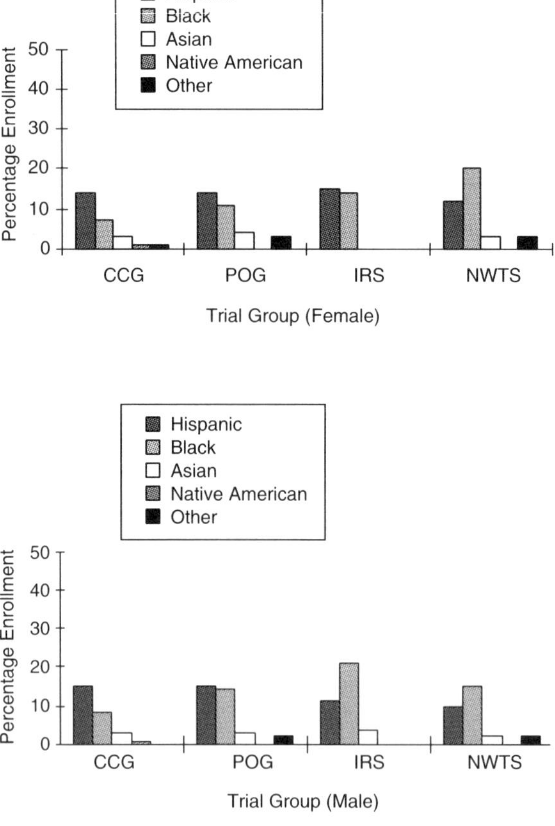

FIGURE 5-1 Percent minority accrual for 1997 cooperative pediatric groups. SOURCE: National Cancer Institute.

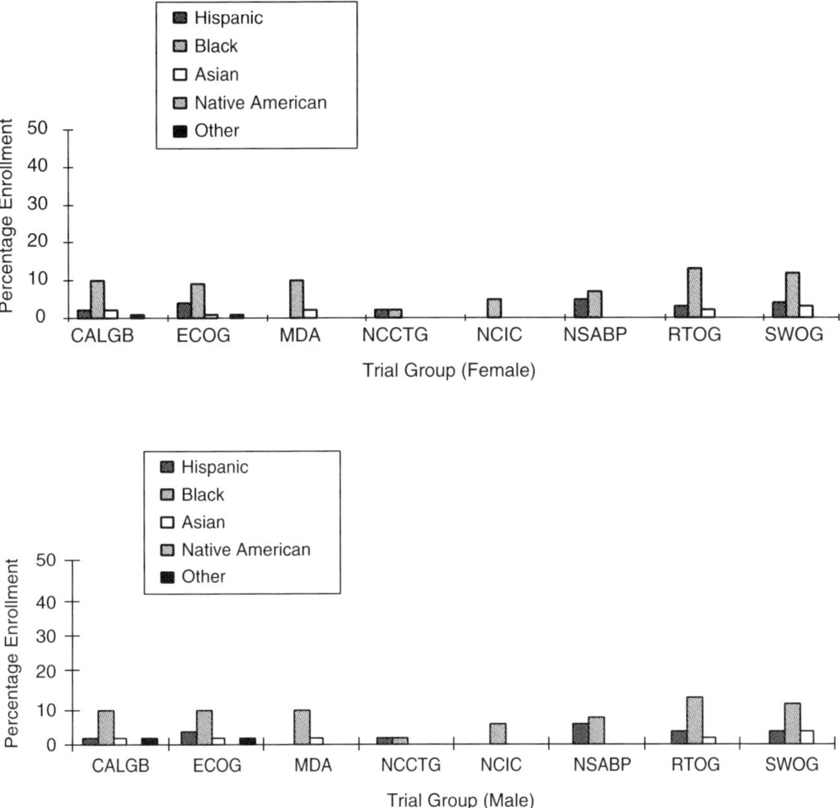

FIGURE 5-2 Percent minority accrual for 1997 cooperative groups. SOURCE: National Cancer Institute.

30 percent are ethnic minority patients. Significantly, 14 percent are Hispanic, whereas 7 percent of the participants are African American. POG enrolls 31 percent minority females and 34 percent minority males, including 14 and 15 percent female and male Hispanics, respectively; 11 and 14 percent female and male African Americans, respectively; and 4 and 3 percent female and male Asian Americans, respectively (Figure 5-1). Bleyer et al. (1997) published a report supporting the conclusion that the accrual of ethnic minorities in POG and CCG is proportional to the incidence of cancer among ethnic minority group children, using enrollment data for nearly 30,000 children enrolled in these trials from January 1991 through June 1994. This study found that 11.6 percent of patients were Hispanic, 10.4 percent were African American, and 4.7 percent were from

other racial groups. On the basis of SEER program data (1989 to 1991 crude incidence data), the expected distribution of patients of the same age in the United States was 9.1 percent for Hispanic children, 10.7 percent for African-American children, and 4.3 percent for other ethnic groups. The authors found that the level of ethnic minority enrollment was equal to or greater than the rate of cancer for 24 of 27 subgroups.

Among the pediatric specialty clinical trial groups, NWTS and IRS appeared to have a high level of representation of ethnic minority patients, with 38 percent of females and 34 percent of males enrolled in NWTS identified as ethnic minorities and 30 percent of females and 36 percent of males enrolled in IRS identified as ethnic minorities. More than half of the ethnic minority females in NWTS were African American (20 percent overall), whereas less than 4 percent each were Asian American, American Indian, or other groups.

Among the adult specialty clinical trial groups, GOG enrolled 21 percent minority women. Of the 1,604 women accrued in 1997, 5.4 percent were Hispanic, 12.8 percent were African American, 2.3 percent were Asian American, and 0.2 percent were American Indian. NSABP reported data on enrollment to 5 treatment trials, including breast, colon, and rectal cancer treatment protocols. Among the colon and rectal cancer trials, 86 percent of the 267 males enrolled in this trial were identified as white, 5.2 percent were identified as Hispanic, 7.1 percent were identified as African American, and 0.3 percent were identified as Asian American. No American Indian men were accrued in these trials. Among the 240 women enrolled in these trials, 85 percent were identified as white, whereas 1.7, 10.4, and 1.2 percent were identified as Hispanic, African American, and Asian American, respectively. One American Indian woman was recruited into this trial. Similarly, of the 2,175 women recruited into NSABP's breast cancer treatment trials, 1,842 (85 percent) were white and 175 (9.0 percent) were African American. NSABP did not collect more detailed data on ethnicity in two of its breast cancer treatment protocols (instead, data were collected on the basis of a former categorization system), but reported that 5.4 percent of women in these trials were of "other" ethnic minority groups. Three newer breast cancer treatment trials did include detailed ethnicity data in accordance with NIH guidelines and revealed that 2.6 percent of the women enrolled were Hispanic, 1.0 percent were Asian American, 0.3 percent were American Indian, and 1.5 percent were of other ethnic minority backgrounds.

The small, regional clinical trial groups experienced low ethnic minority accrual overall. NCCTG was able to enroll only 11 percent female ethnic minority and 4 percent male ethnic minority patients, whereas MDA enrolled 12 percent ethnic minority patients overall. Among NCCTG's patient population, 3.1 percent of females and 1.5 percent of males were

Hispanic, 5.5 percent of females and 1.5 percent of males were African American, 1.5 percent of females and 0.4 percent of males were Asian American, and less than 0.3 percent of both the male and female populations were American Indian. MDA reported the accrual of no Hispanic individuals, whereas 9.2 percent (4 of 42) and 9.6 percent (5 of 52) of the enrolled patient population were African-American females and males, respectively. Only one Asian-American male was accrued to this trial group.

Among the large, nonspecialty clinical trial groups, the level of ethnic minority accrual appeared to be slightly less than those for the other clinical trial groups. The Cancer and Acute Leukemia Group B trial reported that in 1997, 16 percent of the enrolled patient population were ethnic minorities, whereas ECOG reported that 12 percent of females and 15 percent of males were ethnic minorities. RTOG and the Southwest Oncology Group (SWOG) fared similarly, as 16 percent of the females and 19 percent of the males enrolled in RTOG were ethnic minorities, whereas 17 percent of the females and 19 percent of the males enrolled in SWOG were ethnic minorities.

SWOG has conducted an analysis of its accrual to therapeutic trials between 1993 and 1996, comparing accrual rates to the percentage of cancer diagnoses in the U.S. among women, African Americans, and elderly people (ages 65 and older) at four cancer sites. As in the analysis of Tejeda et al. (1996), Unger and his colleagues (Unger et al., 1998) calculated expected values based on 1992 to 1994 SEER program incidence data and U.S. census data. Unger et al. (1998) found that the overall SWOG accrual rate for African Americans (10.2 percent) was almost identical to the estimated percentage of African Americans among U.S. cancer cases (10.1 percent). Similarly, the accrual rate for women (41 percent) was comparable to the estimated percentage of women among all cases of cancer in the U.S. (43 percent). The elderly, however, were substantially under-accrued, as 25 percent of SWOG's trial population was 65 or older, whereas 63 percent of cancer diagnoses occur among this population in the U.S. When examined by cancer site, Unger et al. (1998) found that the elderly were significantly under-accrued in breast, colon and rectal, and lung cancer trials, while African Americans were significantly under-accrued in lymphoma trials (7 percent accrual in SWOG, compared with 11 percent of African Americans among all lymphoma cases during the same period).

Similarly, Chamberlain et al. (1998) report on the sociodemographic characteristics of more than 4,000 patients enrolled in RTOG studies between January 1991 and June 1994, using SEER program and U.S. census data to determine the representativeness of the study sample to the overall U.S. population of cancer patients who have received radiation therapy. Using chi-square analyses, investigators determined that the educational characteristics of older African Americans enrolled in RTOG were not significantly different from those of African Americans in all other age groups except the youngest age group (20 to 54 years), according to data from the U.S. census. African Americans in the youngest age group were two to three times less likely to have completed high school (45.3 percent of African-American males and 52.3 percent of African-American females who were in this age group and who were enrolled in the trial did not complete high school, whereas the expected rates are 18.9 and 17.5 percent, respectively). Chamberlain et al. (1998) also found that the proportion of African-American men (11.9 percent) and women (16.3 percent) enrolled in RTOG significantly exceeded the proportion of patients who were African American and received radiation therapy as a primary treatment (10.4 and 8.7 percent, respectively, on the basis of SEER program data). Similarly, for prostate and cervical cancers, enrollment of African Americans significantly exceeded the expected proportions of African Americans with cancer at those sites. The level of enrollment of African Americans diagnosed with cancers of the brain, head and neck (among females only), and lung (among females only) did not differ significantly from the expected incidence. Enrollment of African-American men with lung cancer, however, fell significantly below the percentage of African-American men with lung cancer who received radiation therapy (7.9 percent enrolled versus 13.2 percent expected). As is the case with Tejeda et al. (1996), Chamberlain et al. (1998) do not provide data on ethnic minority groups other than African Americans, because the stratification of the sample by age and education precluded an analysis of the small number of individuals of other ethnic backgrounds enrolled in RTOG. Similarly, the report provides no socioeconomic data for other populations. It is important that comparable studies be done for low-income whites as well as for other populations.

Overall, the Clinical Trials Cooperative Groups appear to accrue ethnic minority populations in clinical trials at rates proportional to the rates of cancer among those groups. When examined by specific trial groups and types of cancers, however, there appear gaps in accrual that serve to suppress overall ethnic minority accrual.

CCOPs and MBCCOPs

As noted above, 51 CCOPs were funded in FY 1997 to enroll patients in prevention and treatment trials. NCI provided raw data on patient accrual to these trials between June 1996 and February 1997 but did not provide information on accrual by specific ethnic minority groups. These data indicate that of the 4,363 patients enrolled in treatment protocols, 664 (15.2 percent of the total) were ethnic minorities. As is the case with the Clinical Trials Cooperative Groups, accrual of ethnic minorities varied considerably with the site of the CCOP. Compared with the percentage of ethnic minorities residing in the state in which the CCOP is located, it was found that only 12 of the 51 CCOPs met or exceeded this percentage of accrual of ethnic minorities. (It should be noted that the percentage of ethnic minority residents in a state is only a crude standard for accrual, given that cancer incidence rates for various ethnic groups within a population may not be equivalent to their percentages within the total population. Data on the percentage of ethnic minority residents within a CCOP catchment area were not available for all CCOPs.) Of those CCOPs that reported high rates of accrual of ethnic minorities, those in the Oakland, California; Tampa, Florida; Miami Beach, Florida; and Manhassett, New York, reported accrual rates of 32 to 50 percent. Data on patient accrual in four of the CCOPs were unavailable.

In CCOP prevention trials, the rate of accrual of ethnic minorities was poor. Data provided by NCI revealed that of the 4,172 patients enrolled in prevention trials, 289 (6.9 percent of the total) were ethnic minorities. Only 5 of the 51 CCOPs were able to enroll ethnic minority patients at rates equivalent to the proportion of ethnic minorities living in the states in which CCOPs were located. Furthermore, only the Miami Beach and Tampa sites were able to enroll ethnic minority subjects at rates of one-third or more of the total subject population. Data on patient accrual from four CCOP sites were missing.

The eight MBCCOPs appear to have increased the numbers of ethnic minority patients in the overall CCOP pool, yet in some cases they have not performed better than the CCOPs accruing the highest numbers of ethnic minorities. One trial group (in Richmond, Virginia) did not recruit a greater proportion of ethnic minorities in treatment (31 percent) and prevention (24 percent) trials than the proportion of ethnic minorities in the catchment area (38 percent). Two other MBCCOPs reported less than 50 percent ethnic minority enrollment in treatment and prevention trials. In addition, the numbers of ethnic minorities brought into clinical trials via MBCCOPs between June 1996 and February 1997 are small: although data are missing for one of the eight MBCCOPs, the seven remaining groups brought only an additional 215 ethnic minority patients into treatment trials and 102 ethnic minority patients into prevention trials. Overall, 79 percent of the patients enrolled in MBCCOP treatment trials were ethnic minorities, whereas 58 percent of the subjects enrolled in prevention trials were ethnic minorities.

Cancer Prevention Trials

As noted above and in Chapter 3, NCI sponsors five large cancer prevention trials to test the effectiveness of various chemoprevention strategies and cancer screening methodologies in reducing cancer incidence and mortality. The ALTS cervical cancer screening trial assesses the screening and management of minor Pap smear abnormalities. Four sites are involved in this trial, including the University of Pittsburgh, the University of Alabama at Birmingham, the University of Washington, and the University of Oklahoma. The PLCO screening trial is a large-scale, prospective randomized study to determine whether screening for these types of cancers will reduce the rate of associated morbidity (all four types of cancers account for nearly half of all cancer deaths in the United States). Ten centers around the United States are participating in this trial. To increase the rate of accrual of ethnic minorities, two screening centers focused on the recruitment of ethnic minorities were to be added in 1998, in addition to a new center cosponsored by the Centers for Disease Control and Prevention (CDC) to focus on the recruitment of African Americans. CDC is also working with the Henry Ford Health System in Michigan and the University of Pittsburgh PLCO screening trial center to identify effective methods for increasing the rate of recruitment of ethnic minorities and reducing barriers to participation. PCPT includes 222 sites across the United States and is coordinated by SWOG; its purpose is to test whether the drug finasteride will prevent prostate cancer in a randomized trial involving 18,000 men. Finally, BCPT is a randomized, double-blind trial that will assess whether the drug tamoxifen can prevent breast cancer in women at increased risk of developing the disease. More than 13,000 women were recruited from nearly 180 sites for this trial, managed by the National Surgical Adjuvant Breast and Bowel Project.

Data provided by NCI on the rates of accrual of subjects as of February 1998 for these trials indicate that only one trial, ALTS, experienced success in recruiting ethnic minorities. ALTS reports that of the 1,910 women enrolled, 1,102 (57.7 percent) are non-Hispanic whites, whereas 629 (32.9 percent) are African American. Recruitment of other minority groups into this trial, however, is inconsistent: of the women enrolled in the trial, only 65 individuals (3.4 percent) are identified as "white Hispanic" (no data are provided for non-white Hispanic groups), an additional 3.7 percent are Asian, and 2.25 percent are identified as American Indian or Alaska Natives. Figure 5-3 depicts these accrual patterns.

The PLCO trial screens patients for three cancers simultaneously, including prostate, lung, and colorectal cancers for male patients and lung, colorectal, and ovarian cancers for female patients. Of the more than 80,000 participants in this trial, 72,000 (88.9 percent) are white, 3,546 (4.4 percent) are African American, 1,135 (1.4 percent) are Hispanic, 3,505 (4.3 percent) are Asian American, 439 (0.5 percent) are Pacific Islander, and 151 (0.2 percent) are American Indian or Alaska Natives. The rate of

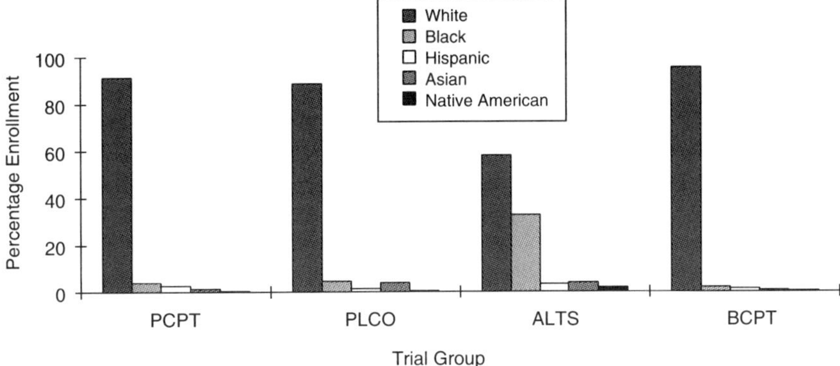

FIGURE 5-3 Enrollment in prevention trials by race/ethnicity.
SOURCE: National Cancer Institute.

accrual of all ethnic minority groups, with the exception of Pacific Islanders, lags behind the percentage of these individuals diagnosed with prostate, lung, colorectal, and ovarian cancers in the United States, according to figures from NCI. NCI reports that among Americans ages 55 to 74 years, the proportion of African Americans diagnosed with prostate, lung, colorectal, and ovarian cancer is 8.7 percent; similarly, the proportions for Hispanics, Asian Americans, and American Indians/Alaska Natives are 3.3, 8.6, and 0.5 percent, respectively. Thus, the rate of accrual of most ethnic minority groups in this trial is two- to threefold lower than the respective incidence of these cancers among these groups.

Similarly, PCPT suffers from a disproportionately low rate of accrual of ethnic minorities. Of the 18,861 patients randomized in this trial as of February 1998, 17,367 (92.1 percent) are white, 709 (3.8 percent) are African American, 500 (2.7 percent) are Hispanic, 157 (less than 0.1 percent) are Asian American, 59 (less than 0.1 percent) are Native American, and 21 (less than 0.01 percent) are Pacific Islander. According to SEER program data (Miller et al., 1996), 10.1 percent of cases of prostate cancer in the United States occur among African Americans. The rate of accrual of this population in PCPT is therefore 2.5 times lower than the national incidence of prostate cancer for this population.

PCPT did, however, provide data on the characteristics of other participants, such as levels of education and income, that may be relevant for targeting cancer control interventions. Of the total sample, 4 percent reported that they had some high school education or less, 15 percent reported only a high school degree, 30 percent reported vocational training or some college education, 16 percent reported a college (bachelor's) degree, and 35 percent reported postgraduate education. The median annual income reported by the sample is $32,000, with 42 percent reporting incomes of $30,000 or less, 49 percent reporting incomes of between $30,000 and $50,000, and 9 percent reporting incomes of greater than $50,000.

BCPT recently yielded data suggesting that tamoxifen may be an effective chemopreventive agent for women at increased risk of breast cancer. This trial, however, which included more than 13,000 women, performed extremely poorly with respect to the accrual of ethnic minorities. Of the 13,266 women enrolled in the trial, 12,630 (95.2 percent) were white, 275 (2.1 percent) were African American, 163 (1.2 percent) were Hispanic, 112 (0.8 percent) were Asian or Pacific Islander, and 33 (0.2 percent) were Native American. According to SEER program data (Miller et al., 1996), African-American women make up 8.2 percent of the population with breast cancer, and Hispanic women make up 3.2 percent of the population with breast cancer. Therefore, for African Americans and Hispanics, the rates of accrual to BCPT were fourfold and almost threefold less, respectively, than the national breast cancer incidence. Asian Americans, Pacific Islanders, and Native Americans were slightly underrepresented in this study, according to national incidence data.

As is the case with the CCOP and MBCCOP prevention trials, the committee finds that the rate of accrual of ethnic minorities into large NIH-sponsored prevention trials in most cases lagged behind that into treatment trials. Especially for African-American and Hispanic populations, the rate of accrual of these groups appeared to be severalfold less than the incidence of the various types of cancer in these groups.

HOW CAN LOW ETHNIC MINORITY ACCRUAL BE ADDRESSED?

The data presented above indicate that NCI has done well in ensuring the proportional representation of ethnic minority individuals in clinical treatment trials. NCI has not enjoyed the same success, however, in accrual the of ethnic minorities in prevention trials. These data underscore the difficulties that researchers face in recruiting and retaining ethnic minority research participants. As noted above, issues of community mistrust of the medical and scientific establishments, researcher reluctance to extend extra effort to recruit ethnic minority and medically underserved populations, and greater costs associated with recruitment are all significant factors in the low rates of accrual. The same difficulties may apply to the recruitment of medically underserved populations, but data are lacking to draw appropriate conclusions. According to NCI's analyses and the experiences of other researchers, several additional factors may contribute to these disparities.

Comorbidity appears to be an important factor that potentially limits enrollment of ethnic minorities in some trials. For example, NCI reports that between 1990 and 1994 there was an overall protocol availability of 20 to 30 percent for adults with newly diagnosed cancers. Eligibility varied by ethnic group, however, because only 33 percent of Hispanics and 40 percent of African Americans were eligible for participation, whereas more than 50 percent of whites were eligible. Ethnic group differences in eligibility were related to the rates of occurrence of comorbid diseases, such as higher rates of hypertension among African Americans. However, after taking into consideration the differences in the extent of comorbidities among the eligible patients, entrance rates did not differ among African Americans (60 percent), whites (62 percent), and Hispanics (70 percent).

Other important factors affecting the rates of recruitment into clinical trials include convenience, costs, conflicts with patient care, complexity, and effect on the patient-physician interaction, including the effects of third-party reimbursement. For example, studies with long-term survivors of pediatric cancers require patients to obtain third-party reimbursement for diagnostic tests such as cardiac echocardiography, which limits accrual of ethnic minorities and low-income populations into these long-term studies. In addition, Medicare and Medicaid health maintenance organization coverage of costs associated with enrollment in a clinical trial is poor and inconsistent, limiting the ability of populations covered by these plans to enter clinical trials.

For prevention trials, researchers face many ethical and practical concerns in recruiting ethnic minority and low-income individuals, especially those who lack insurance coverage or who have inadequate insurance coverage. A patient in whom an abnormality is detected in a screening trial, for example, should receive immediate and appropriate follow-up care. NIH funding for prevention protocols cannot be used for follow-up care of indigent patients. As noted earlier, NCI is attempting to address such downstream costs associated with prevention trials by coordinating with other federal agencies. The committee encourages these efforts and urges greater federal coordination to ensure that downstream costs do not limit the accrual of ethnic minority and low-income individuals.

Recommendation 5-1: NIH and other federal agencies (particularly the Health Care Financing Administration) should continue to coordinate to address funding for clinical trials, particularly to address the additional diagnostic and therapeutic costs associated with prevention trials and third-party payment barriers associated with clinical treatment trials.

Mistrust of biomedical research among many in ethnic minority communities may exacerbate the difficulties associated with their recruitment into prevention trials. Minority individuals who believe themselves to be healthy may experience a greater reluctance to participate in prevention trials, especially if they have no immediate experience with cancer among their family and friends. This wariness may again be traced to the history of medical abuse and exploitation of ethnic minority group members. Despite the considerable patient protections present in human subjects research today, many ethnic minorities, especially older individuals, have firsthand experience with civil rights violations that occurred despite the existence of legal protections that supposedly applied to all Americans. Lessons from these experiences are not likely to be altered, despite the institution of lengthy informed consent procedures (indeed, such procedures may heighten suspicion), especially for individuals who are asymptomatic.

As noted in several of the presentations at the NCI conference on recruitment and Retention of Minority Participants in Clinical Cancer Research (Box 5-1), the informed-consent process should not be seen as a "barrier" to the recruitment of ethnic minority and underserved populations into clinical trials. The informed-consent process is the first step in developing a bond of trust between the researcher and the patient. Improvements in the informed-consent process, particularly alternative means of obtaining consent (e.g., oral consent methods), may help to clarify the research process for potential subjects and help define roles and expectations for both the patient and the researcher. Such alternate means of obtaining consent may also help improve the accrual of populations with low levels of literacy, which may disproportionately include ethnic minority and medically underserved individuals. The committee urges NCI to continue to encourage examination of the informed-consent process.

Recommendation 5-2: NCI should continue to work with other appropriate federal agencies and institutional review boards to explore creative approaches to improving patients' understanding of research and encouraging them to provide consent to participate in research. These approaches should address cultural bias, mistrust, literacy, and other issues that may pose barriers to the participation of ethnic minority and medically underserved groups.

Another potential reason for the low rate of accrual of ethnic minorities in prevention trials is that the physicians who recruit subjects into prevention trials are different from those who recruit subjects into treatment trials. For example, many oncologists are not involved in prevention and screening trials, whereas they are more likely to participate in treatment trials. In addition, investigators with some of the large NCI-supported screening studies, such as the PLCO study, are constrained by the U.S. Office of Management and Budget mandate that a collaborating site must have adequate numbers of patients with all four diseases included as part of the PLCO study. This eliminates centers such as the Veterans Affairs Hospital system as a potential partner, despite the large numbers of people eligible for the prostate, lung, and colon cancer part of the study.

These barriers point to the need for NIH-supported researchers to form partnerships with community-based health service providers and community leaders. In an extensive review of the literature regarding recruitment of ethnic minorities into clinical trials, Swanson and Ward (1995) emphasize the need for researchers to develop community networks, provide community outreach services and programs, establish bonds with community leaders, and recruit as investigators ethnic minority physicians and other health service providers who serve primarily an ethnic minority clientele. Involving community members early in research design and implementation plans can also yield benefits for subject recruitment, as well as for ensuring the smooth operation of a study. Some researchers, for example, have enlisted the cooperation of churches and pastors in African American communities to overcome suspicion of research goals, generate referrals, train lay health workers, and generally promote awareness of healthy behavior. Swanson and Ward, however, note that "contrary to pervasive beliefs about this approach, it is not a panacea for achieving high participation rates of African Americans in clinical trials" (Swanson and Ward, 1995, p. 1753). Multiple approaches and strategies are necessary, they note, to ensure the "buy-in" of community members.

Community-based health care providers and community health clinics, such as the federally supported Community Health Centers (CHCs), offer great potential to researchers as sites to recruit patients and health care providers, to bridge cultural and linguistic gaps between researchers and target populations, and to train new researchers. CHCs serve as primary care providers for more than 9 million low-income patients, many of whom are ethnic minority. NCI support for training, research, and data collection in these settings should be explored not only as a means of increasing the accrual of ethnic minority and medically underserved populations in clinical trials, but also as a point of information dissemination regarding cancer prevention and treatment.

Finally, greater education of researchers is an important component of an overall strategy to improve the rate of recruitment of ethnic minority and medically underserved individuals into clinical trials. Some researchers may not be aware of the importance, from scientific and ethical perspectives, of demographically diverse subject pools; others may reject such goals as "political" or "inconvenient." However, anticipation of when interventions are expected to affect subpopulations differently is critically important. Although it is not known what data are needed to suggest that treatments are likely to affect ethnic minority individuals differently from the ways in which they affect whites, attention to this consideration is needed. More research into the biological, genetic, and pathophysiological considerations of differences in certain cancers among ethnic groups would be helpful in this regard.

Data on the retention of ethnic minorities and medically underserved individuals in treatment and prevention trials have not been addressed in prior NCI reports. Retention in trials, however, is also likely to be problematic for many ethnic minority groups and medically underserved populations. The committee urges routine collection and analysis of data for patients who have dropped out of clinical trials, as well as for those who have been retained, to determine if there are patterns among these groups that may lead to better prediction of who is more likely to drop out and to potential intervention strategies. In addition, the committee urges that NCI require clinical trial investigators to report on the accrual of medically underserved patient populations, including rural residents, low-income individuals, individuals with low levels of literacy, and medically indigent populations. This information should be reported publicly by NCI as part of its effort to inform scientists, health advocates, policy makers, and the general public of progress in clinical trial accrual.

Recommendation 5-3: NCI should report on the accrual and retention of ethnic minority and medically underserved populations in clinical trials using a consistent definition for medically underserved populations, including such characteristics as rural versus urban population, insurance status, socioeconomic status, and level of literacy.

DISSEMINATION OF RESEARCH FINDINGS TO ETHNIC MINORITY AND MEDICALLY UNDERSERVED COMMUNITIES

As noted above, the committee is charged with reporting on "how well research results are communicated and applied to cancer prevention and treatment for minorities." The term *research results* is very vague, ranging from poster sessions at a conference and publications available through a MEDLINE search to clinical practice guidelines. Similarly, the term *dissemination* covers both health care providers and consumers at large. Therefore, for the purposes of this report, the committee interpreted both terms very broadly as the dissemination of scientific information with regard to standards of care. The committee did not separate among cancer prevention, screening and diagnosis, or treatment and follow-up. The committee also looked at literature related to a variety of cancer sites and did not attempt to distinguish between what may be more useful for addressing different types of cancer. For background, the committee reviewed documents provided by NIH, primarily from NCI (these documents are listed in Appendix E). The committee also directed specific questions to NCI and reviewed related research literature.

The remainder of this chapter comprises that report, which is divided into three sections. The first section reviews pertinent research literature. The second section describes examples of dissemination practices by NCI and racial and ethnic patterns of use of the Cancer Information Service (CIS). The third section concludes with recommendations by the committee.

Related Literature on Ethnic Minority and Medically Underserved Populations

The committee's review of the literature reveals that historically, federal, state, and local public health officials have failed to establish specific programs, guidelines, or initiatives to improve health service delivery for minority and medically underserved populations. Significantly, the literature also consistently reveals that ethnic minority and medically underserved individuals are more likely to receive less appropriate or less aggressive treatment for cancer once in the health care system, a fact that may contribute to disparities in cancer survival and mortality.

Studies of disparities in health service delivery indicate that ethnic minority patients, especially African Americans, are less likely to receive appropriate screening, diagnostic, and treatment services for cancer. Some evidence suggests that while "race" and income both predict differences in clinical treatment, "race" may serve as the "overriding determinant of disparities in care" (Geiger, 1996, p. 816). Many such studies have controlled for age, gender, insurance status, income, disease severity, concomitant morbid conditions, and underlying incidence and prevalence rates in the population groups under study. For example, Gornick et al. (1996), in a study of health service delivery to a multi-ethnic population of Medicare beneficiaries, found that African-American patients were less likely than whites to receive mammography. This difference was attenuated modestly when patient income was controlled, although it did not eliminate "racial" differences. While further study is needed to determine whether some of the differences in clinical care are due to other potential confounding factors, such as patient preferences and lack of information about the need for care, the presence of such systemic disparities suggests that racial discrimination by health care providers and institutions, perhaps operating at "unconscious" levels (Gieger, 1996), may be the more likely explanation.

How Can Care Be Improved for Ethnic Minority and Underserved Groups?

The U.S. Preventive Services Task Force is an expert panel established by the federal government in 1984 to develop evidence-based practice guidelines on screening tests and other preventive services (Woolf et al., 1996). The second edition of the *Guide to Clinical Preventive Services* (U.S. Preventive Services Task Force, 1996) does not address multicultural or minority health issues. In the context of patient education, the physician is advised, "In considering a patient's belief system, the provider is challenged to facilitate the bridging of cross-culture gaps as well. Culturally sensitive education and counseling requires that clinicians assess their own cultural beliefs and be aware of local ethnic, regional, and religious beliefs and practices. Such knowledge aids the development of culturally specific health teaching" (U.S. Preventive Services Task Force, 1996, p. 77).

In one study, researchers examined 21 major health data systems of the U.S. Department of Health and Human Services and concluded that data on Hispanics are not included in several departmental national health data collection systems and that even when such data are collected, data on Hispanic subpopulations are found in few of the systems. When available, the databases often do not collect sample sizes adequate for analyzing any one of the four major Hispanic subpopulation. The researchers therefore support the call to collect data on Hispanics in all systems, to provide samples and subsamples large enough for statistical analysis, to support researchers and a research infrastructure for the Hispanic populations, and to support the broad dissemination of findings from the data that are presented in formats that are useful to Hispanic community-based organizations (Delgado and Estrada, 1993). Although the researchers do not address cancer per se, one researcher notes that hypertension is difficult to detect among groups such as Hispanics, for whom an array of impediments, including language and degree of acculturation, may retard the dissemination of information, making it difficult to detect and treat hypertension (Martinez-Maldonado, 1995).

In a survey of chronic disease directors in 50 states, only 16 states (32 percent) reported that they had sponsored or directly supported cancer prevention and cancer control services specifically targeted to American-Indian and Alaska-Native populations. Few state public health agencies had developed culturally relevant cancer education materials for American Indians and Alaska Natives. Although the respondents directed chronic disease or cancer prevention and control programs in their states, many were unfamiliar with the cancer patterns or general health problems among American Indians and Alaska Natives (Michalek and Mahoney, 1994).

The Problem with Guidelines

Legitimate differences of opinion exist, for example, regarding the effectiveness of clinical practice guidelines (e.g., frequency of prostate cancer screening, for which the benefits remain theoretical [Collins and Barry, 1996; Collins et al., 1997]). Several issues are related to efforts to make guideline material useful for patient-specific decision support: (1) incongruity of cancer screening guidelines with local standards, (2) insufficient specificity, (3) insufficient comprehensiveness, and (4) use and dissemination in today's health care environment (Zielstorff et al., 1996).

Despite encouragement from physicians and other health care providers, primary care physicians often do not comply with cancer screening guidelines (Burnett et al., 1995; Greenberg et al., 1996; Guerra et al., 1994; Hovell et al., 1996; Kripalani et al., 1996; Shapira and Levine, 1996). In private-practice settings, the use of preventive medicine services in general has not always been successful. Patient education materials may not be used after they have been ordered and made available to patients. However, several factors that seem to affect the successful implementation of preventive medical services in a clinical setting are often under the control of the physician, such as support from upper levels of administration, "stakeholding" by all of the staff, designation of an individual to manage implementation of a program offering such services, and provision of continuous auditing and feedback to participants (Dickey et al., 1994; Griffith and Rahman, 1994). Although systems for effective physician office-based preventive services can be implemented, they often are not, and strategies for their dissemination may require the involvement of professional medical organizations and managed care companies (Leininger et al., 1996; Simmons and Goforth, 1997).

In fact, it is not clear what factors are both necessary and sufficient to effect change in physician behavior. One 4-year study targeted health care providers in a community receiving an intervention and two control communities. The intervention included the formation of local physician planning groups, mailing of a series of informational packets, provision of medical office staff training sessions, and use of reminder system support. However, the study found no significant postintervention differences in the self-reported ordering of mammographies by physicians practicing in the intervention and control areas. Indeed, over the 4-year study period, routine ordering of mammographies across both groups increased by 36 percent, such that it was ordered for 80 percent of the respondents. The researchers attribute the increase to secular trends resulting from the diffusion of strategies that promoted the use of mammography in general (Taylor et al., 1996). In another study, researchers classified 2,357 Medicaid outpatient barium enemas and 896 outpatient colonoscopic examinations as appropriate, inappropriate, equivocal, or miscoded on the basis of current guidelines in the medical literature. Significantly more colonoscopic examinations were rated as inappropriate, suggesting that more stringent criteria need to be used by physicians in ordering diagnostic examinations of the colon, particularly colonoscopy. The researchers encourage further investigation of the appropriateness, development, and dissemination of such guidelines (Levine et al., 1997).

Physicians are apparently more likely to comply with treatment guidelines than with guidelines related to prevention and screening (Katterhagen, 1996; Olivotto et al., 1997). For instance, negative publicity regarding fraudulent data from a large clinical trial of breast-conserving surgery (BCS) versus modified radical mastectomy apparently did not result in a decline in the rate of use of BCS (Polednak, 1996). However, the only region with an increase in the rate of BCS use from 1986 to 1990 was New England, and in general, use of the guidelines tended to increase only in hospitals that were large and in urban areas, that had higher patient volumes or a cancer center, or that were already using more BCS (Nattinger et al., 1996). In a different study, more disturbing findings indicated that the use of a lumpectomy versus a mastectomy was associated with younger age, private health insurance, and treatment in urban hospitals. Only 45.3 percent of women with Medicaid coverage who had a lumpectomy during the study period received the requisite follow-up radiation therapy, whereas 77.5 percent of private insurance subscribers and 88.1 percent of Medicare beneficiaries had the requisite follow-up radiation. The investigators concluded that research that uses data other than administrative claims data and practice patterns is necessary to determine the reasons for the lack of compliance with treatment protocols by women or physicians (Young et al., 1996).

In fact, significant differences in compliance with practice guidelines can be found between two large hospital providers of cancer services within the same medical community. In one study, a university hospital followed the guidelines more than a community hospital did both before and after publication of an NCI Clinical Alert regarding adjuvant therapy after primary treatment for node-negative breast cancer. The investigators concluded that physician referral patterns influenced the provision of adjuvant therapy, but they also concluded that the process of developing guidelines should include strategies for enhancing compliance with them (Studnicki et al., 1993).

Guidelines themselves must provide more than just a summary of scientific findings; they must make clear recommendations, and their diffusion into general medical practice must involve regional medical groups and their opinion leaders (Starreveld, 1997). The dissemination of standards of treatment may be facilitated (or impeded) by physician and practice setting characteristics such as specialty, affiliation with a CCOP hospital, time in practice, professional centrality (level of participation in cancer information networks), solo practice, and number of colon cancer patients (McFall et al., 1996).

Health behavior is complex, however, and any given behavior often exists among a constellation of other behaviors. One study looked at this relationship in two ways. The researchers compared women 50 to 70 years of age who had received three screening examinations—a clinical breast examination (CBE), mammography, and Pap smear—in the previous 2 years with those who had not received all three examinations. They also compared women who had a Pap smear and at least one breast screening examination (i.e., a mammogram or a CBE) in the previous 2 years with women who were underscreened. Black women were more likely to use screening services in the office setting (i.e., CBE and Pap smear), without a corresponding use of mammography. Nevertheless, more black women than white women received a routine Pap smear in combination with a CBE, a very positive trend with respect to the successful diffusion of at least two screening procedures among older black women. The data suggest that barriers to mammography screening remain even among women who are screened by a CBE and a Pap smear. The researchers point out the need to educate both primary care physicians and their patients that the various components of preventive health are equally necessary and interrelated (Pearlman et al., 1996).

What Works

Many different dissemination and implementation strategies are available; however, traditional passive dissemination methods (for example, publication in professional journals or mailing of practice recommendations to health care professionals) are generally ineffective. Greater attention needs to be given to coordinating active dissemination and implementation strategies to ensure effective professional practice (Grimshaw, 1996). A variety of methods, such as the use of letters of invitation, community mobilization, and mobile service delivery, can be used to increase levels of participation in screening programs (Bryant, 1996). Long-term, ongoing community participation and coalition building in all phases of the research are essential to generating community acceptance of innovative and effective interventions (Matsunaga et al., 1996; Suarez et al., 1993; Ward et al., 1993).

In an example not related to cancer per se (i.e., nursing education and the use of enteral feeding catheters), nurses' primary source of knowledge about the subject was clinical practice (56.9 percent) and consultation with peers (21.7 percent); only 19 percent had received in-service training on the topic. Although written guidelines from the agency varied considerably, two factors significantly associated with use of the guidelines were (1) assistance from pertinent ancillary and support staff and (2) attendance at a relevant seminar or in-service training program. Among their conclusions, the researchers note that research-based guidelines and a more formal means of dissemination of information to clinical staff are needed (Belknap et al., 1997).

The diffusion of new technology is significantly affected by coverage and reimbursement decisions. Medical innovation may improve the quality of health care but may also increase the cost of health care delivery. The Medicare program has a significant influence on the coverage policies of public and private third-party payers. This influence is especially visible in coverage and reimbursement decisions for cancer-related diagnostic procedures and systems. Coverage for these procedures and systems is not widespread because payers have not been convinced of the clinical usefulness of the assays (Logue, 1993).

Clinical practice guideline dissemination or implementation processes have had mixed results. Variables that affect the adoption of guidelines include the quality of the guidelines, the characteristics of the targeted health care professionals, the characteristics of the practice setting, incentives, regulations, and patient-related factors. Specific strategies fall into two categories: primary strategies involving mailing or publication of the actual guidelines and secondary interventional strategies that reinforce the guidelines. Such interventions can be weak (e.g., didactic, traditional continuing medical education and mailings), moderately effective (e.g., audit and feedback, especially concurrent feedback, targeted to specific providers and delivered by peers or opinion leaders), and relatively strong (e.g., reminder systems, academic detailing, and multiple interventions). The evidence shows serious deficiencies in the adoption of clinical practice guidelines in practice. Future implementation strategies must overcome this failure by considering the forces and variables that influence practice and by using methods that are practice and community based rather than didactic (Davis and Taylor-Vaisey, 1997).

Following implementation of a legislative mandate requiring the dissemination of practice guidelines regarding deliveries by cesarean section to obstetric physicians, one study found that the guideline certification program did not accelerate the consistent but gradual downward trend in deliveries by cesarean section that had already been evident in the 3 prior years. The data did suggest a possible greater effect on repeat cesarean deliveries more than on primary cesarean deliveries. The date of guideline implementation reported by hospitals was not related to any systematic change in observed cesarean delivery rates. The researchers conclude that the mere dissemination of practice guidelines by a state agency may not achieve either the magnitude or the specificity of the desired results without an explicit and thorough guideline implementation program. Simple legislative mandates may therefore be ineffective when multiple initiatives are already achieving the desired outcomes (Studnicki et al., 1997).

What Is Needed

In the area of clinical trials, formal overviews or meta-analyses are now widely accepted as reliable means of evaluating the evidence from multiple trials that have assessed a particular form of therapy. Such analyses can have many benefits: the results are particularly clear and therefore have substantial public health impact, the areas of statistical and medical agreement on the evidence can be defined, and the areas of uncertainty (and hence future research priorities) can be clarified prior to the dissemination of the results (Sandercock, 1993).

It has been argued that cancer has lagged behind many other areas of medicine in pursuing outcomes research and management (Weeks and Pfister, 1996). For more than 20 years, studies have documented the substantial geographic variability in medical practice around the United States and have found that such variability is often driven by nonmedical factors. Outcomes management has several key components: the development and implementation of guidelines; measurement, pooling, and dissemination of clinical and outcomes data; and refinement of guidelines on the basis of an analysis of those data. In the case of the National Comprehensive Cancer Network (NCCN), the goal of outcomes research within NCCN member institutions is to pool and analyze selected patterns of care and outcomes data, ultimately creating a uniform outcomes measurement system to monitor guideline compliance (Weeks and Pfister, 1996). Further research, however, is required to determine optimal dissemination strategies and evaluate the impacts of these guidelines (Levine et al., 1996). In workplace environments, there is also a need for better assessment of the effectiveness of information dissemination, along with greater understanding of the barriers to implementation of the information by workers and management and improved hazard surveillance (Fine, 1995).

From the perspective of theory, several gaps regarding diffusion and dissemination should be considered: (1) research, in terms of better understanding of efficacious treatment and alternative treatments as well as prevention; (2) clinical practices, in that practitioners may not be up to date on diagnostic practices, which can be addressed through medical and continuing medical education; and (3) communication, both from the doctor's perspective and from that of the patient, such that health consumers need to be trained in how the medical system works and on how to participate actively in their own care (Bourque, 1996). Arguably, the epidemiologic knowledge of health care workers, media, decision makers, and the general public has improved, and all groups are aware of the main cancer risk factors. Direct assessment of primary prevention activities has proved to be very difficult because many years may pass between the time that the level of exposure to a carcinogen is reduced and the time that the consequences in terms of public health are observed (Hill, 1996).

Although the development of treatment guidelines has evolved a somewhat systematic framework, further research is required to determine optimal dissemination strategies and to evaluate the impacts of these guidelines (Levine et al., 1996). Dissemination and diffusion are complex, long-term endeavors, even within a single institution with multiple sites. In one study that used the context of continuous quality improvement, the intervention arms of the study were training, consultation, networking, and reinforcement for internal multidisciplinary teams as they work through a structured process to understand and improve their clinic's process for providing preventive services. Training alone lasted up to 9 months (Solberg et al., 1996). Given the danger of overloading health care providers with new guidelines, there needs to be a timed strategy for their introduction. Dissemination of guidelines alone is not enough without an appropriate implementation strategy that may require marketing of new ideas to change practice (Forrest et al., 1996).

NCI Cancer Information Dissemination Practices

Of the information supplied to the committee, ethnic minority or medically underserved populations were rarely the targets of specific dissemination activities. The information in general reflect a varied picture of the dissemination process. For instance, consensus development panels are convened to expedite transfer of new knowledge and "medical technologies into the practice of medicine for the benefit of patients." However, one study related to follow-up of a consensus conference on prostate cancer treatment failed to note any consequent change in recommended therapies (Sherman et al., 1992). Clinical Alerts can have an immediate impact on the treatment of certain segments of patient populations (Johnson et al., 1994). Community Clinical Trials Networks can also be used to increase access to cancer care. However, success rates vary with organizational and management styles, the clarity of the goal statement, adequacy of funding, and so forth (Kaluzny et al., 1995b).

The Cancer Information Service as a Dissemination Tool

NCI's CIS is a successful mechanism for cancer information dissemination. According to NCI, the service received 500,000 calls in 1996. In one survey, users tended to be generally very satisfied with the communications from their treating physicians, had strong information needs, and preferred to participate in their treatment plans (Manfredi et al., 1993). However, in that study, 80 percent of the respondents were patients; that is, it was not clear how well CIS disseminates cancer prevention, screening, and early detection guidelines before diagnosis. In addition, no data on the minority status of the users were available.

In addressing these questions, CIS provided the information presented in Tables 5-1 and 5-2. It should be noted that the committee did not formally analyze these data statistically. However, Table 5-1 indicates that less than 15 percent of calls to the CIS telephone service were from minor-

TABLE 5-1 Race or Ethnicity of Callers to CIS Telephone Service (1997)

Race or Ethnic Category	Percentage of Callers	Percentage of U.S. Population
Asians or Pacific Islanders	2.1	3.6
Black (non-Hispanic)	6.0	12.1
Hispanic	4.5	10.7
Native American/Alaska Native	0.9	0.9
White (non-Hispanic)	85.0	72.3
Other/mixed	1.6	

NOTE: Data are for calls to the CIS telephone service (1-800-4-CANCER) in 1997. SOURCE: National Cancer Institute.

TABLE 5-2 Subjects of Inquiry to CIS Telephone Service

Subject	Percentage of Callers
Prevention/risk	4.9
Screening/diagnosis	6.2
Treatment	35.1
Psychosocial	3.3
Site information	19.8
Organizations	5.5
Health professionals	8.1
Support Services	8.5
Other	8.6

NOTE: Data are for calls to the CIS telephone service (1-800-4-CANCER) in 1997. SOURCE: National Cancer Institute.

ities, proportionately less than the proportions of calls from whites. Given the disproportionate incidence of cancer among minority populations, one would hope for appropriately increased numbers of calls from affected groups. For instance, prostate cancer incidence and mortality rates are higher among African-American men than among white men. Compared with white women, African-American women have a lower incidence of breast cancer but higher rates of mortality from breast cancer (American Cancer Society, 1997, 1998). Table 5-2 indicates that treatment topics are addressed much more than are prevention and screening (C. Thomsen, CIS, personal communication, 1998).

Scientific Journal Publications as a Tool for Dissemination

NIH provided a list of 888 scientific journal publications related to cancer among minorities and medically underserved populations that have resulted from awards of programs of NIH in 1985. Having neither the actual publications nor their abstracts in hand, it was difficult to tell how much the articles were in fact related to cancer among ethnic minority and medically underserved populations. The committee therefore analyzed only the titles of the articles listed to determine the distribution of publications across racial and ethnic groups and the number of publications related to dissemination. It should be noted that the categorizations may underestimate references to ethnic minority and medically underserved populations in the articles listed.

The committee examined whether the following specific terms actually appeared in the title:

- *Multicultural:* "race," "racial," "ethnic," "cultural," "multicultural"
- *Not multicultural:* no reference to any such terms at all or clearly indicating only a sample of white, Caucasian, or Anglo individuals.
- *African American:* "African American," "black."
- *Hispanic:* "Hispanic," "Latin/Latino/Latina," "Mexican," "Mexican American," or "Puerto Rican."
- *Asian/Pacific:* "Asian Islander," "Oriental," "Chinese," "Japanese," "Viet-namese," "Hawaiian."
- *American Indian/Alaska Native:* "Native American," "Alaska Native," "tribal."
- *Related to dissemination:* "screening," "education," "guidelines," "media," "disseminate/diffuse."

An article was listed in more than one column if its title included more than one appropriate term, for example, "Hispanic" and "American

Indian." As shown in Table 5-3, starting in 1995, there was a large increase in both the number of publications and the number of titles with some relation to dissemination compared with those in previous years. The reasons for these increases are not clear. For instance, more projects may have been funded, researchers may more frequently have published multiple articles that were based on the same numbers of projects, community and political activism may have increased pressure for both, or there may be other less obvious reasons worth investigating.

Other Sources of Cancer Information

NCI also made available approximately 600 publications and other informational resources. In its response to the Institute of Medicine, NCI listed several examples that are targeted to African-American, Hispanic, Native American, and multiethnic populations. However, no data on the proportion of all materials that are targeted to minority and medically underserved groups were available. The committee did not find any publication comparable to ACS's *Cancer Facts & Figures—1997* (American Cancer Society, 1997), which provided a general comparison of the cancer-related needs of different racial and ethnic groups.

NCI's computerized information systems have been designed to help physicians cope with the information explosion by translating the medical literature into usable forms that are accessible by computer and fax. Systems developed by NCI's International Cancer Information Center provide access to a comprehensive source of bibliographic citations on cancer research (the CANCERLIT database) and to current, peer-reviewed syntheses of state-of-the-art clinical information on cancer (the PDQ database [Hubbard et al., 1995]). However, programs such as the NIH Consensus Development Program and Physician Data Query system have not been shown to have major impacts on treatment patterns (Kosecoff et al., 1987; Lomas et al., 1989). A method that assesses how usage patterns for these programs and systems may vary between minority and nonminority physicians does not seem to exist.

Admitting its lack of experience reaching high-risk populations, particularly those characterized by high proportions of socioeconomically disadvantaged individuals, ACS has begun to fund and provide technical assistance to community demonstration projects, followed by dissemination of model projects to selected ACS divisions with various resources and capabilities (e.g., outreach to high-risk populations, planning, program development, and evaluation) for replication (Corcoran and Robinson, 1994). Since January 1996, NCI has sponsored a series of regional conferences on the recruitment and retention of minorities in clinical trials, in part to promote interaction between community groups and researchers

TABLE 5-3 Articles from NIH-Sponsored Programs Relative to Cancer and Cancer Information Dissemination Among Minority and Medically Underserved Populations by Key Terms in Title

	No. of Articles	Key Term in Title	
Year	Total	Not Multicultural	Multicultural
1997	110	50	28
1996	129	42	20
1995	119	55	13
1994	83	22	12
1993	62	27	27
1992	66	40	10
1991	63	33	2
1990	50	29	3
1989	38	15	5
1988	32	24	2
1987	33	16	2
1986	39	19	3
1985	64	31	8
Total	888	403	135

SOURCE: National Cancer Institute.

to share strategies. There are plans for a future publication about what has been learned through this process. However, it is not clear how NCI identifies successful intervention programs and models or supports their replication. Also, it is not clear whether or how NCI addresses the problem of studying subgroups of target populations.

RECOMMENDATIONS

In Chapter 1 of this report, the committee poses a fundamental question: Is there a strategic plan for reducing the numbers of deaths from cancer among minority and medically underserved populations? If there is a plan, when can results be expected? On the basis of the documentation that the committee reviewed, the committee concludes that such a strategic plan and schedule do not exist. Although NIH has devoted resources to the needs of special populations, with regard to dissemination there is a difference between the delivery of information and the impact of information. The committee could find little to no dissemination research or activ-

African American	Hispanic	Asian/ Pacific	Native American/ Alaska Native	Dissemination
22	7	10	5	26
25	9	11	16	38
17	20	10	4	35
17	9	6	6	2
31	24	12	10	4
22	3	7	2	6
3	5	11	1	
6	4	6		6
5	3	6	5	3
1	2	3		
4	3	3		2
3	6	7	2	
3	6	14	4	1
159	101	106	57	123

ities specifically targeting health care providers who come from minority and medically underserved groups or who, regardless of their own backgrounds, serve those groups. As might be expected, much published research simply describes the results of specific projects or studies. There is little to no documentation of the long-term impacts of these studies for either health care providers or consumers at large. As a result, in the research literature, some investigators have begun to call for the use in dissemination of studies outcomes measurement approaches like those used in clinical studies. This may evolve into something like "clinical guidelines" for dissemination and diffusion.

The overall recommendation of the committee is that NCI and NIH should develop a strategic plan and timetable to address the issues raised in this chapter. The strategic plan should use established cancer guidelines and recommendations in the areas of cancer prevention, screening and early detection, diagnosis, treatment, and follow-up. The strategic plan should provide a "gold standard" against which knowledge, attitudes, and behaviors can be benchmarked across various target populations of health care consumers and providers, regardless of racial, ethnic, or socioeconomic status.

> **Recommendation 5-4: NCI should continue to assess its dissemination practices to identify effective cancer information delivery strategies among ethnic minority and medically underserved populations, revise and implement the strategic dissemination plan on the basis of the results of that research, and institute an ongoing system of monitoring to assess its effectiveness.**

As part of the strategic planning process, NCI and NIH should:

- Establish a formal reporting mechanism, perhaps through the National Cancer Advisory Board or the President's Cancer Panel, on the formulation and achievement of the strategic plan.
- Establish baseline data regarding dissemination research for both researchers and their target populations. For instance, ethnic group and gender data should be recorded regarding (1) the principal investigators submitting research proposals, (2) the principal investigators eventually funded to do research, (3) the populations targeted in research, and (4) the practical impact of funded research on those populations. This process should use scientifically appropriate methods that would not bias the application review process.
- Establish a more structured framework for disseminating cancer guidelines and recommendations both to health care consumers in ethnic minority and medically underserved communities and to the health care professionals who serve them. Among health care professionals, dissemination should target the continuum from undergraduate through postgraduate training and continuing education for those already in practice.
- Establish a more structured framework for monitoring the knowledge and application of cancer guidelines and recommendations by health care consumers and providers, noting differences in minority, nonminority, and medically underserved populations.
- Establish a framework in which implementation of guidelines by both consumers and providers can be planned.

SUMMARY

The committee finds that the inclusion of minority and medically underserved populations in clinical trials and that the dissemination of information to minority and medically underserved communities and their health care providers is a critical link connecting scientific innovation with improvements in health and health care delivery. Enhancing this link is clearly within the purview of NCI and NIH. While many factors pose challenges to improvement (e.g., community mistrust), without a concerted effort to enhance this process, minority and medically underserved communities will continue to lag behind the American "majority" in benefiting from the tremendous recent scientific advancements and medical breakthroughs in cancer prevention, treatment, and control. The following recommendations were offered in this chapter:

Recommendation 5-1: NIH and other federal agencies (particularly the Health Care Financing Administration) should continue to coordinate to address funding for clinical trials, particularly to address the additional diagnostic and therapeutic costs associated with prevention trials and third-party payment barriers associated with clinical treatment trials.

Recommendation 5-2: NCI should continue to work with other appropriate federal agencies and institutional review boards to explore creative approaches to improving patients' understanding of research and encouraging them to provide consent to participate in research. These approaches should address cultural bias, mistrust, literacy, and other issues that may pose barriers to the participation of ethnic minority and medically underserved groups.

Recommendation 5-3: NCI should report on the accrual and retention of ethnic minority and medically underserved populations in clinical trials using a consistent definition for medically underserved populations, including such characteristics as rural versus urban population, insurance status, socioeconomic status, and level of literacy.

Recommendation 5-4: NCI should continue to assess its dissemination practices to identify effective cancer information delivery strategies among ethnic minority and medically underserved populations, revise and implement the strategic dissemination plan on this basis of the results of that research, and institute an ongoing system of monitoring to assess its effectiveness.

6

Cancer Survivorship

The preceding chapter provided an overview of the National Institutes of Health's (NIH's) efforts to apply new knowledge to address the needs of individuals living with or at risk for cancer, whether through research applications in clinical trial settings or through efforts to disseminate information to affected communities and their providers. These efforts would be fruitless, however, without sensitivity to the needs of individuals living with cancer and their families and the unique needs of ethnic minority and medically underserved communities. In this chapter, the committee addresses this aspect of the committee charge: to report on "the adequacy of [NIH's] understanding of survivorship issues that uniquely impact on minority and medically underserved communities."

The term *survivorship* is complex. The literature on cancer survivorship ranges from issues of drug efficacy, clinical trials, and 5-year survival rates to pain management, psychosocial needs, quality of life, religion, and spirituality. Furthermore, the last set of issues often involves the cancer patient's family, friends, and significant others. Consequently, for the purposes of this report, the committee did not attempt to define the term either narrowly or precisely. However, it should be noted that survivorship issues may be considered to exist on a continuum, with quantity of life at one end and quality of life at the other

This chapter is divided into three sections. The first section reviews pertinent research literature on cancer survivorship. The second section describes NIH programs and research relevant to cancer survivorship and information that the committee received from representatives of cancer survivorship groups and community organizations. The final section provides the committee's recommendations.

REVIEW OF RELATED LITERATURE

Improved prevention and detection methods coupled with advances in medical treatment have resulted in increasing numbers of cancer survivors. Today, there are more than 8 million cancer survivors, and for 5 million of these survivors their cancers were diagnosed 5 or more years ago (Beyer, 1995). The term *cancer survivor* means different things to different people, from a minimum—a person who has been free of cancer for 5 or more years—to a maximum—anyone with a history of cancer—beginning at the point of diagnosis and continuing through the rest of life. The latter definition carries with it a range of experiences and interventions that include a variety of programs in patient education, peer support services, exercise modalities, counseling employment services, and long-term follow-up clinics (Johnson, 1995). For example, there is a growing body of discussion regarding the development of free-standing survivor clinics for children and adults (Hollen and Hobbie, 1995). In addition, late effects of multimodality treatments may result in organ compromise or new primary cancers for a growing population of long-term survivors of cancer (Konsler and Jones, 1993).

Cancer survivors often face a range of health-related, financial, social, and psychological needs and concerns that may affect treatment and that may even persist well after diagnosis. One study surveyed the current physical, psychological, and social functional status of a sample of breast cancer survivors 16 months to 32 years from their original surgery for breast cancer. The results revealed that length of survivorship is not necessarily associated with a diminishment of concerns about the cancer. Chronic physical problems, continued thoughts about recurrence, nervousness associated with medical follow-up, concerns regarding health insurance coverage, and other social concerns remain significant issues for many long-term survivors (Polinsky, 1994). In addition, pain due to cancer or its treatment can undermine rehabilitative efforts and detract from quality of life. Pain and pain relief, however, are often overlooked in breast cancer survivors (Newman et al., 1996).

The growing cancer survivorship movement explores the various levels of involvement that cancer patients may choose and provides resources to help individuals and their families improve their survival skills. As a result, many cancer patients are taking more active, assertive roles, demanding second opinions and treatment option information, and seeking partnerships with their physicians in making decisions and managing their overall health care programs (Leigh, 1994, 1996).

Quality of Life

As a research topic, quality of life has evolved over 40 years from early narrative and cross-sectional studies to simple quantitative measures of various parameters, and later by longitudinal studies of greater complexity, to inclusion in randomized clinical trials. Quality of life has become a standard means of assessing clinical outcomes and in clinical trials is an accepted endpoint measurement that is considered alongside patient survival and side effects or complications (Morton, 1995). Measurement of health-related quality of life among cancer survivors is important, but comparison of quality-of-life measurement instruments is needed to clarify which questionnaires are preferable for particular populations or situations (Ferrell et al., 1995; Osoba et al., 1995). In general, however, studies indicate that although cancer survivors experience long-term changes in their overall quality of life after the completion of treatment, many positive benefits that help to balance the worst outcomes may also be gained (Dow et al., 1996).

Cancer affects not only the patient but the entire family unit. Yet, very little research on the impact of cancer and cancer therapy on the family members of patients has been performed (Rivera, 1997). Professionally led support groups are increasing in number, and participation in such groups seems to enhance the quality and possibly even quantity of the patient's survival. However, there has been little research on what type of group may be appropriate for which patients and when in the course of their care that it might be appropriate (Krupnick et al., 1993).

Psychosocial and spiritual factors influence a broad spectrum of medical and surgical disorders, yet the results of studies described in the research literature are inconsistent and the studies themselves are beset with major methodologic problems (Creagan, 1997). One study has shown that for some survivors, the cancer experience elicits a search for meaning, which is significantly associated with self-blame, although well-being scores were not significantly related to this search for meaning (Dirksen, 1995). Other researchers have found that long-term survivors of breast cancer are challenged to redirect their energy from issues of cancer treatment and early side effects toward quality-of-life issues related to long-term survivorship, such as menopause, infertility, fear of recurrence, family distress, and uncertainty (Ferrell and Dow, 1996; Ferrel et al., 1997). These can be categorized into four domains, each with particular areas of concern. In the domain of physical well-being, the areas of worst outcome were in menstrual changes and fertility, fatigue, and pain. In the domain of psychological well-being, predominant needs were in the areas of fear of the spread of cancer, distress from surgery, fear of recurrence, fear of second cancer, impact on self-concept, and fear of future tests. Concerns regarding social well-being are largely related to disruption in the area of family distress, and feelings of uncertainty touch the domain of spiritual well-being. The researchers conclude that there is a need for further research, assessment, and intervention across each of the quality-of-life domains (Ferrell et al., 1996).

Similar issues are raised for long-term gynecologic cancer survivors. There is little information in the literature, however, regarding the clinical issues faced by gynecologic cancer patients who have been free of disease for a period of months to years, especially younger patients (Auchincloss, 1995).

Key variables influencing a patient's response to a cancer diagnosis include cultural views of illness, understanding of the role of medicine, theological and spiritual worldviews, and the sense of identity as expressed in religious ritual practice. Attention to the ethnic and cultural characteristics of the patient with cancer has been shown to enhance the quality of professional intervention (Mark and Roberts, 1994). Although conventional treatments for cancer have been proven to lower mortality rates significantly, patients continue to look for and use alternative therapies. There is little in the literature describing the actual frequency of use of such therapies, nor are there published data regarding the actual popularity of such therapies. One study reanalyzed data for 2,970 patients from the Cancer Survivorship Questionnaire of the 1992 National Health Interview Survey and found that use of additional therapies such as self-healing and psychosocial techniques increased by 63.9 percent after 1987 (Abu-Realh et al., 1996).

Clinical Practice Guidelines

Clinical practice guidelines are usually considered from the perspectives of physicians and other health care providers regarding the management of specific cancers. Ethical questions surrounding their use need to be resolved, however, especially regarding what constitutes quality cancer care and who will define it. The National Coalition of Cancer Survivorship (NCCS) has identified three elements essential to quality cancer care: (1) access to services, (2) appropriate, timely referrals, and (3) access to clinical trials. NCCS makes the case that (1) a goal of practice guidelines should be to help empower patients by educating them about what questions to ask as informed health care consumers, (2) well-researched quantitative and qualitative data on the patient's experience should be used to inform the guideline development process, and (3) guideline developers need to keep in mind that the focus of clinical guidelines is not the disease itself but, rather, the patient with that disease (Stovall, 1996).

Clinical practice guidelines are presented in terms of treatment; however, cancer survivorship is a process rather than a stage or time point. It involves a continuum of events from the time of diagnosis to a time long after treatment has been completed. Although there is little consensus about what underlying processes explain different levels of long-term functioning, health care practitioners can foster consumer empowerment and should incorporate advocacy training into care plans (Clark and Stovall, 1996). Cancer survivors themselves can serve as models to promote cancer prevention and screening. In one example, cancer survivors participated as models in a cancer survivors' fashion show. They tended to report that the experience was very positive for themselves and for their families and friends in attendance, although it was not demonstrated that the participants were effective lay advocates for cancer prevention and screening (Kottke et al., 1996).

NIH AND NCI PROGRAMS AND RESEARCH OUTCOMES RELEVANT TO CANCER SURVIVORSHIP

In preparing this report, the committee reviewed documents provided by NIH, primarily from the National Cancer Institute (NCI). Documentation from NCI indicates a number of activities related to survivorship, including efforts targeted to ethnic minority and medically underserved populations. It is not clear, however, how proportionate the samples are in terms of subgroups, and it is not clear how the research attempts to address issues that may be peculiar to the targeted groups. It is also not clear how NIH specifically addresses or prioritizes the issues raised by the research literature.

In response to a request from the committee, the following program information related to cancer survivorship was provided by NCI:

- A description of the Office of Cancer Survivorship (OCS), which was established in August 1996. The document indicates that 126 grants deal with special and medically underserved populations and that 80 percent of these are investigator-initiated grants (R01 grants). No data on the actual breakdown of the minority and medically underserved populations targeted in funded grants are available, however. For instance, virtually all breast cancer research targets women. However, it is not clear to what degree such research targets ethnic minority and medically underserved women.
- A description of NCI activities with advocacy and voluntary organizations.

• A current program announcement entitled *Cancer Survivorship Studies in Established Epidemiologic Cohorts* (National Cancer Institute, 1998j).

• Agenda for a conference entitled Research Issues in Cancer Survivorship, sponsored by the Division of Cancer Control and Population Sciences of OCS and held on March 9 and 10, 1998.

• Background information from the NCI home page on the World Wide Web, "Creating the Director's Consumer Liaison Group" (DCLG) (National Cancer Institute, 1998f), established in 1997. It is not clear from the information provided how DCLG addresses the needs of ethnic minority and medically underserved groups.

• A list of more than 850 scientific journal publications resulting from awards or programs of NIH relative to cancer among ethnic minority and medically underserved populations since 1985.

NCI Office of Cancer Survivorship

OCS was established in 1996 to serve as a focal point for research and program activities related to the issues faced by cancer survivors. The objectives of OCS were established through a series of workshops and include the following:

• to develop an agenda for the continuous acquisition of knowledge concerning the problems facing cancer survivors, including the medical, psychological, and economic late effects of treatment;

• to support studies that aim to increase the length of survival for cancer patients, including those that involve prevention of subsequent disease and disability;

• to enable the dissemination of information to professionals who provide treatment concerning the problems and needs of cancer survivors;

• to assist in providing information to the public regarding the issues of concern to survivors; and

• to improve the quality of survival of all individuals diagnosed with cancer.

Shortly after the office was established, OCS hosted four workshops to assess the state of research information on cancer survivorship and articulate areas of needed emphasis. Conferees at the first such meeting concluded that the levels of research support then available were inadequate to address the range of survivorship-related research needs in areas such as quality of life, physiological outcomes, second malignancies, reproduction and sexuality, and the economic impact of cancer survival.

These priority areas of emphasis have evolved to shape OCS's current research activities, which include research on the following:

- physiological late effects in cancer survivors 5 or more years after receiving a diagnosis of cancer, including cardiac, renal, and cognitive complications;
- development of long-term follow-up studies of survivors, in concert with cooperative groups, cancer centers, and the Surveillance, Epidemiology, and End Results program registries;
- factors that predispose cancer survivors to the development of second malignancies;
- reproduction and fertility problems following treatment;
- economic issues and questions concerning ongoing medical care; and
- quality-of-life issues, especially among medically underserved populations and long-term survivors.

To assess the state of research in these areas and to make recommendations for future work, OCS sponsored a national scientific meeting on March 9 and 10, 1998. More than 100 investigators and consumers were invited to the conference. An analysis of research findings from abstracts of 64 speaker presentations and poster sessions indicates that only 5 presentations addressed research issues specific to ethnic minority women or offered inter-ethnic group analyses. None of the abstracts was found to address issues specific to medically underserved populations.

In response to a request from the study committee for information regarding cancer survivorship research among ethnic minority and medically underserved populations, OCS staff wrote, "NCI's portfolio is currently looking at issues relevant to all cancer survivors regardless of race. They include quality of life, cancer pain management, the management of side effects due to treatment, rehabilitation, psychological and problem solving, and training for coping with cancer" (National Cancer Institute, Office of Cancer Survivorship, 1998, p. 1).

As noted above, OCS also provided the study committee with a list of 126 current NIH-supported research grants that address survivorship issues among special and medically underserved populations. Only 11 of these research grant titles specifically include terms such as "rural," "black," "Hispanic," "multiethnic," "American Indian," "minority," or "Spanish translation." These research projects appear to be directed toward issues such as cancer pain management, adapting quality-of-life measures for special populations, promotion of self-help, genetic testing and counseling, clinical trials participation, nurse interventions, and coping with cancer risk.

Director's Consumer Liaison Group

As noted in Chapter 4, NCI recently established DCLG for the purpose of establishing a formal mechanism to receive input from cancer survivors and consumer advocates on the NCI cancer research agenda. DCLG advises the NCI Advisory Committee to the Director and provides input in the planning of programs and the establishment of future research directions, in addition to providing NCI with advice and feedback from the consumer community on a broad range of issues. As such, DCLG is expected to participate in providing input to the NCI research priority-setting process, helping to shape the research agenda regarding cancer survivorship, and helping the Institute better inform and receive information from the cancer survivor community. DCLG therefore serves as a conduit between the advocacy and scientific communities.

Also as noted in Chapter 4, the DCLG Planning Group consciously considered ethnic and multicultural diversity among the criteria for the selection of DCLG members (in addition to representation by individuals with cancer at a broad mix of different sites, etc.). NCI appears to have succeeded in this effort, because one-third of the members of the group are ethnic minorities. In its November 6, 1997, press release, NCI notes:

> The majority of the newly appointed DCLG members are cancer survivors, but family members of cancer patients and health professionals involved in cancer advocacy are represented. The cancer experience of the group includes prostate, breast, kidney, ovarian, cervical, lung, bladder, and brain cancer, Hodgkin's disease, leukemia, sarcoma, and myeloma. The group includes Asian American, Native American, Hispanic, African American, and non-Hispanic white persons, the young and the old, men and women, and people from all geographic areas of the country, both rural and urban (National Cancer Institute, 1997c).

Although at least one of the DCLG members appears to be from a non-urban community (Missoula, Montana), it is unclear whether other rural or medically underserved populations are represented. Nonetheless, DCLG's composition suggests that the panel may prove to be an effective mechanism for highlighting the research and program needs of ethnic minority and medically underserved cancer survivors. Furthermore, as noted in Chapter 4, the conscious attention to diversity and the inclusion of ethnic minority and medically underserved individuals on the panel serves as an excellent model for addressing the compositions of other scientific and review panels at NIH.

Dissemination of Information to Cancer Survivors

As noted in Chapter 3, NCI has established a number of offices, programs, and mechanisms for outreach to cancer survivors and consumers, including several programs and services tailored to the needs of ethnic minority and medically underserved communities. These will not be described in detail here (see Chapter 3 for a full description of these programs). NCI's Cancer Information Service (CIS), however, deserves greater attention, given its prominence as a primary source of information for many cancer survivors.

CIS is a successful avenue for cancer information dissemination. According to NCI, the service received 500,000 calls in 1996. In one survey, in which 80 percent of the respondents were patients, users tended to be generally very satisfied with communication from their treating physicians, had strong information needs, and preferred to participate in their treatment plans (Manfredi et al., 1993). However, no data on the ethnic minority status of the users were provided.

CIS provided information on calls to its toll-free telephone service. These data are summarized in Tables 5-1 and 5-2 in Chapter 5. It should be noted that the committee did not formally analyze these data statistically (i.e., it did not compare the observed patterns of calls with the expected frequencies on the basis of an analysis of cancer incidence among the U.S. population). However, Table 5-1 indicates that approximately 15 percent of calls to the CIS telephone service were from ethnic minorities. Because ethnic minorities make up about 28 percent of the U.S. population, however, it appears that ethnic minorities are proportionately less likely to use CIS services than whites. Given the disproportionate incidence of cancer among some ethnic minority populations, one would hope for appropriately increased numbers of calls from affected groups.

Published Research Related to Survivorship

NIH provided a list of more than 850 scientific journal publications related to cancer among minority and medically underserved populations that have resulted from awards or programs of NIH since 1985. The committee analyzed only the titles of the articles listed to determine the distribution of publications across racial and ethnic groups and the number of publications related to cancer survivorship. It should be noted that the categorizations may underestimate references to ethnic minority and medically underserved populations in the articles listed. The committee examined whether the indicated specific terms in the following categories actually appeared in the title:

• *Multicultural:* "race," "racial," "ethnic," "cultural," "multicultural."

• *Not Multicultural:* no reference to any such terms at all or clearly indicating only a sample of white, Caucasian, or Anglo individuals.

• *African American:* "African American," "black."

• *Hispanic:* "Hispanic," "Latin/Latino/Latina," "Mexican," "Mexican American," or "Puerto Rican."

• *Asian/Pacific:* "Asian Islander," "Oriental," "Chinese," "Japanese," "Vietnamese," "Hawaiian."

• *American Indian/Alaska Native:* "Native American," "American Indian," "Alaska Native," "tribal."

• *Related to dissemination:* "screening," "education," "guidelines," "media," "disseminate/diffuse."

An article was listed in more than one column in Table 6-1 if its title included more than one appropriate term, for example, "Hispanic" and "American Indian." As indicated in Table 6-1, starting in 1995, there were large increases in both the number of publications and the number of titles with some relation to dissemination compared with the numbers in previous years. The reasons for these increases are not clear, but several possibilities are apparent: since the mid-1980s NCI has funded an increasing number of research projects related to ethnic minority and medically underserved populations, resulting in an increase in the number of related publications; researchers may have published at a greater frequency multiple articles that were based on the same numbers of projects performed in previous years; and community and political activism may have increased the pressure for both. Other, less obvious reasons may also be worth investigating.

NEEDS OF ETHNIC MINORITY AND MEDICALLY UNDERSERVED CANCER SURVIVORS

As noted in Chapter 4, the committee sought to better understand the needs of ethnic minority and medically underserved cancer survivors and the perceptions of NIH programs and research activities among individuals in these communities by holding a public meeting at which testimony was received from representatives of several community-based cancer prevention and health promotion organizations. These individuals are identified and their comments are summarized in Chapter 4. However, some of the testimony presented at that meeting relates directly to the experience of cancer survivors (two of the panelists were breast cancer survivors, and another experienced the loss of a close family member due to cancer). These comments, along with the panelists' recommendations, are summarized below.

TABLE 6-1 Articles from NIH-Sponsored Programs Relative to Cancer Among Minority and Medically Underserved Populations by Key Terms in Title

	No. of Articles	Key Term in Title	
Year	Total	Not Multicultural	Multicultural
1997	110	50	28
1996	129	42	20
1995	119	55	13
1994	83	22	12
1993	62	27	27
1992	66	40	10
1991	63	33	2
1990	50	29	3
1989	38	15	5
1988	32	24	2
1987	33	16	2
1986	39	19	3
1985	64	31	8
Total	888	403	135

SOURCE: National Cancer Institute.

1. Dissemination of cancer information to ethnic minority and medically underserved groups requires more than a simple translation of materials.

Venus Gines and Lucy Young noted that when they were first diagnosed with breast cancer, they had a difficult time finding information in their native languages (Spanish and Chinese, respectively) that addressed concerns particular to their cultural groups. Gines noted that what she did find was merely translated from English. Such translations, she noted, often fail to address specific concerns that may be more common among some ethnic groups (such as the fatalism regarding a cancer diagnosis that exists among some Hispanic populations) or that fail to take into account cultural differences in the ways in which information is best communicated. In response, Gines, in collaboration with the American Cancer Society, developed Mi Nueva Esperanza (My New Hope) to provide information regarding breast cancer among Hispanic women. The booklet is written in clear, simple Spanish but also uses pictures to convey information.

2. Cancer education materials must be made available in languages other than English and Spanish.

African American	Hispanic	Asian/ Pacific	Native American/ Alaska Native	Related to Survivorship
22	7	10	5	9
25	9	11	16	15
17	20	10	4	5
17	9	6	6	4
31	24	12	10	8
22	3	7	2	1
3	5	11	1	2
6	4	6		2
5	3	6	5	1
1	2	3		
4	3	3	2	1
3	6	7	2	
3	6	14	4	
159	101	106	57	48

On the basis of information provided to the study committee, it appears that most non-English-language NCI publications for cancer survivors are in Spanish. The committee found few examples of materials printed in other languages that are increasingly spoken in multiethnic America, such as Asian and Southeast Asian languages. This observation was supported by Lucy Young, who expressed frustration at the lack of Chinese-language cancer education materials. Her organization (the Chinese American Cancer Society) has had to import Chinese-language cancer education materials or provide resources for the translation of information generated in English.

3. Members of ethnic minority and medically underserved communities, especially cancer survivors, can serve as a valuable resource in reaching other members of their communities.

Barbara Clinton noted that research on the efficacy of lay community health workers is lacking. These individuals, she stated, often have experience in dealing with cultural aspects of the disease (e.g., fear of public acknowledgment of a cancer diagnosis), but they can also help patients deal with the maze of treatment options, providers, and other medical choices. Cancer survivors from ethnic minority and medically underserved communities may be especially helpful at destigmatizing the disease, providing social support, and "normalizing" psychological reactions following diagnosis.

The following recommendations were summarized in Chapter 4 but are relevant for the consideration of survivorship needs and are therefore restated here:

4. Greater sensitivity to culturally appropriate outreach efforts is needed.

All of the panelists noted that problems of stigmatization, fatalism, isolation and lack of social supports following a diagnosis of cancer, and mistrust of the medical and scientific establishment, although present in the majority population, may be especially prevalent and problematic among ethnic minority and medically underserved communities. These issues affect almost all aspects of cancer treatment and control among these populations, including cancer screening behavior, decisions to seek treatment, compliance with medical regimens, and so forth. More research is needed to understand the nature of these social and belief systems and to develop appropriate interventions. For example, as noted earlier in this report, community-based health centers may serve an invaluable function in reducing isolation and increasing social support among ethnic minorities diagnosed with cancer; the role of such centers as vehicles for increasing social support (and other behavioral interventions) should be studied. An adequate understanding of these issues will also help to shape efforts at outreach to minority and underserved communities.

5. NCI should develop a strategic plan to address the survivorship needs of ethnic minority communities.

This recommendation cuts across all of the recommendations put forth by the panel. As Young noted, such a strategic plan would begin with an assessment of the needs of specific ethnic and cultural groups and would be followed by a proposal to better tailor research efforts and to serve members of affected communities and their health care providers. Working closely with grassroots organizations, according to Young, is a key component of such an effort.

RECOMMENDATIONS

Cancer survivors are, in the committee's view, perhaps the most underused resource in the War on Cancer. This is especially true among ethnic minority and medically underserved populations, who face numerous cultural, socioeconomic, and in some cases, institutionalized racial barriers to cancer prevention and treatment services (i.e., poor or less adequate medical treatment and services are provided to minorities than to whites [Sullivan, 1991]). As noted by the panel of representatives of community group and cancer survivorship organizations that appeared before the committee, ethnic minority cancer survivors are often painfully aware of the lack of services and information that might assist neighbors, friends, and relatives with either avoiding or coping with a cancer diagnosis. Perhaps more importantly, however, they possess critical expertise in how to reach members of their communities with cancer education information. This expertise should be tapped to the fullest extent possible.

To its credit, NCI has established an impressive infrastructure of programs and resources to assist cancer survivors. The OCS, as noted above, has convened a conference to delineate research issues related to cancer survivorship and to coordinate NCI's survivorship-related activities. The newly established DCLG advises the NCI director on a number of consumer-related issues that affect NCI's survivorship research portfolio. In addition, NCI's Office of Cancer Information, Communication, and Cancer Education has performed a number of outreach efforts tailored to specific communities. Greater attention must be paid, however, to the unique needs of ethnic minority and medically underserved communities. As highlighted by the panel of representatives of community group and cancer survivorship organizations that appeared before the committee, NCI's outreach efforts must address problems such as fatalism regarding a cancer diagnosis in some ethnic minority communities; isolation and lack of social supports, especially among individuals who are diagnosed with cancer and who live in rural or other medically underserved communities; mistrust of medical research by many ethnic minorities who retain memories of abusive and unethical research; a lack of visibility among NCI-sponsored researchers in ethnic minority and medically underserved communities; financial and time constraints and a lack of reinforcement for researchers who seek to work in and with underserved communities; a perception that community-based organizations are discouraged from applying for research funding from NCI; and many other issues.

The overall recommendation of the committee is that NCI and NIH should develop a strategic plan and timetable to address proactively and systematically the cancer survivorship issues raised in this report. The strategic plan should provide a "gold standard" against which to benchmark knowledge, attitudes, and behaviors across various target populations of health care consumers and providers.

Recommendation 6-1: NCI should establish a strategic plan to address the cancer survivorship needs of ethnic minority and medically underserved groups, including coordination of an overall re-

search agenda on survivorship and a more structured framework for monitoring knowledge, attitudes, and behavior regarding cancer survivorship.

As part of the strategic planning process, NCI and NIH should:

- Establish a research agenda to elucidate the issues related to cancer survivorship. This research agenda should at least aim to distinguish between and clarify the relationship between physical therapeutics and quality-of-life issues and the degree to which those issues may be generic for all cancer patients or may vary according to factors unique to ethnic minority and medically underserved populations.
- Develop a plan to improve the development and dissemination of cancer information to ethnic minority and medically underserved groups. Such a plan should increase the participation of cancer survivors from ethnic minority and medically underserved groups in outreach efforts. In addition, NCI should improve its efforts at the development of printed information about cancer by expanding the number of materials translated into languages other than Spanish (e.g., Asian and Southeast Asian languages) and ensuring that straight translation is not performed without attending to the possible loss of information and the cultural appropriateness of the translation.
- Establish baseline data regarding cancer survivorship research as it targets and affects ethnic minority and medically underserved populations. As noted in previous chapters, this will require a consistent definition of "medically underserved" groups and active efforts to collect data on these populations.
- Establish a more structured framework for the dissemination of cancer survivorship research findings, targeting health care consumers, survivors, and the significant others of survivors in minority and medically underserved communities as well as the health care providers who serve them.
- Establish a more structured framework for monitoring the knowledge, attitudes, and behaviors regarding cancer survivorship among health care consumers, survivors, and the significant others of survivors in ethnic minority and medically underserved communities, as well as the health care providers who serve them. As noted above and in Chapter 5, some of this can be accomplished through the cancer supplement of the National Health Interview Survey, which asks individuals who have been diagnosed with cancer questions regarding the use of psychosocial support systems (e.g., "After your cancer was diagnosed, did you receive any counseling or join any support groups to help you cope?") and sources of information to learn more about the disease (e.g., "Did a doctor, nurse, or social worker

give you written information about your cancer or its treatment?"). Ethnic group differences in response to these and other questions may be useful in obtaining an understanding of the unique needs of ethnic minority and medically underserved communities and tailoring survivorship-related research and programs.

7

Monitoring and Reporting

In addition to the specific aspects of the study charge addressed in earlier chapters of this report, this committee was charged with making recommendations on the creation of an annual reporting mechanism on the status of cancer research among ethnic minority and medically underserved populations. This chapter offers a discussion of the different measures of process (e.g., the number of research grants targeted to the study of cancer in ethnic minority and medically underserved populations) and outcomes (e.g., cancer incidence and mortality statistics) that could be included in such a report and provides relevant recommendations.

The committee first reviewed prior congressional requests relevant to the reporting of cancer research in general. A prior Senate Committee on Appropriations had expressed concern about the increasing incidence of cancer and rates of mortality from cancer, especially among people ages 55 and older (U.S. Congress, Senate, 1990). Although the Senate committee commended the National Cancer Institute (NCI) for its "success in generating information and understanding of many fundamental biological processes at the cellular and molecular levels" (p. 89), it was concerned that the translation of this information into better prevention and treatment had not resulted in decreased rates of mortality. It requested that NCI convene a special committee to recommend the most appropriate measures for assessing progress against cancer.

In appropriating funds for the National Institutes of Health (NIH) for fiscal year 1997 (P.L 104-208), the Senate Appropriations Subcommittee on Labor, Health and Human Services, and Education focused on cancer in ethnic minority and medically underserved populations. The legislation stated that "cancer crosses all groups in America, but often takes its deadliest toll among minorities and the medically underserved." As examples, it quoted a higher rates of cervical cancer among Hispanic women and prostate cancer among African-American men, and lower rates of survival from lung cancer among Native Americans. The latter Senate committee expressed similar concern about cancer among ethnic minority and medically underserved populations that the prior Senate Committee on Appropriations had expressed about cancer among older members of the general population. It recognized that NIH support for research, training, recruitment, and information dissemination regarding minority health issues had improved; but it was concerned that this segment of the population continued to experience disproportionately higher risks for cancer. The Senate committee believed that "the gravity of this issue demands that every appropriate effort be taken to ensure that the programs and the activities of the Nation's chief medical research institution produce long-term gains against cancer that will benefit all Americans."

Both Senate committees sought a better mechanism for monitoring and reporting of results that will affirm a commitment to equity. For this reason the Institute of Medicine Committee on Cancer Research Among Minorities and the Medically Underserved reviewed the response to the previous Senate Committee on Appropriations request for information on cancer among older Americans, with the hope that the mechanisms suggested for reporting on ethnic minority and medically underserved populations would be consistent with the mechanism for reporting on the rest of the population. In accordance with the Senate request for information on older Americans, the Extramural Committee, chaired by Lester Breslow, was formed to assess measures of progress against cancer (Extramural Committee to Assess Measures of Progress Against Cancer, 1990). That committee approached the problem of reporting from the perspective of linking the population with the problem of cancer and linking the processes of cancer intervention with measurable results. Similarly, this chapter first discusses the reporting of results and then discusses the reporting of certain processes in cancer research that relate specifically to ethnic minority and medically underserved populations. The committee distinguishes between monitoring and reporting, the former being a continuous activity, and the latter serving an intermittent activity.

REPORTING OF RESULTS

Ethnic Minority Groups

At the beginning of the 20th century, health statistics classified the U.S. population into two groups: the white population and everyone else, who were simply non-white. By about the middle of the century, African Americans were recognized as a specific group. During the civil rights movement, however, there was not consensus, even among African Americans, about the use of racial designations. Some felt that racial designations would be used to support racism, but others thought that the use of racial designations was useful for purposes of health planning and assessing the improvement of health status. At this time, the cancer mortality rate among African Americans was just beginning to exceed that among whites. Classification schemes were totally based on race, and Hispanics were not identified. There was a further problem of classification when Hispanics were identified, because they did not fit the usual racial designations. As a result it was necessary to further identify Hispanic whites and non-Hispanic whites. The classification then became racial and ethnic. All other ethnic groups were included in the "Other" category.

With the increasing diversity of the U.S. population, it has become clear that racial designations are inadequate, confusing, and misleading. At the same time there is increasing demand to recognize the identities of the various ethnic groups included in the U.S. population. Until recently there was no routine reporting on cancer among ethnic minorities other than African Americans. This was corrected by the Surveillance, Epidemiology, and End Result (SEER) program monograph entitled *Racial/Ethnic Patterns of Cancer in the United States 1988–1992* (Miller et al., 1996). That report, however, does not include data on the medically underserved population, and the source documents from which reports such as that of Miller et al. (1996) are prepared do not provide such information. The problem, then, is to find a method of reporting on cancer information that routinely includes data on ethnic minority and medically underserved populations without at the same time producing an excessive amount of data.

Health statistics are usually described as rates that are calculated from a numerator (numbers of people affected) and a denominator (the numbers of people in the population at large). The denominator is discussed first. In classifying the population, the committee has taken into account the fact that the census and all government agencies must conform to U.S. Office of Management and Budget (OMB) Directive No. 15 (U.S. Office of Management and Budget, 1977) and subsequent revisions. That classification reflects the old notions of four races. An important change would be to discontinue use of the old and divisive racial classifications and to recognize the scientific view that all humans are members of one race. The population would then be classified into ethnic groups. Under this arrangement, Hispanics and whites would not be divided. One may choose to be identified either as Hispanic or as white. Pending this change, NCI could simply omit the term "racial" from its titles without doing any harm to the War on Cancer or acting in violation of OMB Directive No. 15. All Hispanics would then be classified as Hispanics or whites by self-identification. This would also allow NCI to avoid violating another important principle of classification: that the categories be mutually exclusive and totally exhaustive. It should not be possible for a person to be placed into two different groups simultaneously, and the system should accommodate the entire population.

This change would not be merely semantic, because it would avoid some of the ambiguity that currently decreases the reliability of calculations. Data for all ethnic groups could be reported in this way, but because of the increasing diversity of the U.S. population, it would still be necessary to aggregate small population groups into "macro-ethnic" groups. As noted earlier, "macro-ethnic" groups include, for example, Asian-American populations (whose subgroups include individuals of Chinese, Japanese, Korean, Indian, Southeast Asian, and other Asian descent). This becomes important because in the smallest population groups the number of cases of cancer will be small and the calculated rates will be unstable or unreliable. In addition, in reporting on ethnic minorities it is useful to present data on the rest of the population to make the classification complete for purposes of comparison.

The top margin of a summary table on cancer mortality could be as follows:

Ethnic Group A	Ethnic Group B	Ethnic Group C	Ethnic Group D	All Others	Total

Medically Underserved Populations

Data on the medically underserved population are not usually included in cancer statistics reports. The information could be obtained by revision of the source documents to include the necessary data or by special studies. Implementation of the required changes will take time, but the revision of source documents would have a more permanent effect. The source document for calculating incidence could be modified to include this information. Retrieval of the information from the death certificate may be more problematic. For this reason it may be better to obtain the necessary data from the cancer incidence registries. Data may come from other databases such as those that are part of the Medicare program, but in that case, it would also be necessary to extrapolate the data to the general population. There may also be some differences of opinion about what should characterize the status of medically underserved individuals. Possible factors could include socioeconomic status, access to care, or occupation. The National Center for Health Statistics (NCHS) is already exploring ways of providing such information, as reported in *Health United States, 1998* (National Center for Health Statistics, 1998).

Ideally, it would be best if the medically underserved status could be displayed in the same table with the ethnic group status, since the medically underserved status would cut across all ethnic groups. In that case the data for medically underserved and non-medically underserved individuals would be shown for each ethnic group. For the sake of clarity, however, it might be best to show the relationship between the two variables and cancer in separate tables, and until the data for medically underserved individuals can be incorporated into source documents, it may be necessary to obtain the information by performing special studies or by linkage with other databases.

Many Cancer Sites

Cancer is not a single disease, and the complexity of the disease combined with the increasing diversity of the population makes it necessary to group various forms of cancer for purposes of planning and control, in the same way that it is necessary to aggregate smaller ethnic groups into macro-ethnic groups. It is customary to focus on those forms of cancer that present the greatest risk because of the magnitude and severity of the problems involved. In recent years the major causes of death from cancer in the United States among all ethnic groups have been cancers involving the lung, female breast, prostate, and colon-rectum. It is important that these forms of cancer be identified when one attempts to assess progress against cancer for the nation as a whole. If one ranked the top five causes of death for each ethnic group, however, the list would be different for each ethnic group, and herein lies the importance of monitoring and reporting on cancer among different ethnic groups. Cancer of the cervix, for example, is not among the five leading causes of death among white women, but it is among African-American women. It may also be among the top five for white women who are medically underserved, but this group is not currently considered in reports of the causes of death. Cancer of the breast is the leading cause of cancer death among Hispanic women, but cancer of the lung is the leading cause of cancer death among white women. If one groups the categories by giving priority to the burden of cancer, then all the major causes of death for all ethnic groups must be included. Although cancers at many sites are continuously monitored, reporting should routinely focus on the sites associated with the greatest burden of cancer while aggregating data on cancers at other sites.

Aggregation of deaths from cancer from those causing the highest rate of mortality to those causing the lowest rate of mortality is only one approach to the problem. The Breslow Committee suggested consideration of three other alternatives: cancers that can be grouped according to preventable cancers, cancers that can be controlled by timely screening and detection, and cancers against which efficacious treatments exist (Extramural Committee to Assess Measures of Progress Against Cancer, 1990). These alternatives would facilitate easy linkage to the present state of knowledge and practice with respect to prevention, control, and treatment. Whatever aggregation method is used, the objective would be to avoid the overwhelming amount of data that would be accumulated if the data included all possible types of cancer for all ethnic groups. As in the case of the group by ethnic groups, the aggregation should include entries for "all other sites" and for total sites.

The left margin of the table would then appear as follows:

Site A

Site B

Site C

Site D

All other

All sites

Reporting on Mortality

Despite the problems associated with recording and coding of deaths, the mortality data remain the most important measure of success of the efforts being made against cancer. The denominator data for calculation of the rates are derived from the census and the numerator data are derived from death certificates. The mortality data are obtained from NCHS of the Centers for Disease Control and Prevention. Reported data would be the most recent available, which currently means information on events that occurred 2 or more years prior to publication. A separate table could then show changes in mortality, and it is the change or lack of change that becomes the basis for discussions about progress. For those who are intimidated by statistics, presentation of the same trends in graphical form may be important.

Another alternative is to present the data in terms of "potential reduction of deaths." Various ethnic groups experience different rates of mortality from cancer at different sites. The reasons for these differences are not always clear, but one could construct a hypothetical U.S. population based on the lowest rates of each of the leading causes of cancer in any ethnic group. Using this as a reference population, one could compare the number of deaths that now occur in each ethnic group with the number of deaths that would have occurred in the hypothetical population with the best rates at major sites drawn from any ethnic group. The difference between the number of deaths that occurred and the number that would have occurred in the hypothetical population would be the potential reduction. This could also be expressed as the percent potential reduction, and it would be the goal of the cancer program to approach the "all American best rate" for all ethnic groups.

The committee asked NCHS to do such calculations, and their findings are significant (Figure 7-1). The total observed annual numbers of deaths from cancer among men for the period covered (1990 to 1995) was 276,146, but if the rate of cancer among all Americans was the lowest rate of cancer for any ethnic group, the expected number of deaths among men would have been 137,476. This is a potential reduction of 138,670 deaths, or 50 percent. The potential reduction for women was comparable. The white population, because of its majority size, would have experienced the greatest reduction in the number of deaths. The African-American population would have experienced the greatest percent reduction because of its greater burden of cancer. A more rigorous study of cancer among the various ethnic groups of the United States would be of great help in achieving the potential reduction in the numbers of deaths from cancer. Each ethnic group could set its own target on the basis of its own potential reduction and participate fully in the effort to reach the target. In the same manner, targets can be set for the medically underserved population when data are collected for this group.

The entire report (National Center for Health Statistics, 1998) of NCHS is included in Appendix F, but the caveats deserve special consideration, and are fully stated here.

1. Quality of data varies by "race" and ethnicity in both death certificate and Census data. The quality of data for the white and the African-American populations are good in contrast to that for other groups. American Indian data are estimated to be underreported by about 10 percent. With respect to population data, perhaps the most serious problem is the

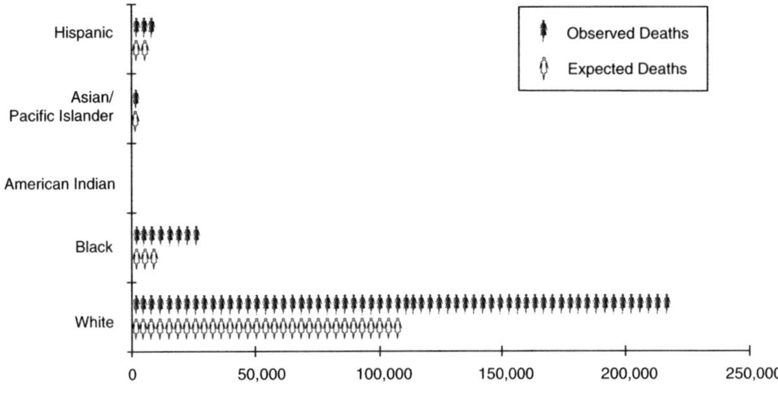

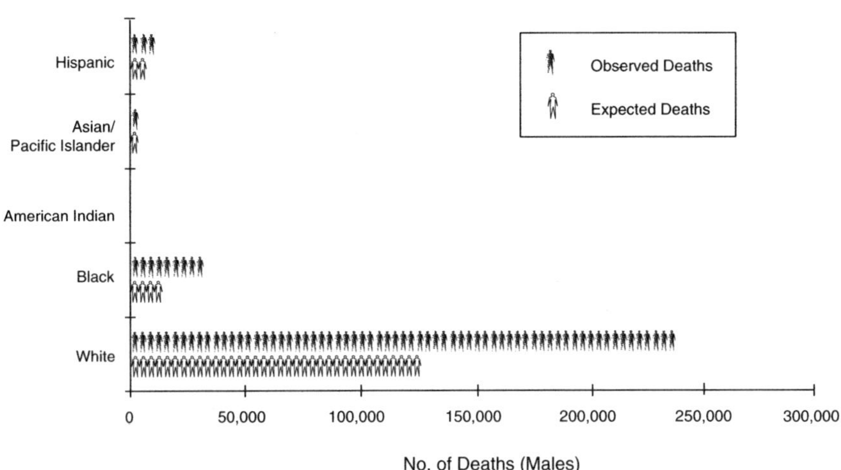

FIGURE 7-1 Estimated average annual excess deaths due to cancer by U.S. ethnic group, 1990–1995. SOURCE: National Center for Health Statistics.

reported 33 percent increase in the American Indian population between 1960 and 1990 that reflects increased preference to self-report as an American Indian.

2. Age-specific death rates, especially those for the elderly, are underreported.

3. Hispanic origin and "race" are separate items. NCHS picked the best rates going across these two variables, but show the deaths for both Hispanic origin and "race."

4. Hispanic origin was not reported on all state death certificates in this time period. The rates used in the calculation were based on 46 states and the District of Columbia. The observed death count was inflated to a national total by using the reciprocal of the fraction of the Hispanic population living in these 46 states and D.C.

5. The number of events, particularly at young ages for certain ethnic minority groups, are small. This would affect the stability of the rates. To counter that tendency, NCHS used data for the 1991-95 time period. In the summary table, NCHS has expressed the number of deaths in terms of a single year of data.

6. The reduction for all cancer sites combined differs depending on whether the values are summed across specific sites or is done separately. The reduction is greater when the values are summed.

These cautions are valid regardless of the approach that is used and serve to indicate the limitations of the data that one continuously faces. Any or all of the methods could be used whether the primary focus is on the general population, on ethnic minority groups, or on the medically underserved population.

It may be useful to present the information in several forms. Another method would be to measure progress against the objectives defined for the nation, such as the objectives outlined in *Healthy People 2000* (U.S. Public Health Services, 1991) or Healthy People 2010. The national objectives are set on the basis of what is known to be preventable. Objectives were set for total cancers and for cancers of the lung, breast, cervix, and colon-rectum. The objectives were based on the assumptions of improved tobacco control, increased rates of use of mammography and the Pap smear, and both the early detection of and improvements in treatments for colorectal cancer. Goals were not set for prostate cancer, awaiting evidence of methods of effective prevention or treatment. In some cases Healthy People has set specific targets for some ethnic minority groups.

The summary data can be refined and presented in separate tables on the distribution of cancer by age and sex for each ethnic group, averages over a specific period, annual rates, and trends over a prolonged period. The trends in mortality are very important because this is a matter of prime interest to Congress and to the public at large. For example, Congressman Louis Stokes has repeatedly asked at appropriations hearings about the rate of mortality from cancer among African Americans. He is quoted as having recently asked the director of NCI the following question on behalf of the American people: "Last year, you told us that African American men had the highest rate of prostate cancer in the world. Is that still the situation?" (Cancer Letter, 1998). This is one reason why the trends in mortality should be the primary basis of reports to Congress. A graph showing trends is often more powerful than a large display of numbers. The trends may show progress, no progress, or a worsening of the cancer problem.

Other Measures of Progress

In addition to mortality it is important to include information on trends in incidence and survival. If either prevention or treatment has not been able to be affected, the mortality rate will be unchanged. Under these circumstances it is helpful to be able to explain that even though the case fatality rate is unchanged, there has been an improvement in the length of survival. Sometimes this improvement is small, measured in days to a few months, but sometimes differences in lengths of survival provide clues to patterns of cancer treatment and access to cancer care, and increased lengths of survival may be important, especially if the quality of life is good. In the attempt to explain changes in the rates of mortality from cancer among the various ethnic groups, it is therefore necessary to present evidence not only on mortality but also on incidence and survival.

The incidence and survival data are provided by the SEER program at NCI and are usually presented in the same format as the mortality data, in which the rates for various cancer sites and ethnic groups are presented, and the data are refined to show distributions by age and gender. The Breslow Committee indicated that the SEER program's system is of very high quality but did "not provide sufficient data about the occurrence of cancer in important segments of the population" (Breslow et al., 1990, p. 827). This would have been true with respect to ethnic minority and medically underserved populations. This problem has been partially addressed by a report that appeared in 1996, *Racial/Ethnic Patterns of Cancer in the United States 1988-1992* (Miller et al., 1996). In discussing the incidence data, it is necessary to emphasize what progress in increasing the efficacy of prevention efforts has been made and how this progress could influence the incidence of cancer reported for each ethnic group. This would relate the knowledge to the statistical findings and especially to the mortality data.

It is then helpful to provide information on early detection, treatment, and survival. This could be related to current knowledge about carcinogenesis, early detection, and treatment and to steps that could alter the outcome. As in the case of mortality data, the incidence and survival data report events that may be 2 or 3 years older than current knowledge. These data are associated with their own set of problems that are different from those for the mortality data and require explanation. For example, an increase in incidence could mean a real increase in the rate of occurrence of the disease, or it might reflect an increase in the aggressiveness of screening.

Despite these problems, an explanation for the occurrence of progress is not difficult when in fact there is progress. The problems that have arisen in the past have largely been due to a lack of improvement in the measures that one usually considers strong evidence of progress. Previously, the mortality data did not coincide with the impressive reports of progress reported in scientific articles and press releases. Members of the public and their representatives expected better results, but some scientists appeared to confirm the idea that real progress had been made. This confusion was understandable in view of the fact that the mortality rate from cancer was increasing 0.4 percent per year from 1973 to 1990. The evidence of progress was easily accepted when there was evidence of a significant decrease of 0.5 percent per year from 1990 to 1995. However, differences with respect to the causes of the decline were expressed. According to John Bailar, the government had no role in directing the improvements. In his opinion the improvements were due to the decisions of millions of individuals to improve their lifestyles (Bailar and Gornik, 1997). The decline in the rate of mortality from cancer at all sites combined was greater for blacks and Hispanics than it was for whites, whereas the rate of mortality from cancer among Asians and Pacific Islanders was unchanged.

The problem is more difficult when no progress with respect to mortality can be reported. Under these circumstances it is most critical to consider additional measures, but consideration of all available measures helps to clarify the rates of mortality from cancer and may suggest additional areas where improvements are possible. In addition to the direct measures of the rate of mortality from cancer, the incidence rate, the survival rate, and quality of life, the Breslow Committee recommended the inclusion of indirect measures (Extramural Committee to Assess Measures of Progress Against Cancer, 1990). Examples included smoking rates, levels of alcohol consumption, rates of use of the Pap smear and mammography, treatment by protocol, quality of laboratory tests, patterns of care, and psychosocial factors such as time hospitalized, levels of drug use, and time to return to work after the occurrence of cancer. These measures of progress would be used where relevant. In this way the reports are both outcome and process oriented.

SPECIAL PROCESS ITEMS

The U.S. Congress has been interested in results, but it is also interested in the process. In the case of ethnic minority and medically underserved populations, it is aware that unless there is a specific focus on their problems, they are likely to be ignored. Congress is therefore seeking a reporting mechanism that will permit members to be assured that issues of research on cancer among ethnic minority and medically underserved populations are not ignored. The dominant strategy of NIH of supporting investigator-initiated research is a perfect mechanism for ignoring ethnic minority and medically underserved populations. It is commendable that NCI plans to be more inclusive in its research activities and include ethnic minority and medically underserved populations as part of the general research program, but that is not enough. The Senate Committee report suggests that it wants to know about an NIH strategy for specifically targeting the cancer research needs of these groups over and above a general statement of inclusion. For this reason the Senate is not likely to be impressed by statistical analyses that ignore the questions concerning the relative share of NIH resources allocated to cancers disproportionately affecting medically underserved and ethnic minority populations.

A section added to specific reports should include the following statements:

- a statement of research programs *specifically targeted* toward ethnic minority and medically underserved populations;
- a list of ethnic minority scientists who have participated in decision making and performed research in the programs that have been outlined
- a list of ethnic minority scientists and researchers who have proposed concepts that might be the basis of research activities; and
- a statement of the method by which communication has been established between NCI and ethnic minority and medically underserved communities and the extent to which the communication is two-way and effective. The statement should include some of the major issues of discussion, including issues of survivorship.

This opens for NCI a more democratic process that should increase NCI's effectiveness with ethnic minority and medically underserved populations.

Linking Research Findings

Another approach to reporting is to assume that the overall strategic objective of the research program is to reduce rates of mortality from cancer. The objective is achieved by research that focuses on understanding the mechanisms of cancer development, testing the efficacies of interventions for prevention and treatment, and testing the effectiveness of interventions in the general population. The results of such research can be reported by providing such quantitative measures as mortality rates, incidence rates, survival rates, and qualitative measures such as quality of life. This can be followed by a discussion of the new knowledge related to the findings. It may be that despite the improvements in knowledge there is no improvement in results because that knowledge has not yet had time to be applied or is not being applied to the extent possible. The discussion would also explain where there are gaps in knowledge that hinder progress. These gaps become the basis for the future research agenda, which could include a modification of the present strategy. There may also be gaps in the research process, such as the availability of adequately trained investigators in prevention research.

Regardless of what research is done, the War on Cancer cannot be won by NCI. This war will require much work at the individual level, and NCI can claim neither all of the credit nor all of the blame.

The linking of progress to advances in research has several consequences. It becomes clear that progress against cancer depends not only on good research but also on the application of the knowledge derived from that research. The use of that knowledge goes beyond the domain of the research community. Much of it depends on the actions of individuals, but the research community can help by doing a more effective job of educating professionals and the public and analyzing the reasons for the failure to put knowledge into practice. It would appear that NCI has not given enough attention to this matter and that it may be necessary for some other entity to fill this gap, especially for ethnic minority and medically underserved populations. This method of reporting would emphasize both results and process and would suggest possible changes in strategy. Without the linkage it is easy to understand the suspicion among ethnic minority and disadvantaged individuals that NCI is more interested in describing than in improving. Furthermore, stating the necessary change in strategy, if any, that results from the findings would permit the U.S. Congress to understand NCI's priorities and would support requests for funding.

TYPES AND TIMING OF REPORTS

Reports on the incidence of cancer among ethnic minority and medically underserved populations may be presented in several forms, depending on the purposes and the audience for which they are intended. The most important report would be a summary report intended for the U.S.

Congress and the public. Such a report would not attempt to describe the status of each of the more than 100 diseases classified as cancer, nor would it attempt to describe all possible ethnic groups. Ethnic groups and cancer sites would be aggregated. The five cancer sites responsible for the highest rates of mortality from cancer and the macro-ethnic groups representing the largest segments of the population would be included. These macro-ethnic groups would be white, African American, Hispanic, Asian American (including Pacific Islanders), and Native American. Data for medically underserved individuals may be included as subgroups of data for all ethnic groups in the same table or may be included in a separate table. The report would include all the features mentioned above, including rates, explanations of rates on the basis of current knowledge, gaps in knowledge, and changes in strategy. This summary report would be issued every year.

Another type of report, a special report, would focus on one macro-ethnic group including the medically underserved population. This would permit expanded coverage of a specific ethnic group and its components in comparison with other ethnic groups. This coverage would be summarized but would also include data for a larger range of cancer sites. For example, it could report on data for Asian Americans but would include data for the subgroups of Asian Americans not included in the summary reports. The report would cover the same results and process areas as the summary report. It would also be a report to Congress and the public but would have a more limited circulation since it would be especially targeted to the one or two macro-ethnic groups involved. Because some of the ethnic groups have small populations in terms of the overall U.S. population, it is less likely that there would be statistically observable and reliable differences over a short time. For this reason, a 5-year period would be appropriate for any one group, but the reports may appear annually and may feature a different ethnic group, with the different ethnic groups covered in some form of rotation.

SUMMARY

The reporting to the U.S. Congress and the public should first focus on results and trends primarily by use of mortality data. Progress will not be dramatic but it should be steady. The statistics can be presented in a variety of ways to increase their clarity to a wider audience. One can also examine the processes of early detection, prevention, and treatment as contributing factors. Two kinds of reports have been suggested to be submitted annually. To address the additional concerns of Congress with respect to ethnic minority and medically underserved populations, it has been suggested that a special section of the appropriate reports include specific statements about strategies, targeted programs, participation by ethnic minority and medically underserved populations in the process, and communication between these communities and NCI. Although the Senate report refers to NIH, most suggestions have been directed toward NCI as the principal focus for cancer research. At the same time, it is clear that progress against cancer is not totally dependent on NCI and the research that it funds.

Recommendation 7-1: The committee recommends a regular reporting mechanism to increase NIH accountability to the U.S. Congress and public constituencies. Such reports should

- **report on data on progress against cancer using the nomenclature "ethnic groups" rather than "racial" groups and include data on medically underserved populations with ethnic group data;**

- **provide data on the incidence of cancer at several cancer sites, including those cancers that disproportionately affect ethnic minority and medically underserved populations;**

- **consider as one alternative reporting of mortality data in terms of "potential reduction of deaths," a statistic that is based on the lowest mortality rate among U.S. ethnic groups and that emphasizes the need for cross-cultural studies to ascertain optimal strategies for cancer prevention, treatment, and control;**

- **link research findings to reductions in cancer incidence and mortality and identify any gaps that may occur in this linkage; and**

- **report on "process" developments, such as the number and type of research programs specifically targeted to ethnic minority and medically underserved groups and the contributions of ethnic minority scientists and community groups to the research priority-setting process.**

References

Abu-Realh MH, Magwood G, Narayan MC, Rupprecht C, and Suraci M. 1996. The Use of Complementary Therapies by Cancer Patients. *Nursing Connections* 9:3–12, 1996.

Ad Hoc Working Group of the National Cancer Advisory Board. *A Review of the Intramural Program at the National Cancer Institute.* Bethesda, MD: National Cancer Institute, 1995.

Adler NE, Boyce T, Chesney MA, Cohen S, Folkman S, Kahn RL, and Syme SL. Scioeconomic Status and Health: The Challenge of the Gradient. *American Psychologist,* 49:15–24, 1994.

Altshuler D, Kruglyak L, and Lander E. Genetic Polymorphisms and Disease. *New England Journal of Medicine* 338:1626, 1998.

American Anthropological Association. *AAA Response to OMB Directive 15: Race and Ethnic Standards for Federal Statistics and Administrative Reporting.* Arlington, VA: American Anthropological Association, 1997.

American Anthropological Association. American Anthropological Association Statement on "Race." [www document]. URL http://www.ameranthassn.org/ombdraft.htm (accessed July 28, 1998).

American Cancer Society, Subcommittee on Cancer in the Economically Disadvantaged. *Cancer in the Economically Disadvantaged.* New York American Cancer Society, 1986.

American Cancer Society. *Cancer and the Socioeconomically Disadvantaged* Atlanta, GA: American Cancer Society, 1990.

American Cancer Society. *Cancer Facts & Figures—1997.* Atlanta, GA: American Cancer Society, 1997.

American Cancer Society. *Cancer Facts & Figures—1998.* Atlanta, GA: American Cancer Society, 1998a.

American Cancer Society. *Progress Against Cancer: A Report to the Nation.* Atlanta, GA: American Cancer Society, 1998b.

Auchincloss SS. After Treatment. Psychosocial Issues in Gynecologic Cancer Survivorship. *Cancer* 76(Suppl.10):2117–2124, 1995.

Bacquet C and Ringen K. *Cancer Among Blacks and Other Minorities.* Washington, DC: National Institutes of Health, 1986.

Bailar JC III and Gornik HL. Cancer Undefeated. *New England Journal of Medicine* 336:1569–1574, 1997.

Bailar JC III and Smith EM. Progress Against Cancer? *New England Journal of Medicine* 314:1226–1232, 1986.

Ballard-Barbash R, Taplin SH, Yankaskas BC, Ernester VL, Rosenberg RD, Carney PA, Barlow WE, Geller BM, Kerlikowske K, Edwards BK, Lynch CF, Urban N, Chrvala CA, Key CR, Poplack SP, Worden JK, and Kessler LG. Breast Cancer Surveillance Consortium: A National Mammography Screening and Outcomes Database. *American Journal of Roentgenology* 169:1001–1008, 1997.

Belknap DC, Seifert CF, and Petermann M. Administration of Medications Through Enteral Feeding Catheters. *American Journal of Critical Care* 6:382–392, 1997.

Beyer DA. Cancer Is a Chronic Disease. *Nurse Practitioners Forum* 6:201–206, 1995.

Bleyer WA. The U.S. Pediatric Cancer Clinical Trials Programmes: International Implications and the Way Forward. *European Journal of Cancer* 33:1439–1447, 1997.

Bleyer WA, Tejeda HA, Murphy SB, Brawley OW, Smith MA, and Ungerleider RS. Equal particicpation of minority patients in U.S. national pediatric cancer clinical trials. *Journal of Pediatric Hermatologic Oncology* 19:423–427, 1997.

Bodenhimer TS. Regional Medical Programs: No Road to Regionalization. *Medical Care Reviews* 26:1125–1166, 1969.

Bourque NM. Searching for the Knowledge to Heal: Improving the Links Between Medical Research and the Consumer. *Canadian Journal of Public Health* 87:S68–S70, 1996.

Breen N and Ching A. Race, Class, Gender, and Cancer. In *Proceedings of the 25th Public Health Conference on Records and Vital Statistics.* Hyattsville, MD: National Center for Health Statistics, 1995.

Breen N and Figueroa JB. Stage of Breast and Cervical Cancer Diagnosis in Disadvantaged Neighborhoods: A Prevention Policy Perspective. *American Journal of Preventive Medicine* 12:319–326, 1996.

Breen N, Kessler LG, and Brown ML. Breast Cancer Control Among the Underserved—An Overview. *Breast Cancer Research and Treatment* 40:105–115, 1996.

Brown N, Evans R, and Kramer W. *The Reality of Socioeconomic Status in American Society.* [www document] URL: http://www.miavx1.muohio.edu/~psybersite/stero] (accessed July 29, 1998).

Bryant H. Breast Cancer Screening in Canada: Climbing the Diffusion Curve. *Canadian Journal of Public Health.* (*Revue Canadienne de Sante Publique*) 87(Suppl. 2):S60–S62, 1996.

Burhansstipanov L. Native American Data Limitations and Home Care. *Alaska Medicine* 37:133–138, 1995.

Burnett CB, Steakley CS, and Tefft MC. Barriers to Breast and Cervical Cancer Screening in Underserved Women of the District of Columbia. *Oncology Nurses Forum* 22:1551–1557, 1995.

(The) Cancer Letter. Black Men Face Disparate Cancer Burden: Minority Rates Vary, Klausner Tells House. *The Cancer Letter,* vol.24, no. 13, pp. 1–5. Washington, DC: The Cancer Letter, Inc., 1998.

Centers for Disease Control and Prevention. *The National Program of Cancer Registries at-a-Glance 1998.* Atlanta, GA: Centers for Disease Control and Prevention, 1998.

Chamberlain RM, Winter KA, Vijayakumar S, Porter AT, Roach M III, Streeter O, Cox JD, and Bondy ML. Sociodemographic analysis of Patients in Radiation Therapy Oncology Group Clinical Trials. *International Journal of Radiation Oncology and Biological Physics* 40:19–15, 1998.

Chen M. Behavioral and Psychosocial Cancer Research in the Underserved: An Agenda for the Future. *Cancer,* 74:1503–1508, 1994.

Chevarley F and White E. Recent Trends in Breast Cancer Mortality Among White and Black US Women. *American Journal of Public Health* 87:775–781, 1997.

Clark EJ and Stovall EL. Advocacy: The Cornerstone of Cancer Survivorship. *Cancer Practice* 4:239–244, 1996.

Cobb N and Paisano RE. *Cancer Mortality Among American Indians and Alaska Natives in the United States: Regional Differences in Indian Health, 1989–1993.* Rockville, MD: Indian Health Service, 1997.

Collins FS, Guyer MS, and Chakravarti A. Variations on a Theme: Cataloging Human DNA Sequence Variation. *Science* 278:1580–1581, 1997.

Collins MM and Barry MJ. Controversies in Prostate Cancer Screening. Analogies to the Early Lung Cancer Screening Debate. *Journal of the American Medical Association* 276:1976–1979, 1996.

Cooper, RD. A Note on the Biologic Concept of Race and its Application in Epidemiologic Research. *American Heart Journal,* 108:715–723, 1984

Corcoran RD and Robinson RG. Community Demonstration Project Initiative: Technical Support for Program Development at the Community Level. *Cancer Practice* 2:222–228, 1994.

Coyne CA, Hohman K, and Levinson A. Reaching Special Populations with Breast and Cervical Cancer Public Education. *Journal of Cancer Education* 7:293–303, 1992.

Crane LA, Kaplan CP, and Bastani, R. Determinants of Adherence Among Health Department Patients Referred for a Mammogram. *Women and Health* 24 (2):43–64, 1996.

Creagan ET. Attitude and Disposition: Do They Make a Difference in Cancer Survival? *Mayo Clinic Proceedings* 72:160–164, 1997.

Cron T. *Historic Overview: Cancer Research Among Minorities and the Medically Underserved.* Unpublished document. Washington, DC: National Academy of Sciences, 1998.

Davis DA and Taylor-Vaisey A. Translating Guidelines into Practice. A Systematic Review of Theoretic Concepts, Practical Experience and Research Evidence in the Adoption of Clinical Practice Guidelines. *Canadian Medical Association Journal* 157:403–404, 408–416, 1997.

Delgado JL and Estrada L. Improving Data Collection Strategies. *Public Health Reports* 108:540–545, 1993.

Dickey LL, Griffith HM, and Kamerow DB. Put Prevention into Practice: Implementing Preventive Care. *Journal of the American Academy of Nurse Practitioners* 6:257–266, 1994.

Dirksen SR. Search for Meaning in Long-Term Cancer Survivors. *Journal of Advances in Nursing* 21:628–633, 1995.

Dow KH, Ferrell BR, Leigh S, Ly J, and Gulasekaram P. An Evaluation of the Quality of Life Among Long-Term Survivors of Breast Cancer. *Breast Cancer Research and Treatment* 39:261–273, 1996.

Durso TW. Health Care Inequalities Lead to a Mistrust of Research. *The Scientist.* [www document]. URL http://www.the-scientist.library.u...du/yr1997/feb/durso_p1_970217.html (accessed November 14, 1997).

Extramural Committee to Assess Measures of Progress Against Cancer. Special Report: Measurement of Progress Against Cancer. *Journal of the National Cancer Institute,* 82:825–835, 1990.

Fearon ER. Human Cancer Syndrome: Clues to the Origin and Nature of Cancer. *Science* 278:1043–1050, 1997.

Ferrell BR, Dow KH, and Grant M. Measurement of the Quality of Life in Cancer Survivors. *Quality of Life Research* 4:523–525, 1995.

Ferrell BR and Dow KH. Portraits of Cancer Survivorship: A Glimpse Through the Lens of Survivors' Eyes. *Cancer Practice* 4:76–80, 1996.

Ferrell BR, Grant M, Funk, Garcia N, Otis-Green S, and Schaffner ML. Quality of Life in Breast Cancer. *Cancer Practice* 4:331–340, 1996.

Ferrell BR, Grant M, Funk B, Otis-Green S, and Garcia N. Quality of Life in Breast Cancer Survivors as Identified by Focus Groups. *Psycho-Oncology* 6:13–23, 1997.

Fine LJ. The Importance of Information Dissemination in the Prevention of Occupational Cancer. *Environmental Health Perspective* 103:217–218, 1995.

Forrest D, Hoskins A, and Hussey R. Clinical Guidelines and Their Implementation. *Postgraduate Medical Journal* 72:19–22, 1996.

Freeman HP. Cancer in the Socioeconomically Disadvantaged. Pp. 4–26 in *Cancer and the Socioeconomically Disadvantaged.* Atlanta, GA: American Cancer Society, 1990.

Frey CM, McMillen MM, Cowan CD, Horm JW, and Kessler LG. Representativeness of the Surveillance, Epidemiology, and End Results Program Data: Recent Trends in Cancer Mortality Rates. *Journal of the National Cancer Institute* 84:872–877, 1992.

Friedell GH, Tucker TC, McManmon E, Moser M, Hernandez C, and Nadel M. Incidence of Dysplasia and Carcinoma of the Uterine Cervix in an Appalachian Population. *Journal of the National Cancer Institute* 84:1030–1032, 1992.

Friedell, GH. Personal communication with the IOM Committee on Cancer Research Among Minorities and the Medically Underserver, September 22, 1998.

Friedell GH, Linville LH, and Hullet S. Cancer Control in Rural Appalachia. *Cancer (Supplement),* 83:1868–1871, 1998.

Frost F, Tollestrup K, Hunt WC, Gilliland F, Key CR, and Urbina CE. Breast Cancer Survival Among New Mexico Hispanic, American Indian, and Non-Hispanic White Women (1973–1992). *Cancer Epidemiology, Biomarkers, and Prevention* 5:861–866, 1996.

Geiger, HJ. Race and Health Care: An American Dilemna? *The New England Journal of Medicine,* 335:815–816.

Giachello, AL. Access to Health Care Among Hispanics in the Midwestern States. Presentation at the U.S. Surgeon General's Midwest Meeting on Hispanic-Latino Health, Chicago, March 1993.

Giachello, AL. Issues of Access and Use. In CW Molina and M Aguirre-Molina (eds.), *Latino Health in the United States: A Growing Challenge.* Washington, DC: American Public Health Association, 1994.

Gilliland FD and Key CR. Prostate Cancer in American Indians, New Mexico, 1969 to 1994. *Journal of Urology* 159:893–898, 1998.

Gilliland FD, Hunt WC, and Key CR. Trends in the Survival of American Indian, Hispanic, and Non-Hispanic White Cancer Patients in New Mexico and Arizona, 1969–1994. *Cancer* 82:1769–1783, 1998.

Gimenez M. Latino/Hispanic—Who Needs a Name? The Case Against a Standardized Terminology. *International Journal of Health Services* 19:557–571, 1989.

Good BJ and DelVecchio GM. The Meaning of Symptoms: A Cultural Hermeneutic. Model for Clinical Practice. Pp. 165–196 in L Eisberg and A Kleinman (eds.), *The Relevance of Social Science for Medicine.* Dordrecht, The Netherlands: D. Reidel Publishing Company, 1981.

Gornick ME, Eggers PW, Reilly TW, Mentnech RM, Fitterman LK, Kucken LE, Vladeck, BC. Effects of Race and Income on Mortality and Use of Services Among Medicare Beneficiaries. *New England Journal of Medicine,* 335:791–799, 1996.

Greenberg B, Richter S, Feltes M, Gross E, Holton-Smith D, Pryor B, and Ross-Russell D. Cancer Screening in Primary Care: Strategies for Your Office. A Program of the Connecticut Division of the American Cancer Society. *Connecticut Medicine* 60:709–716, 1996.

Greenwald HP, Borgatta EF, McCorkle R, and Polissar N. Explaining Reduced Cancer Survival Among the Disadvantaged. *Milbank Quarterly* 74:215–238, 1996.

Greenwald, HP. Presentation to the IOM Committee on Cancer Research Among Minorities and the Medically Underserved, June 12, 1998.

Griffith HM and Rahman MI. Implementing the Put Prevention into Practice Program. *Nurse Practioner* 19:15–19, 1994.

Grimshaw JM. Towards Effective Professional Practice. *Therapie* 51:233–236, 1996.

Guerra LG, Meza AD, Ho H, Casner PR, and Moldes O. Medicine Residents Practices in Cancer Screening in a Hispanic Population. *Southern Medical Journal* 87:631–633, 1994.

Hahn RA. The State of Federal Health Statistics on Racial and Ethnic Groups. *Journal of the American Medical Association,* 267:268–271, 1992.

Hahn RA. *Sickness and Healing: An Anthropological Perspective.* New Haven, CT: Yale University Press, 1995.

Harlan L, Brawley O, Pommerenke F, Wali P, and Kramer B. Geographic, Age, and Racial Variation in the Treatment of Local/Regional Carcinoma of the Prostate. *Journal of Clinical Oncology* 13:93–100, 1995.

Harris JR, Lippman ME, Veronesi U, and Willett W. Breast Cancer. *New England Journal of Medicine* 327:319–328, 390–398, 1992.

Harvard Center for Cancer Prevention. Harvard Report on Cancer Prevention, Volume 1: Causes of Human Cancer. *Cancer Causes and Control* 7(Suppl.): 1996. [www document]. URL http://www.hsph.harvard.edu/Organizations/canprevent/conhtml (accessed May 14, 1998).

Health C. Special Section: Racial and Ethnic Patterns. In *Cancer Fact & Figures—1997.* Atlanta, GA: American Cancer Society, 1998.

Heckler MM. *Report of the Secretary's Task Force on Black and Minority Health, 1985.* Washington, DC: U.S. Department of Health and Human Services, 1985.

Hill C. 20 Years of Cancer Epidemiology. The Epidemiologist's Viewpoint. *Revue Epidemiologie Sante Publique* 44:547–555, 1996.

Hoffman-Goetz L, Breen NL, and Meissner H. The Impact of Social Class on the Use of Cancer Screening Within Three Racial/Ethnic Groups in the United States. *Ethnicity & Disease* 8:43–51, 1998.

Hollen PJ and Hobbie WL. Establishing Comprehensive Specialty Follow-Up Clinics for Long-Term Survivors of Cancer. Providing Systematic Physiological and Psychosocial Support. *Supportive Care Cancer* 3:40–44, 1995.

Hovell MF, Slymen DJ, Jones JA, Hofstetter CR, Burkham-Kreitner S, Conway TL, Rubin B, and Noel D. An Adolescent Tobacco-Use Prevention Trial in Orthodontic Offices. *American Journal of Public Health* 86:1760–1766, 1996.

Hubbard SM, Martin NB, and Thurn AL. NCI's Cancer Information Systems—Bringing Medical Knowledge to Clinicians. *Oncology* 9:302–306, 1995.

Institute of Medicine. *Inclusion of Women in Clinical Trials: Policies for Population Subgroups.* Washington, DC: National Academy Press, 1993

Institute of Medicine. *Scientific Opportunities and Public Needs: Improving Priority Setting and Public Input at the National Institutes of Health.* Washington, DC: National Academy Press, 1998.

Intercultural Cancer Council. *Group Gives Government "Incomplete" on Cancer Report Card* (press release), March 13, 1998.

Johnson J. Cancer Survivorship: A Systematic Approach for Providing Psychosocial Interventions (meeting abstract). *In 7th International Symposium on Supportive Care in Cancer,* September 20–23, 1995, Luxembourg, 1995.

Johnson TP, Ford L, Warnecke RB, Nayfield SG, Kaluzny A, Cutter G, Gillings D, Sondik E, and Ozer H. Effect of a National Cancer Institute Alert on Breast Cancer Practice Patterns. *Journal of Clinical Oncology* 12:1783–1788, 1994.

Kaluzny AD, Konard TR, and McLaughlin CP. Organizational Strategies for Implementing Clinical Guidelines. *Joint Commission Journal of Quality Improvement* 21:347–351, 1995a.

Kaluzny AD, Warnecke R, Lacey LM, Johnson T, Gillings D, and Ozer H. Using a Community Clinical Trials Network for Treatment, Prevention, and Control Research: Assuring Access to State-of-the-Art Cancer Care. *Cancer Investigation* 13:517–525, 1995b.

Katterhagen G. Physician Compliance with Outcome-Based Guidelines and Clinical Pathways in Oncology. *Oncology* 10(Suppl.):113–121, 1996.

Klausner RD. Presentation to the IOM Committee on Cancer Research Among Minorities and the Medically Underserved at public meeting, National Academy of Sciences, Washington, D.C., June 12, 1998.

Kleinman A, Eisenberg L, and Good B. Culture, Illness, and Care: Clinical Lessons From Anthropologic and Cross-Cultural Research. *Annals of Internal Medicine,* 88:251–258, 1978.

Kleinman A. *Patients and Healers in the Context of Culture. An Exploration of the Borderland Between Anthropology, Medicine and Psychiatry.* Berkeley, CA: University of California Press, 1980.

Knoppers BM, Hirtle M, and Lormeau S. Ethical Issues in International Collaborative Research on the Human Genome: The HGP and the HGDP. *Genomics,* 34:272–282, 1996.

Knoppers BM, Hirtle M, Lormeau S, Laberge CM, and Laflamme M. Control of DNA Samples and Information. *Genomics,* 50:385–401,1998.

Konsler GK and Jones GR. Transition Issues for Survivors of Childhood Cancer and Their Healthcare Providers. *Cancer Practice* 1:319–324, 1993.

Kosecoff J, Kanouse DE, Rogers WH, McCloskey L, Winslow CM, and Brook RH. Effect of the National Institutes of Health Consensus Development Program on Physician Practice. *Journal of the American Medical Association* 258:2708–2713, 1987.

Kottke TE, Trapp MA, Spittal P, Panser L, and Novotny P. The Psychological Impact of Modeling in a Cancer Survivors' Fashion Show. *American Journal of Preventive Medicine* 12:203–207, 1996.

Kripalani S, Weinberg AD, and Cooper HP. Screening for Breast and Prostate Cancer: A Survey of Texas Primary Care Physicians. *Texas Medicine* 92:59–67, 1996.

Krupnick JL, Rowland JH, Goldberg RL, and Daniel UV. Professionally-Led Support Groups for Cancer Patients: An Intervention in Search of a Model. *International Journal of Psychiatry Medicine* 23:275–294, 1993.

Leigh S. Cancer Survivorship: A Consumer Movement. *Seminars in Oncology* 21:783–786, 1994.

Leigh S. Survivorship and Pancreatic Cancer: The Role of Advocacy. *Oncology* 10(Suppl. 9):38–39, 1996.

Leininger LS, Finn L, Dickey L, Dietrich AJ, Foxhall L, Garr D, Stewart B, and Wender R. An Office System for Organizing Preventive Services: A Report by the American Cancer Society Advisory Group on Preventive Health Care Reminder Systems. *Archives of Family Medicine* 5:108–115, 1996.

Lenfant C. Communication with IOM Committee on Cancer Research Among Minorities and the Medically Underserved, April 22, 1998

Lerman C, Rimer B, and Glynn T. Priorities in Behavioral Research in Cancer Prevention and Control. *Preventive Medicine* 26(Pt. 2):S3–S9, 1997.

Leslie C. *Asian Medical Systems: A Comparative Study*. Berkeley, CA: University of California Press, 1976.

Levine A and Nidiffer J. *Beating the Odds: How the Poor Get to College.* San Francisco: Jossey-Bass, 1996.

Levine M, Browman G, Newman T, and Cowan DH. The Ontario Cancer Treatment Practice Guidelines Initiative. *Oncology* 10(Suppl.):19–22, 1996.

Levine MS, Sor S, Yin D, Langlotz CP, and Bachwich D. Barium Enema and Colonscopy: Appropriateness of Utilization in a Medicaid Population. *Abdominal Imaging* 22:41–44, 1997.

Lillie-Blanton M, and LaVeist T. Race/Ethnicity, the Social Environment, and Health. *Social Science and Medicine,* 43:83–91, 1996.

Lin-Fu JS. Asian and Pacific Islander Americans: An Overview of Demographic Characteristics and Health Care Issues. *Asian American and Pacific Islander Journal of Health* 1(1):20–26, 1993.

Logue LJ. Reimbursement of Tumor Marker Tests. *Clinical Chemistry* 39(Pt. 2):2435–2438, 1993.

Lomas J, Anderson GM, Domnick-Pierre K, Vayda E, Enkin MW, and Hannah WJ. Do Practice Guidelines Guide Practice? The Effect of a Consensus Statement on the Practice of Physicians. *New England Journal of Medicine* 321:1306–1311, 1989.

Mahoney MC and Michalek AM. Health Status of American Indians/Alaska Natives: General Patterns of Mortality. *Family Medicine* 30:190–194, 1998.

Manfredi C, Czaja R, Buis M, and Derk D. Patient Use of Treatment-Related Information Received from the Cancer Information Service. *Cancer* 71:1326–1337, 1993.

Mark N and Roberts L. Ethnosensitive Techniques in the Treatment of the Hasidic Patient with Cancer. *Cancer Practice* 2:202–208, 1994.

Martinez-Maldonado M. Hypertension in Hispanics. Comments on a Major Disease in a Mix of Ethnic Groups. *American Journal of Hypertension* 8 (Pt. 2):120S–123S, 1995.

Matsunaga DS, Enos R, Gotay CC, Banner RO, DeCambra H, Hammond OW, Hedlund N, Ilaban EK, Issell BF, and Tsark JA. Participatory Research in a Native Hawaiian Community. The Wai'Anae Cancer Research Project. *Cancer* 78:1582–1586, 1996.

McFall SL, Warnecke RB, Kaluzny AD, and Ford L. Practice Setting and Physician Influence on Judgements of Colon Cancer Treatment by Community Physicians. *Health Services Research,* 31:5–19, 1996.

Michalek AM and Mahoney MC. Provision of Cancer Control Services to Native Americans by State Health Departments. *Journal of Cancer Education* 9:145–147, 1994.

Midwest Latino Health Research, Training and Policy Center. Minorities and Women in Cancer Clinical Trials—Recruitment, Enrollment and Retention. Unpublished document. Midwest Latino Health Research, Training and Policy Center, University of Illinois at Chicago, 1996.

Miller BA, Kolonel LN, Bernstein L, Young JL Jr., Swanson GM, West D, Key CR, Liff JM, Glover CS, Alexander GA, et al. (eds.). *Racial/Ethnic Patterns of Cancer in the United States 1988–1992.* Bethesda, MD: National Cancer Institute, 1996.

Morton RP. Evolution of Quality of Life Assessment in Head and Neck Cancer. *Journal of Laryngology and Otology* 109:1029–1035, 1995.

Naranjo D. *Health in the Hispanic Community: A Summary of Health-Related Activities and Needs of NCLR Affiliates.* Washington, DC: National Council of La Raza, 1992.

National Cancer Institute. *Measures of Progress Against Cancer, Vols. I–VII.* Bethesda, MD: National Cancer Institute, 1993.

National Cancer Institute. *Documentation of the Cancer Research Needs of American Indians and Alaska Natives.* Bethesda, MD: National Cancer Institute, 1994.

National Cancer Institute. *NCI Progam Activities Related to Minority/Special Populations: Recommendations of the NCI Special Action Committee.* Bethesda, MD: National Cancer Institute, 1996a.

National Cancer Institute. *Extramural Funds, Fiscal Year 1996.* Bethesda, MD: National Cancer Institute, 1996b.

National Cancer Institute. *National Cancer Institute 1997/1998 Bypass Budget Request Principal Budget Components.* Bethesda, MD: National Cancer Institute, 1996c.

National Cancer Institute. *Program Structure Fiscal Year 1996.* Bethesda, MD: National Cancer Institute, 1996d.

National Cancer Institute. *Proceedings of the Conference on Recruitment and Retention of Minority Participants in Clinical Cancer Research.* Publication No. 96-41820. Bethesda, MD: National Cancer Institute, 1996e.

National Cancer Institute. *A New Agenda for Cancer Control Research: Report of the Cancer Control Review Group.* Bethesda, MD: National Cancer Institute, 1997a.

National Cancer Institute. *Research Dollars by Various Cancers.* Bethesda, MD: National Cancer Institute, 1997b.

National Cancer Institute. Press release, November 6, 1997. Bethesda, MD: National Cancer Institute, 1997c.

National Cancer Institute. *NCI Selects First Members of New Director's Consumer Liaison Group.* Press release, December 10, 1997. Bethesda, MD: National Cancer Institute, 1997d.

National Cancer Institute. *Breast Cancer Prevention Trial Shows Major Benefit, Some Risk,* press release dated April 6, 1998. Bethesda, MD: National Institutes of Health, 1998a.

National Cancer Institute. *NCI Initiatives for Special Populations, 1998.* Bethesda, MD: National Cancer Institute, 1998b.

National Cancer Institute. *Background Information from SEER Expansion Report.* Document provided to the study committee by Dr. Brenda Edwards of NCI, April 23, 1998. 1998c.

National Cancer Institute. *The Nation's Investment in Cancer Research. A Budget Proposal for Fiscal Year 1999.* Bethesda, MD: National Cancer Institute, 1998d.

National Cancer Institute. *Total NCI Dollars by Mechanism.* Bethesda, MD: National Cancer Institute, 1998e.

National Cancer Institute. *NCI Extramural Research and Program Activities Targeted to Minorities.* Bethesda, MD: National Cancer Institute, 1998f.

National Cancer Institute. *Priority Setting at the National Cancer Institute.* Bethesda, MD: National Cancer Institute, 1998g.

National Cancer Institute. *Clinical Trials.* Bethesda, MD: National Cancer Institute, 1998h.

National Cancer Institute, Office of Cancer Surviorship. Communication to the Institute of Medicine Committee on Cancer Research Among Minorities and the Medically Underserved. Office of Cancer Survivorship, National Cancer Institute, Bethesda, MD, 1998i.

National Cancer Institute. *Cancer Survivorship Studies in Established Epidemiologic Cohorts.* Publication No. PA-98-0270. Bethesda, MD: National Cancer Insitute, 1998j.

National Center for Health Statistics, U S. Department of Agriculture, and Human Nutrition Information Service. *Nutrition Monitoring in the United States: An Update Report on Nutrition Monitoring.* Hyattsville, MD: Life Sciences Research Office, Federation of American Societies for Experimental Biology, 1989.

National Center for Health Statistics. *Health, United States, 1998 With Socioeconomic Status and Health Chartbook.* Hyattsville, MD: National Center for Health Statistics, 1998.

National Institues of Health. *Outreach Notebook for the NIH Guidelines on Inclusion of Women and Minorities as Subjects in Clinical Research.* Bethesda, MD: National Institutes of Health, 1994.

National Institutes of Health. *Setting Research Priorities at the National Institutes of Health.* Bethesda, MD: National Institutes of Health, 1997.

National Institutes of Health, Office of Research on Minority Health. Minority Programs: Fact Finding Team Recommendations. Bethesda, MD: Office of Research on Minority Health, National Institues of Health, 1992.

National Institutes of Health. Cancer Research Initiative, Estimates for FY 1999. Bethesda, MD: National Institutes of Health, March, 1998.

National Institutes of Health, Office of Research on Minority Health. ORMH Budget Prepared at the Request of the IOM Commitee on Cancer Research Among Minorities and the Medically Underserved. Office of Research on Minority Health, National Institutes of Health, Bethesda, MD, 1998a.

National Institutes of Health, Office of Research on Minority Health. Budget Information. Office of Research on Minority Health, National Institutes of Health, Bethesda, MD, 1998b.

Nattinger AB, Gottloeb MS, Hoffman RG, Walker AP, and Goodwin JS. Minimal Increase in Use of Breast-Conserving Surgery from 1986 to 1990. *Medical Care* 34:479–489, 1996.

Newman ML, Brennan M, and Passik S. Lymphedema Complicated by Pain and Psychological Distress: A Case with Complex Treatment Needs. *Journal of Pain Symptom Management* 12:37–6379, 1996.

North American Association of Central Cancer Registries. *Cancer in North America, 1990–1994*. Sacramento, CA: North American Association of Central Cancer Registries, 1998.

Nutting PA, Freeman WL, Risser DR, Helgerson SD, Paisano R, Hisnanick J, Beaver SK, Peters I, Carney JP, and Speers MA. Cancer Incidence Among American Indians and Alaska Natives, 1980 Through 1987. *American Journal of Public Health* 83:1589–1598, 1993.

Olivotto A, Coldman AJ, Hislop TG, Trevisan CH, Kula J, Goel V, and Sawka C. Compliance with Practice Guidelines for Node-Negative Breast Cancer. *Journal of Clinical Oncology* 15:216–222, 1997.

Osoba D, Till JE, Pater JL, and Young JR. Health-Related Quality of Life: Measurement and Clinical Application. A Workshop Report. *Canadian Journal of Oncology* 5:338–343, 1995.

Pearlman DN, Ehrich B, and Rakowski W. Mammography, Clinical Breast Exam, and Pap Testing: Correlates of Combined Screening. *American Journal of Preventive Medicine* 12:52–64, 1996.

Penn V. Overview of the NIH Policy on Inclusion of Women and Minorities in Clinical Research. In *Recruitment and Retention of Minority Participants in Clinical Cancer Research*. Washington, DC: U.S. Department of Health and Human Services, 1996.

Pincus T and Callahan LF. What Explains the Association Between Socioeconomic Status and Health: Primary Access to Medical Care or Mind-Body Variables. *The Journal of Mind-Body Health* 11:4–35, 1995.

Polednak AP. Trends in Breast-Conserving Surgery in Connecticut: No Effect of Negative Publicity. *Connecticut Medicine* 60:527–530, 1996.

Polinsky ML. Functional Status of Long-Term Breast Cancer Survivors: Demonstrating Chronicity. *Health and Social Work* 19:165–173, 1994. (Erratum, 19:297).

President's Cancer Panel. *Report of the President's Cancer Panel: The Meaning of Race in Science—Considerations for Cancer Research.* Highlights and Recommendations for the President's Cancer Panel Meeting, April 7, 1997, New York, NY. Bethesda, MD: National Cancer Institute, 1997.

The President's Commission on Heart Disease, Cancer, and Stroke. *Report to the President. A National Program to Conquer Heart Disease, Cancer and Stroke.* Washington, DC: U.S. Government Printing Office, 1964.

Reiman J. *The Rich Get Richer and the Poor Get Prison: Ideology, Class, and Criminal Justice.* Needham Heights, MA: Viacom Company, 1997.

Rivera LM. Blood Cell Transplantation: Its Impact on One Family. *Seminars in Oncological Nursing* 13:194–199, 1997.

Robert Wood Johnson Foundation. *To Improve Health and Health Care, 1997: The Robert Wood Johnson Foundation Anthology,* SL Isaacs and JR Knickman (eds.). San Francisco: Jossey-Bass, 1997.

Robinson SB, Ashley, M, and Haynes, MA. Attitudes of African-Americans Regarding Prostate Cancer Clinical Trials. *Journal of Community Health,* 21:77–87, 1996.

Ruffin J. ORMH Assistance in Funding Special NIH Institute and Center. Minority Health/Training Initatives. Memorandum to NIH Institute and Center Directors, November 25, 1996.

Salazar MK. Hispanic Women's Beliefs About Breast Cancer and Mammography, *Cancer Nursing* 19:437–446, 1996.

Samet JR, Key CR, Hunt WC, and Goodwin JS. Survival of American Indian and Hispanic Cancer Patients in New Mexico and Arizona, 1969–1982. *Journal of the National Cancer Institute* 79:457–463, 1987.

Sandercock P. Collaborative Worldwide Overviews of Randomized Trials. *Annals of the New York Academy of Sciences* 703:149–154, 1993.

Saunders L. *Cultural Differences and Medical Care: The Case of the Spanish-Speaking People of the Southwest.* New York: Russell Sage Foundation, 1954.

Schapira DV and Levine RB. Breast Cancer Screening and Compliance and Evaluation of Lesions. *Medical Clinics of North America* 80:15–26, 1996.

Schneider, J. Rewriting the SES: Demographic Patterns and Divorcing Families. *Social Science and Medicine* 23:211–222, 1986.

Scrimshaw S and McMiller W. *What's in a Name? The Meaning and Measurement of Ethnicity for Latinos and African Americans in Health Research.* East Lansing, MI: Population Research Group, 1996.

Sherman CR, Potosky AL, Weis KA, and Ferguson JH. The Consensus Development Program: Detecting Changes in Medical Practice Following a Consensus Conference on the Treatment of Prostate Cancer. *International Journal of Technology Assessment and Health Care* 8:683–693, 1992.

Simmons WJ and Goforth L. The Impact of Managed Care on Cancer Care. Review and Recommendations. *Cancer Practice* 5:111–118, 1997.

Sink L. *Race and Ethnicity Classification Consistency Between the Census Bureau and The National Center for Health Statistics.* Population Division Working Paper No. 17. Washington, DC: U.S. Bureau of the Census, 1997.

Smedley A. *Race in North America: Origin and Evolution of a Worldview,* Second Edition. Boulder, CO: Westview Press, 1999.

Smith DW, Hann NE, Kays CW, and Young L. Native American Supplement–Oklahoma Behavioral Risk Factor Survey. In *Abstracts of the 23rd Annual Meeting of the American Public Health Association.* Washington, DC: American Public Health Association, 1995.

Solberg LI, Kottke TE, Brekke ML, Calomeni CA, Conn SA, and Davidson G. Using Continuous Quality Improvement to Increase Preventive Services in Clinical Practice–Going Beyond Guidelines. *Preventive Medicine* 25:259–267, 1996.

Spielman RS, McGinnis RE, and Ewens WJ. Transmission Test for Linkage Disequilibrium: The Insulin Gene Region and Insulin Dependent Diabetes Mellitus (IDDM). *American Journal of Genetics* 52:506–516, 1993.

Starreveld A. A Surgical Subculture. The Use of Mastectomy to Treat Breast Cancer. *Canadian Medical Association Journal 1*56:25–35; 43–45; 1119, 1121; 1379–1380, 1997.

Stehelin D, Varmus H, Bishop J, et al. DNA Related to the Transforming Gene(s) of Avian Sarcoma Viruses in Normal Avian DNA. *Nature* 260:170–173, 1976.

Stovall EL. Practice Guidelines: Patients' Perspective. *Oncology* 10:255–260, 1996.

Studnicki J, Schapira DV, Bradham DD, Clark RA, and Jarrett A. Response to the National Cancer Institute Alert. The Effect of Practice Guidelines on Two Hospitals in the Same Medical Community. *Cancer* 72:2986–2992, 1993.

Studnicki J, Remmel R, Campbell R, and Werner DC. The Impact of Legislatively Imposed Practice Guidelines on Cesarean Section Rates: The Florida Experience. *American Journal of Medical Quality* 12:62–68, 1997.

Suarez L, Nichols DC, Pulley L, Brady CA, and McAlister A. Local Health Departments Implement a Theory-Based Model to Increase Breast and Cervical Cancer Screening. *Public Health Reports* 108:477–482, 1993.

Suarez L. Pap Smear and Mammogram Screening in Mexican American Women: The Effects of Acculturation. *American Journal of Public Health* 84:742–746, 1994.

Sugarman JR, Warren CW, Oge L, and Helgerson SD. Using the Behavioral Risk Surveillance System to Monitor Year 2000 Objectives Among American Indians. *Public Health Reports* 401:449–456,1992.

Sugarman JR, Holliday M, Ross A, Castorina J, and Hui Y. Improving American Indian Cancer Data in the Washington State Cancer Registry Using Linkages with the Indian Health Service and Tribal records. *Cancer (Supplement)* 78(7):1564–1568, 1996.

Sullivan LW. Effects of Discrimination and Racism on Access to Health Care From the Secretary of Health and Human Services. *Journal of the American Medical Association* 266:2674, 1991.

Swanson GM and Ward AJ. Recruiting Minorities Into Clinical Trials: Toward a Participant-Friendly System. *Journal of the National Cancer Institute,* 87:1747–1759, 1995.

Taylor VM, Taplin SH, Urban N, White E, Mahloch J, Majer K, McLerran D, and Peacock S. Community Organization to Promote Breast Cancer Screening Ordering by Primary Care Physicians. *Journal of Community Health* 21:277–292, 1996.

Tejeda HA, Green SB, Trimble EL, Ford L, High JL, Ungerleider RS, Friedman MA, and Brawley OW. Representation of African-Americans, Hispanics, and Whites in National Cancer Institute Cancer Treatment Trials. *Journal of the National Cancer Institute,* 88:812–816, 1996.

Unger J, Hutchins L, Crowley J, Coltman C, and Albain K. Southwest Oncology Group (SWOG) Accrual by Sex, Race, and Age, Compared to US Population Rates. In *Abstracts of the American Society of Clinical Oncology,* 17:1596. Alexandria, VA: American Society: American Society of Clinical Oncology, 1998.

U.S. Bureau of the Census. *Income, Poverty and Health Insurance.* Washington, DC: U.S. Bureau of the Census, 1997.

U.S. Bureau of the Census. *Poverty in the United States: 1996.* Series P60-198. Washington, DC: U.S. Government Printing Office, 1997.

U.S. Bureau of the Census. Census Bureau to Release Results of Research on Questions on Race and Hispanic Origin. Press release, May 15, 1997. From U.S. Bureau of the Census webpage URL: http://www.census.gov/Press-Release/cb97-83.html (accessed October 20, 1998). 1998a.

U.S. Bureau of the Census. *USA Statistics in Brief: Population,* Washington, DC: U.S. Bureau of the Census, 1998b.

U.S. Congress. National Cancer Act of 1971. Public Law 92-218. Washington DC: U.S. Government Printing Office, 1971.

U.S. Congress. Office of Technology Assessment. *Health Care in Rural America.* OTA-H-434. Washington, DC: U.S. Government Printing Office, 1990.

U.S. Congress. Senate Report No. 100-189. Washington, DC: U.S. Government Printing Office, 1990.

U.S. Department of Health and Human Services. *Report of the Secretary's Task Force on Black & Minority Health, Vol. 1.* Washington, DC: U.S. Government Printing Office, 1985.

U.S. Department of Health and Human Services. NIH Guidelines for the Inclusion of Women and Minorities as Subjects in Clinical Research. *Federal Register* 59:14508–14513, 1994.

U.S. General Accounting Office. *Hispanic Access to Health Care: Significant Gaps Exist.* GAO/PEMD 92-96. Washington, DC: U.S. Government Printing Office, 1992.

U.S. Office of Management and Budget. Revisions to the Standards for the Classification of Federal Data on Race and Ethnicity, *Federal Register* 62 (131):36847–36946, July 9, 1997.

U.S. Preventive Services Task Force. *Guide to Clinical Preventive Services,* 1977. xxvii. Baltimore, MD: The Williams & Wilkins Co., 1996.

U.S. Public Health Service. *Healthy People 2000: National Health Promotion and Disease Prevention Objectives.* Washington, DC: U.S. Department of Health and Human Services, 1991.

Valdez RB, Giachello A, Rodriguez-Trias H, Gomez P, and de la Rocha C. Improving Access to Health Care in Latino Communities. *Public Health Reports,* 108:534–539, 1993.

Valway S. *Cancer Mortality Among Native Americans in the United States: Regional Differences in Indian Health, 1984–1988, and Trends Over Time, 1968–1987.* Washington, DC: Indian Health Service, U.S. Department of Health and Human Services, 1990.

Ward J, Collins G, and Walmsley J. A Model for Implementing Healthy People 2000 Objectives in African-American Communities in California. *Ethnic Diseases* 3:158–168, 1993.

Warnecke RB, Johnson TP, Kaluzny AD, and Ford LG. The Community Clinical Oncology Program: Its Effect on Clinical Practice. *Journal of Community Quality Improvement* 21:336–339, 1995.

Weeks J and Pfister DG. Outcomes Research Studies. *Oncology* 10(Suppl.):29–34, 1996.

Weinberg, RA. *Racing to the Beginning of the Road.* New York: Harmony Books, 1996.

Wilcox LS and Mosher WD. Factors Associated with Obtaining Health Screening Among Women of Reproductive Age. *Public Health Reports* 76–86, 1993.

Williams DR, Lavizzo-Mourey R, Warren, RC. The Concept of Race and Health Status in America. *Public Health Reports,* 109:26–41, 1994.

Wingo PA, Ries LAG, Rosenberg HM, Miller DS, and Edwards BK. *Cancer Incidence and Mortality, 1973–1995: A Report Card for the United States.* Atlanta, GA: American Cancer Society, National Cancer Institute, and Centers for Disease Control and Prevention, 1998.

Woolf SH, DiGuiseppi CG, Atkins D, and Kamerow DB. Developing Evidence-Based Clinical Practice Guidelines: Lessons Learned by the US Preventive Services Task Force. *Annual Review of Public Health* 17:511–538, 1996.

Young WW, Marks SM, Kohler SA, and Hsu AY. Dissemination of Clinical Results. Mastectomy Versus Lumpectomy and Radiation Therapy. *Medical Care* 34:1003–1017, 1996.

Zenner W. Ethnicity. Pp. 393–395 in *Encyclopedia of Cultural Anthropology.* New York: Henry Holt and Co., 1996.

Zielstroff RD, Barnett GO, Fitzmaurice JB, Estey G, Hamilton G, Vickery A, Welebob E, and Shahzad C. A Decision Support System for Prevention and Treatment of Pressure Ulcers Based on AHCPR Guidelines. Pp. 562–566 in *Proceedings of the AMIA Annual Fall Symposium.* Bethesda, MD: American Medical Informatics Association, 1996.

Appendixes

A

Methodology

To assist the committee in addressing its charge, the committee gathered information from several resources both within and outside of the National Institutes of Health (NIH). This appendix describes the committee's charge and briefly addresses the types of information that the committee requested and received from those resources.

COMMITTEE CHARGE

The Committee on Cancer Research Among Minorities and the Medically Underserved was charged with evaluating and critiquing the efforts of NIH's cancer research agenda for minority and medically underserved populations. The committee was charged with three specific tasks: (1) review the status of cancer research relative to minorities at the various institutes, centers, and divisions of NIH to evaluate the relative share of resources allocated to cancer in minorities (including a review of NIH's ability to prioritize its cancer research agenda for minorities and the role of minority scientists in decision making on research priorities); (2) examine how well research results are communicated and applied to cancer prevention and treatment programs for minorities and the adequacy of understanding of survivorship issues that uniquely affect minority communities; and (3) obtain an understanding of the adequacy of NIH procedures for equitable recruitment and retention of minorities in clinical trials.

SOURCES OF INFORMATION PROVIDED TO THE COMMITTEE

At the onset of the study, the committee found that it needed data that would provide an inclusive overview of the research enterprise at NIH as it pertains to minority and medically underserved populations. Data were therefore collected from the following sources:

- Institutes of NIH: National Cancer Institute (NCI); National Institute of Allergy and Infectious Diseases (NIAID); National Heart, Lung, and Blood Institute (NHLBI); National Institute of Environmental Health Sciences (NIEHS); National Human Genome Research Institute; and the National Institute of Diabetes and Digestive and Kidney Diseases (NIDDKD).
- Other federal and nongovernmental health agencies and organizations: the Centers for Disease Control and Prevention's (CDC's) National Cancer Registry, the North American Association of Central Cancer Registries (NAACCR), the California Cancer Registry, and the Georgia Cancer Registry.

The requests were for information covering the three core areas of the committee's charge.

DATA

The information that the committee received is described briefly. Copies of letters from the committee requesting information are listing at the end of this appendix.

NIH Priority-Setting Processes

To address aspects of the charge related to a review of NIH priority setting and the mechanisms for input from NIH constituencies, the committee requested and received the following information from NIH:

- information on priority setting at NIH (e.g., National Institute of Health, 1997)
- copies of testimony and reports to the U.S. Congress, and
- information regarding NIH and NCI advisory panels.

NIH Research Programs

To facilitate review of NIH research programs, the committee requested and received the following information:

Surveillance Activities

- NCI and NIH definitions of "special populations,"
- information regarding national surveillance programs, including data from NAACCR and CDC, and
- information regarding the Surveillance, Epidemiology, and End Results (SEER) program and its coverage areas.

Research Programs

- Summaries of intramural and extramural research programs at NCI, NIDDKD, NIAID, NHLBI, NIEHS, etc., related to the study of cancer among minority and medically underserved populations.
- Information regarding funding for research related to minority and medically underserved populations for fiscal years (fiscal years [FYs] 1985, 1989, 1993, and 1997).
- Program announcements and requests for applications (RFAs) relevant to cancer research among minority and medically underserved populations for FYs 1985, 1989, 1993, and 1997.
- Program announcements and RFAs relevant to cancer research among minority and medically underserved populations for FYs 1985, 1989, 1993, and 1997.
- A list of research grants pertaining to cancer research among minority and medically underserved populations funded in FYs 1985, 1989, 1993, and 1997.

Clinical Trials

- Information regarding accrual and retention of minority and medically underserved populations in NIH-sponsored cancer clinical and prevention trials.
- Information on strategies used by NCI and NIH to recruit and retain these populations.

Training Programs

- Information regarding NIH and NCI training programs for minority scientists.

Dissemination

- Information on NIH and NCI strategies to disseminate cancer research.

- Information to minority and medically underserved communities and their providers.
- Information on publications resulting from NIH grants for research on cancer among minorities and medically underserved populations.

Survivorship

- Information on research grants related to cancer survivorship and supported by the NCI.
- Information on ongoing activities of the Office of Cancer Survivorship.

ADDITIONAL INFORMATION RESOURCES

Computer Retrieval of Information Scientific Projects

To further assist the committee in its review of the NCI and NIH research agenda the Institute of Medicine (IOM) staff conducted a search of the Computer Retrieval of Information on Scientific Projects (CRISP) database. The CRISP database contains information on federally funded research, including grants, contracts, and cooperative agreements conducted primarily by investigators at universities, hospitals, and other research institutions. Projects listed in the CRISP database are funded by a number of US Public Health Services agencies including NIH. This database contains information on special projects, investigators, scientific concepts, and emerging trends. The CRISP database is updated weekly.

The IOM staff search was conducted for projects funded in 1997 only. Specific search terms used included "NIH" or "NCI," "R01," "CA" for cancer, and the wildcard "minorit*." There is no global term in the CRISP database for "underserved" or "medically underserved."

Public Meeting

The committee held a public meeting on June 11–12, 1998, in Washington, D.C. The purpose of this meeting was to provide an opportunity for cancer advocacy groups and community-based health organizations to present their views on the responsiveness of NIH to their concerns and input into cancer research studies. The committee also heard testimony from invited NIH representatives. A copy of the agenda for this meeting is located in Appendix D.

Survey

IOM staff developed and distributed a survey to assess the responsiveness of NCI to minority investigator-initiated research and funding opportunities. More than 850 surveys were mailed to individuals who are members of the following groups or organizations:

- Appalachian Leadership Initiative on Cancer (principal cancer investigators),
- Hispanic Cancer Network,
- Intercultural Cancer Council,
- Society for the Advancement of Chicanos and Native Americans in Science (fields related to cancer only),
- NIH Minority Supplement Trainees, and
- American Association for Cancer Research (members of the minority section only).

The results of the survey are summarized in Chapter 4. A copy of the survey is included in Appendix E.

B
A New Agenda for Cancer Control Research: Report of the Cancer Control Review Group

In 1996, the director of the National Cancer Institute (NCI) and chair of the Board of Scientific Advisors convened a panel of experts "to review the scope of the NCI cancer control research program and to make recommendations regarding the pursuit of research opportunities most likely to accelerate reductions in the nation's cancer burden" (National Cancer Institute, 1997a, p. i). The panel's report, released in 1997, makes a number of recommendations: "To build even stronger cancer control research programs, the new Division of Cancer Control and Population Science should pursue the following goals" (National Cancer Institute, 1997a, p. ii):

- Create a unit focused on basic behavioral and social research in cancer control.
- Create a research focus in informatics and communication.
- Establish programs that recognize the role of behavioral prevention across the lifespan.
- Increase integration of and support for cancer screening research.
- Create a research focus on rehabilitation and survivorship.
- Establish research links to various health care delivery systems.
- Expand cancer surveillance and produce a "cancer report card."
- Maintain strong support of biometry and applied research within the new division.
- Focus research efforts on underserved populations and those with a disproportionate cancer burden.
- Expand training in cancer control research.

C
National Cancer Institute Health Promotion Branch Publications and Public Service Announcements

The National Cancer Institute (NCI) Health Promotion Branch has developed the following publications and public service announcements for "special populations":

AFRICAN AMERICANS

- *Down Home Healthy Cookin'* (booklet)
- *Down Home Healthy* (bookmark)
- *Eat More Fiber at Every Meal* (poster)
- Your Best Body: A Story About Losing Weight (pamphlet)
- Tips on How to Eat Less Fat (brochure)
- Racial Differences in Breast Cancer Survival (cancer facts)
- Chances Are . . . You Need A Mammogram (brochure; a collaborative effort between American Association of Retired Person's, American Cancer Society, and NCI)
- Knowledge: It's Part of the Cure (bookmark)
- Knowledge: It's Part of the Cure (print public service announcement)
- Breast Cancer and Mammography (public service announcement featuring Ruby Dee and Nancy Wilson)
- On Track to Good Health (public service announcement)
- Public service announcement on mammography featuring Angela Bassett
- Smoking Facts and Quitting Tips for Black Americans

HISPANICS

- *Probalemente . . . Usted Necesita Hacerse un Mamogram (Chances Are . . . You Need a Mammogram)*
- *Preguntas para Hacerle a Su Medico sober el Cancer del Zeno (Questions to Ask Your Doctor About Breast Cancer)*
- *El conocimiento: Es parte de la cure* (Knowledge: It's Part of the Cures; print public service announcement)
- *Los mamogramas: No Solomente una Vez, Sino por Toda una Vida* (brochure and bookmark)
- *Datos y Consejos para Dejar de Fumar* (Smoking Facts and Tips for Quitting)
- *Celebre la Cocina Hispana* (Hispanic recipe book)
- ¡Su Familia se Merece los Mejores Alimentos! (booklet and poster)
- *Coma Menos Grasa* (tip sheet)
- *Rompa con el Vicio. Una Guia para Dejar de Fumar*
- *La Prueba Pap: Un Metodo para Diagnosticar Cancer del Cuello del Utero* (brochure)

NATIVE AMERICANS

- *Taking Control of Your Health: The Pap Test and Cervical Cancer* (videotape)
- Traditional Foods Can Be Healthy (booklet)

MULTIETHNIC MAMMOGRAPHY MATERIALS (FEATURING AFRICAN-AMERICAN, ASIAN, HISPANIC, NATIVE AMERICAN, AND WHITE WOMEN)

- *Understanding Breast Changes: A Guide for All Women*
- *The Facts About Breast Cancer and Mammography*
- *Mammograms* . . . Not Just Once, but for a Lifetime (an easy-to-read publication, also available in Spanish)
- Mammograms . . . Not Just Once, but for a Lifetime (bookmark)
- Why Get Mammograms? (a physician's pad with tear-off fact sheets on mammograms to give to their patients)
- Over Age 40? Consider Mammograms (a set of five posters each featuring a women of a different race or ethnicity)
- *Cancer Facts: Breast Cancer and Mammography Facts* (a book that describes rates of incidence, mortality, and mammography screening for women of different races or ethnicities)

D
Survey of Ethnic Minority Researchers and of Researchers Interested in Cancer Among Ethnic Minority and Medically Underserved Groups

The recommendations of respondents to the committee's survey and some representative comments related to each of the recommendations from respondents to the survey, as described in Chapter 4, are presented here.

1. Involve community members and community-based researchers as partners in the research process.

> "Adapt RFP [request for proposal] guidelines to support community-based research—don't assume the research centers and universities are competent at researching communities. Require participation and joint input with community agencies."

> "Support initiatives that involve minority and health care leaders [of organizations that serve these populations] in the development of cancer prevention and control research applications."

> "Speak with these communities, especially the young investigators."

2. Improvements should be made in training and grant programs to increase the capacity for scientific research among minority and medically underserved populations.

"Overall these is a mismatch between training incentives and career transition initiatives. NIH should . . . establish a bonus program to facilitate supplementation of a minority scientist's first grant."

"For younger, promising minority investigators, provide five year grants and funding for salary support and *technical support* (salary support alone is insufficient). If productive, *renew* the grant for an additional five years. Have the same for mid-level (associate professor) investigators also."

"Regional seminars for trainees on these types of issues [research funding] held periodically would heighten awareness, interest, and understanding of availability of funding/research."

"Minority research career development awards, renewable for up to 10+ years."

"Provide more seed grants for new investigators' short-course (three to six months) research. Training opportunities for aspiring clinicians."

"Until minorities make up a larger percentage of those investigators applying for NIH funds . . . we will continue to see low numbers of research proposals focusing on minority-related issues and subsequently low receptivity to these proposals."

3. Scientists from minority and medically underserved communities should be involved in the NIH priority-setting process and in staffing of NIH positions.

"Recruit minorities in NIH Board of Scientific Counselors and peer review committees."

"Increase minority staff at NIH at all levels, particularly in policy positions."

"NIH staff at all levels must be part of cultural competency training. They have too [many] biases against minority investigators."

"Get more minorities on study sections."

"Include more minorities on review panels. Continue work with

HBCUs [historically black colleges and universities] including 1890 institutions."

"Develop an advisory board on addressing research needs of minority and medically underserved communities."

4. Community members and community-based researchers should be partners in research priority setting.

"Hold focus groups with community leaders, primary care doctors, and research scientists to review current priorities with the needs of the community."

"Include members from target populations in committees which discuss and decide priorities."

5. Research issues for minority and underserved populations must be integrated into a national cancer research agenda.

"NIH must take a national approach in funding and develop cancer research in minority and medically underserved communities. This approach must be a part of NIH's national agenda and must be aimed toward the reduction of cancer in these populations."

6. Define special populations research more adequately.

"Much more critical assessment of the nature of 'underserved' and the extent to which minorities are underserved."

"Improve the definition of 'minority' and 'medically underserved' communities. Or better, eliminate the term 'minority' as pejorative, and define better the target populations."

"Do not make race or ethnic background an issue. These have become political issues, and these cloud public and medical judgment."

"Any work with American Indians needs to be regionalized to accommodate the differences among tribes. Most of the work [of NCI] has been focused on Southwestern tribes, and their characteristics are very different from [those of] East Coast, Northwest, Plains Indians, etc."

7. Involve institutions serving minority and medically underserved communities in cancer research.

> "Greater focus on training, translation research in minority and medically underserved communities, support of cancer centers at HBCUs."

> "Networking of research capabilities of minority . . . universities/ research medical centers."

> "Use of black colleges and medical schools."

INSTITUTE OF MEDICINE
NATIONAL ACADEMY OF SCIENCES
2101 CONSTITUTION AVENUE, N.W. WASHINGTON, D.C. 20418

Committee on Cancer Research
Among Minorities and the
Medically Underserved

Phone: (202) 334-1755
Fax: (202) 334-1385
Internet: bsmedley@nas.edu

May 21, 1998

Dear Colleague:

On behalf of the Institute of Medicine's Committee on Cancer Research Among Minorities and the Medically Underserved, I am writing to you to solicit your input for this critically important report. You have been identified as an individual who has expertise in issues related to the study committee's charge, which are:

- to review the status of cancer research relative to minorities and the medically underserved at the various institutes, centers and divisions of NIH to evaluate the relative share of resources allocated to cancer in minority and medically underserved populations (including a review of the NIH's ability to prioritize its cancer research agenda for minorities and the medically underserved and the role of minority scientists in decisionmaking on research priorities);

- to examine how well research results are communicated and applied to cancer prevention and treatment programs for minorities and the medically underserved and the adequacy of understanding of survivorship issues that uniquely impact on minority and medically underserved communities; and,

- to assess the adequacy of NIH procedures for equitable recruitment and retention of minorities and the medically underserved in clinical trials.

The committee will also be asked to make recommendations on an annual reporting mechanism on the status of cancer research among minorities and the medically underserved at the NIH.

We seek your input into any and all of the areas outlined in the charge above, but more specifically, we would like to receive your opinion on specific topic areas in the attached questionnaire.

We would be grateful to receive your input **on or before June 10, 1998**, so that the committee may review this information at its next meeting. Please mail the questionnaire to us at the mailing address listed at the bottom of the questionnaire, or fax it to us at (202) 334-1385. Please return it to the attention of Brian Smedley, Ph.D., Study Director. **Please do not include identifying information on the questionnaire. Committee staff will work to**

Page 2
IOM Cancer Research Survey

ensure that names of respondents remain confidential (e.g., identifying information at the top of received faxes will be removed and return envelopes discarded). If you have any questions regarding this questionnaire, please contact Brian Smedley at (202) 334-1755 by phone, or by email at bsmedley@nas.edu.

Thank you again for your assistance.

Sincerely,

M. Alfred Haynes, M.D., M.P.H.
Chair

IOM Study of Cancer Research Among Minorities and the Medically Underserved

Please do not provide any identifying information other than in response to the questions below. Responses will be presented to the committee to inform the study report.

What is your race/ethnicity?

Please indicate the highest degree you have attained:

What is the nature of your present work?

____ Primarily research (laboratory, clinical, or field-based)
____ Primarily teaching
____ Primarily clinical practice
____ Primarily health policy
____ Other (please indicate): ________________

Your employer is:

____ Federal, state or local Government
____ Non-profit educational or research institution
____ Health care service
____ Other (please indicate): ________________

Have you ever submitted a research proposal to NIH or its Institutes?
Have you ever responded to an NIH Request for Applications or Program Announcement?
Have you ever received funding from NIH or its Institutes for a research program?
If so, please describe the nature of the research:

Have you ever received research training funds from NIH or its Institutes?
If so, please describe the nature of the funding:

If you have applied for funding at NIH (other than training funds), how would you rate the experience (please circle one)?

1	2	3	4	5	6	7
very negative		neutral			very positive	

Please describe your experience:

How familiar are you with the research priority-setting process at NIH?
Have you ever been asked to sit on an NIH advisory body (e.g., Board of Scientific Counselors)?
If so, which one?
Have you ever attempted to provide input into the research priority-setting process at NIH?

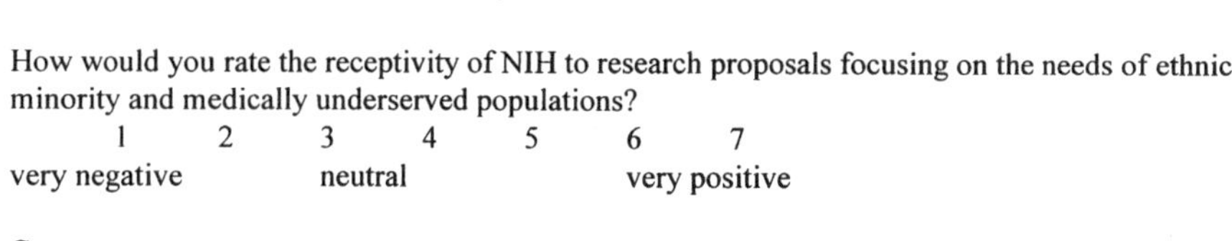

How would you rate the receptivity of NIH to research proposals focusing on the needs of ethnic minority and medically underserved populations?

1 2 3 4 5 6 7

very negative neutral very positive

Comments:

In general, how would you rate the value or priority that NIH places on research relevant to minority and medically underserved populations?

1 2 3 4 5 6 7

very negative neutral very positive

Comments:

In general, how would you rate the value or priority that NIH places on training of minority scientists?

1 2 3 4 5 6 7

very negative neutral very positive

Comments:

Are there examples of NIH activities, programs, or initiatives that you feel have worked well to address the research needs of minority and medically underserved communities?

Do you have recommendations on how NIH might improve its approach to addressing research needs of minority and medically underserved communities?

Can you provide other comments, based on your personal experience, on other areas of the study committee's charge that have not been addressed above? Please support your comments with examples.

Thank you for your assistance. Please mail or fax the questionnaire to: Brian Smedley, Ph.D., Study Director, FO-3014, Institute of Medicine, 2101 Constitution Ave., N.W., Washington, D.C. 20418. Fax: (202) 334-1385

E
National Institutes of Health and National Cancer Institute Background Material

In response to the Institute of Medicine Committee on Cancer Research Among Minorities and the Medically Underserved, the National Institutes of Health (NIH) and the National Cancer Institute (NCI) provide the following background material related to cancer survivorship:

- Description of the Office of Cancer Survivorship, which was established in August 1996. The document indicates that there are currently 126 grants that deal with special populations and the medically underserved, 80 percent of which are R01 investigator-initiated grants. Since 1994, all NCI grants are evaluated in the review process to ensure the inclusion of women and minorities. (Indeed, the PHS 398 form used for NIH grant applications has sections asking investigators to demonstrate inclusion of women and minorities.) However, no data on the actual breakdown of women and minorities targeted in funded grants are available. For instance, virtually all breast cancer research will target women. However, it is not clear to what degree such research targets minority and medically underserved women.
- Activities with advocacy and voluntary organizations.
- A current program announcement entitled Cancer Survivorship Studies in Established Epidemiologic Cohorts (PA-98-027).
- Agenda for a conference entitled Research Issues in Cancer Survivorship, sponsored by the Office of Cancer Survivorship, Division of Cancer Control and Populations Sciences, on March 9–10, 1998.

- Background information from the NCI World Wide Web page on Creating the Director's Consumer Liaison Group, established in 1997. It is not clear how specifically these groups include targeted minority groups.
- A list of 850 scientific journal publications resulting from awards or programs of NIH relative to cancer among minority and medically underserved population since 1985.

F
Information Provided by the National Center for Health Statistics on the Potential Reductions in Mortality from Cancer, by Ethnic Group

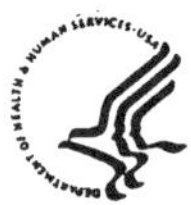

DEPARTMENT OF HEALTH & HUMAN SERVICES

Public Health Service
Centers for Disease Control and Prevention

National Center for Health Statistics
6525 Belcrest Road
Hyattsville, Maryland 20782

September 16, 1998

M. Alfred Haynes, M.D., M.P.H.
Chair, Committee on Cancer Research Among
Minorities and the Medically Underserved
Institute of Medicine
2101 Constitution Avenue, N.W.
Washington, D.C. 20418

Dear Dr. Haynes:

I am writing in response to your letter of July 24, 1998 in which you asked for an analysis of cancer mortality based on race. Please find enclosed a statement of the methodology we used including several caveats, a summary table, and a detailed table demonstrating the reduction in cancer deaths that could be achieved if differences by race or ethnicity could be eliminated.

A few notes on what we've done: You asked us if we could illustrate the number and percent of deaths that would be avoided if all race or ethnic groups shared the same mortality risks for specific cancer sites. You also asked that we consider that the "best" mortality experience be the one that all groups could, at least hypothetically, experience.

We departed somewhat from the methodology you recommended in the letter with respect to sex, rates, and race:

> First, in consultation with NCI, we performed the calculations separately by sex because of the major differences in cancer experience by sex.
>
> Second, we used age-adjusted death rates to select a "best" group, and age-specific death rates to calculate the "excess" deaths.
>
> Third, we combined both the Asian and Pacific Islander and American Indians into a total Asian and Pacific Island group and a total American Indian group. These groups were formed to stabilize estimates, to use groups for which we have estimates of the degree to which race has been misreported, and to use the most recent data available, which is only available for the broad groups.

Even with these steps, we do have some serious reservations about the procedures used and resulting conclusions because race and ethnicity-specific death rates are known to be substantially too low for certain racial/ethnic groups. The consequence is that excess deaths presented here may be substantially greater than would be the case if the rates were not a function of these errors. Indeed, we are most concerned about using the American Indian rates as a baseline or "best rate" group. Given the errors in reporting, it is difficult to believe that other groups could achieve these rates. The two kinds of errors in reported death rates include serious mis-classification of race and ethnicity and misreporting of age, particularly among the elderly. These problems occur on the death certificate and also on censuses and surveys.

Page 2 - M. Alfred Haynes, M.D., M.P.H.

Given our concerns we decided to make two estimates (Method A and Method B). In Method A, for those sites for which the American Indian rates were "best," we chose the race/ethnic group that was the next lowest in death rate for that cancer site. In Method B, we used American Indian rates when they were the "best." Two sets of tables are provided, but we strongly prefer those that are not based on American Indians as the "best" or target rate (Method A).

While Method A are preferred estimates, this method does not make any adjustment for known race misclassification. Overall we expect that the estimated number of "excess" deaths from cancer would be around ten percent fewer for women and closer to twenty percent for men. This percentage would vary by cancer site.

Please note that I strongly believe this exercise can be useful. As I mentioned on the phone, I view differences in cancer mortality risk as, first and foremost, reflecting a variety of cancer causes and differential group responses to risk factors. Illustrating the differences between groups provides clues to form hypotheses on cancer causes, risk factors or biology. Secondly, for some cancer sites, we understand the causes and processes of cancer development sufficiently to be able to say how one group can achieve the lower risk shown by another group. Perhaps the best example I know of in the second case is the low rates of cancer among Mormons in Utah and Los Angeles, which reflect life-style choices that could be replicated in other populations.

All of us at NCHS are appreciative to our NCI colleagues who made available their SEER database and helped us make the calculations.

Please contact Mr. Maurer or Drs. Hoyert or Rosenberg (301-436-8884) if you have any additional questions.

Sincerely,

Edward J. Sondik, Ph.D.
Director
National Center for Health Statistics

Enclosures

cc:
Brian Smedley
Jeff Maurer
Donna Hoyert, Ph.D.
Harry Rosenberg, Ph.D.
Lynn Ries
Brenda Edwards, Ph.D.
Mary Anne Freedman
Jennifer Madans, Ph.D.
Richard Klausner, M.D.

Page 3 - M. Alfred Haynes, M.D., M.P.H.

Methodology and Caveats

The methodology that we used in computing the requested approach is as follows:

1) Our basic data included 1990-95 age-adjusted death rates (using a 1970 population standard), age-specific deaths and death rates, and populations by race and ethnicity following the structure of the 1996 SEER publication cited in your letter (produced by NCI using NCHS and Census data)

2) Method A: For specific cancer sites, we selected the group with the smallest age-adjusted death rate separately by sex. The groups for which the age-adjusted death rates were compared included white, black, Asian and Pacific Islander, Hispanic (total), and Non-Hispanic (total).

   Method B: For specific cancer sites, we selected the group with the smallest age-adjusted death rate separately by sex. The groups for which the age-adjusted death rates were compared included white, black, **American Indian**, Asian and Pacific Islander, Hispanic (total), and Non-Hispanic (total).

3) For each cancer site, we multiplied the age-specific death rate for the "best" group by the population of each of the race or ethnic groups to determine an "expected" number of deaths.

4) For each cancer site, we subtracted the "expected" number of deaths from the "observed" number of deaths to determine a value for deaths that would not have occurred.

5) For each cancer site, we also divided the "expected" number of deaths by the "observed" number of deaths, subtracted 1 from the quotient, and multiply by 100. This yields the percent difference in observed and expected deaths.

6) For all cancers combined (shown in the summary table), we summed the expected and observed deaths by sex and calculated the "excess" and percent difference from the summation for specific sites.

7) The detail table expresses the number of deaths for the full time period. The summary table express the number of deaths per year.

Page 4 - M. Alfred Haynes, M.D., M.P.H.

Caveats of this approach include the following:

1) Quality of data varies by race and ethnicity in both death certificate data and Census data. The quality of data for the white and black populations are good in contrast to that for other groups. American Indian is estimated to be underreported on the death certificate by more than 20% (probably greater than this) and Asian and Pacific Islander is underreported by about 10%. With respect to population data, perhaps, the most serious problem is the 33% increase in the American Indian population between 1960 and 1990 that reflects increased preference to self-report as an American Indian.

2) Age-specific death rates, especially those for the elderly, are underestimates.

3) Hispanic origin and race are separate items. We picked the best rates going across these two variables, but show the deaths for both Hispanic origin and race.

4) Hispanic origin was not reported on all State death certificates in this time period. The rates used in the calculation were based on 46 States and the District of Columbia. The observed deaths count was inflated to a national total by using the reciprocal of the fraction of the Hispanic population living in these 46 States and D.C.

5) The number of events, particularly at young ages for certain minority groups, are small. This would affect the stability of the rates. To counter that tendency, we used data for the 1990-95 time period. In the summary table, we have expressed the number of deaths in terms of a single year of data.

6) The reduction for all cancer sites combined differs depending on whether the values are summed across specific cancer sites or is done separately. The reduction is greater when the values are summed.

Summary table of annual reductions "possible" for cancer
version excluding American Indians as "best" (i.e. Method A)

Men

All cancers

Best group rates (varies by site)

	Expected deaths	Observed deaths
TOTAL	140,449	276,146
White	125,372	239,397
Black	11,479	32,505
American Indian	672	753
Asian Pacific Islander	2,926	3,492
Hispanic	6,916	8,374
Non-Hispanic	133,533	267,772
	Estimated excess deaths	**Percent difference in observed and expected deaths**
TOTAL	135,697	-49
White	114,024	-48
Black	21,026	-65
American Indian	81	-11
Asian Pacific Islander	566	-16
Hispanic	1,458	-17
Non-Hispanic	134,239	-50

Lung and bronchus

Best group rates (Hispanic)

	Expected deaths	Observed deaths
TOTAL	40,971	91,673
White	36,643	79,943
Black	3,296	10,578
American Indian	191	239
Asian Pacific Islander	841	914
Hispanic	1,947	1,947
Non-Hispanic	39,024	89,726
	Estimated excess deaths	**Percent difference in observed and expected deaths**
TOTAL	50,702	-55
White	43,300	-54
Black	7,281	-69
American Indian	48	-20
Asian Pacific Islander	73	-8
Hispanic	(0)	0
Non-Hispanic	50,702	-57

Women

All cancers

Best group rates (varies by site)

	Expected deaths	Observed deaths
TOTAL	126,225	247,702
White	111,714	217,628
Black	11,428	26,456
American Indian	590	716
Asian Pacific Islander	2,492	2,903
Hispanic	6,103	7,358
Non-Hispanic	120,122	240,344
	Estimated excess deaths	**Percent difference in observed and expected deaths**
TOTAL	121,477	-49
White	105,913	-49
Black	15,027	-57
American Indian	126	-18
Asian Pacific Islander	411	-14
Hispanic	1,255	-17
Non-Hispanic	120,222	-50

Lung and bronchus

Best group rates (Hispanic)

	Expected deaths	Observed deaths
TOTAL	19,699	54,951
White	17,526	49,416
Black	1,725	4,890
American Indian	86	149
Asian Pacific Islander	362	495
Hispanic	886	886
Non-Hispanic	18,813	54,065
	Estimated excess deaths	**Percent difference in observed and expected deaths**
TOTAL	35,252	-64
White	31,890	-65
Black	3,165	-65
American Indian	63	-42
Asian Pacific Islander	133	-27
Hispanic	(0)	0
Non-Hispanic	35,252	-65

Pancreas

Best group rates (As & Pac Islander)

	Expected deaths	Observed deaths
TOTAL	9,008	12,610
White	8,062	10,951
Black	721	1,449
American Indian	42	27
Asian Pacific Islander	183	183
Hispanic	424	440
Non-Hispanic	8,584	12,169

	Estimated excess deaths	Percent difference in observed and expected deaths
TOTAL	3,601	-29
White	2,889	-26
Black	728	-50
American Indian	(15)	56
Asian Pacific Islander	(0)	0
Hispanic	16	-4
Non-Hispanic	3,585	-29

Pancreas

Best group rates (As & Pacif Islander)

	Expected deaths	Observed deaths
TOTAL	9,179	13,512
White	8,183	11,664
Black	794	1,650
American Indian	39	34
Asian Pacific Islander	163	163
Hispanic	403	441
Non-Hispanic	8,775	13,071

	Estimated excess deaths	Percent difference in observed and expected deaths
TOTAL	4,333	-32
White	3,481	-30
Black	856	-52
American Indian	(5)	14
Asian Pacific Islander	0	-0
Hispanic	38	-9
Non-Hispanic	4,295	-33

Ovary

Best group rates (As Pacif Islander)

	Expected deaths	Observed deaths
TOTAL	6,403	13,081
White	5,614	11,888
Black	611	1,012
American Indian	33	35
Asian Pacific Islander	146	146
Hispanic	341	413
Non-Hispanic	6,062	12,668

	Estimated excess deaths	Percent difference in observed and expected deaths
TOTAL	6,678	-51
White	6,275	-53
Black	401	-40
American Indian	2	-6
Asian Pacific Islander	(0)	0
Hispanic	72	-18
Non-Hispanic	6,605	-52

Colon/rectum
Best group rates (Hispanic)

	Expected deaths	Observed deaths
TOTAL	16,753	28,310
White	14,964	24,974
Black	1,361	2,910
American Indian	80	66
Asian Pacific Islander	349	360
Hispanic	814	814
Non-Hispanic	15,939	27,495
	Estimated excess deaths	**Percent difference in observed and expected deaths**
TOTAL	11,556	-41
White	10,009	-40
Black	1,550	-53
American Indian	(14)	21
Asian Pacific Islander	11	-3
Hispanic	(0)	0
Non-Hispanic	11,556	-42

Breast
Best group rates (As Pacif Islander)

	Expected deaths	Observed deaths
TOTAL	18,236	43,513
White	15,917	38,045
Black	1,783	4,932
American Indian	98	98
Asian Pacific Islander	438	438
Hispanic	1,017	1,328
Non-Hispanic	17,219	42,184
	Estimated excess deaths	**Percent difference in observed and expected deaths**
TOTAL	25,277	-58
White	22,128	-58
Black	3,149	-64
American Indian	(0)	0
Asian Pacific Islander	0	-0
Hispanic	311	-23
Non-Hispanic	24,966	-59

Colon/rectum
Best group rates (Hispanic)

	Expected deaths	Observed deaths
TOTAL	15,954	28,919
White	14,215	25,303
Black	1,386	3,244
American Indian	69	71
Asian Pacific Islander	284	302
Hispanic	709	709
Non-Hispanic	15,245	28,210
	Estimated excess deaths	**Percent difference in observed and expected deaths**
TOTAL	12,964	-45
White	11,088	-44
Black	1,857	-57
American Indian	2	-2
Asian Pacific Islander	17	-6
Hispanic	(0)	0
Non-Hispanic	12,964	-46

Stomach
Best group rates (White)

	Expected deaths	Observed deaths
TOTAL	7,329	8,198
White	6,539	6,540
Black	599	1,327
American Indian	35	38
Asian Pacific Islander	155	293
Hispanic	362	519
Non-Hispanic	6,967	7,679
	Estimated excess deaths	**Percent difference in observed and expected deaths**
TOTAL	869	-11
White	0	-0
Black	728	-55
American Indian	3	-8
Asian Pacific Islander	138	-47
Hispanic	157	-30
Non-Hispanic	712	-9

Stomach
Best group rates (White)

	Expected deaths	Observed deaths
TOTAL	5,004	5,634
White	4,463	4,463
Black	432	928
American Indian	21	25
Asian Pacific Islander	88	219
Hispanic	220	374
Non-Hispanic	4,784	5,260
	Estimated excess deaths	**Percent difference in observed and expected deaths**
TOTAL	630	-11
White	0	-0
Black	495	-53
American Indian	4	-14
Asian Pacific Islander	131	-60
Hispanic	154	-41
Non-Hispanic	476	-9

Cervix
Best group rates (White)

	Expected deaths	Observed deaths
TOTAL	3,976	4,578
White	3,438	3,439
Black	410	997
American Indian	23	34
Asian Pacific Islander	105	109
Hispanic	245	336
Non-Hispanic	3,731	4,242
	Estimated excess deaths	**Percent difference in observed and expected deaths**
TOTAL	602	-13
White	0	-0
Black	588	-59
American Indian	10	-30
Asian Pacific Islander	4	-4
Hispanic	91	-27
Non-Hispanic	511	-12

Kidney/renal/pel
Best group rates (As Pac Islander)

	Expected deaths	Observed deaths
TOTAL	2,433	6,350
White	2,163	5,715
Black	204	550
American Indian	12	31
Asian Pacific Islander	54	54
Hispanic	127	257
Non-Hispanic	2,306	6,093
	Estimated excess deaths	**Percent difference in observed and expected deaths**
TOTAL	3,917	-62
White	3,552	-62
Black	346	-63
American Indian	19	-61
Asian Pacific Islander	0	-0
Hispanic	130	-51
Non-Hispanic	3,786	-62

Kidney/renal/pel
Best group rates (As Pacif Islander)

	Expected deaths	Observed deaths
TOTAL	1,685	4,099
White	1,501	3,678
Black	146	369
American Indian	7	23
Asian Pacific Islander	30	30
Hispanic	75	150
Non-Hispanic	1,610	3,949
	Estimated excess deaths	**Percent difference in observed and expected deaths**
TOTAL	2,414	-59
White	2,177	-59
Black	222	-60
American Indian	15	-68
Asian Pacific Islander	0	-0
Hispanic	75	-50
Non-Hispanic	2,339	-59

Other
Best group (Asi or Pacif Islander)

	Expected deaths	Observed deaths
TOTAL	43,975	88,231
White	39,044	77,673
Black	3,738	9,352
American Indian	225	238
Asian Pacific Islander	968	968
Hispanic	2,363	3,026
Non-Hispanic	41,612	85,205
	Estimated excess deaths	**Percent difference in observed and expected deaths**
TOTAL	44,256	-50
White	38,629	-50
Black	5,614	-60
American Indian	13	-6
Asian Pacific Islander	0	-0
Hispanic	662	-22
Non-Hispanic	43,594	-51

	Expected deaths	Observed deaths
TOTAL	42,373	75,355
White	37,556	66,372
Black	3,814	7,950
American Indian	196	225
Asian Pacific Islander	808	808
Hispanic	2,036	2,462
Non-Hispanic	40,337	72,893
	Estimated excess deaths	**Percent difference in observed and expected deaths**
TOTAL	32,981	-44
White	28,816	-43
Black	4,136	-52
American Indian	29	-13
Asian Pacific Islander	(0)	0
Hispanic	425	-17
Non-Hispanic	32,556	-45

Prostate

Best group rates (As Pacif Islander)

	Expected deaths	Observed deaths
TOTAL	14,221	34,070
White	12,826	28,261
Black	1,082	5,477
American Indian	59	78
Asian Pacific Islander	254	254
Hispanic	587	917
Non-Hispanic	13,634	33,153
	Estimated excess deaths	**Percent difference in observed and expected deaths**
TOTAL	19,849	-58
White	15,436	-55
Black	4,394	-80
American Indian	19	-24
Asian Pacific Islander	(0)	0
Hispanic	330	-36
Non-Hispanic	19,519	-59

Nasopharynx

Best group rates (Hispanic)

	Expected deaths	Observed deaths
TOTAL	299	450
White	264	312
Black	26	62
American Indian	2	6
Asian Pacific Islander	7	71
Hispanic	17	17
Non-Hispanic	282	433
	Estimated excess deaths	**Percent difference in observed and expected deaths**
TOTAL	151	-33
White	47	-15
Black	36	-58
American Indian	4	-71
Asian Pacific Islander	63	-90
Hispanic	0	-0
Non-Hispanic	151	-35

Nasopharynx

Best group rates (Hispanic)

	Expected deaths	Observed deaths
TOTAL	145	233
White	128	186
Black	13	24
American Indian	1	2
Asian Pacific Islander	3	21
Hispanic	7	7
Non-Hispanic	137	226
	Estimated excess deaths	**Percent difference in observed and expected deaths**
TOTAL	88	-38
White	58	-31
Black	10	-44
American Indian	1	-66
Asian Pacific Islander	18	-86
Hispanic	0	-0
Non-Hispanic	88	-39

Liver & intrahepatic bile Best group rates (White)	Expected deaths	Observed deaths	Liver & intrahepatic bile Best group rates (White)	Expected deaths	Observed deaths
TOTAL	5,340	5,936	TOTAL	3,571	3,829
White	4,759	4,759	White	3,174	3,174
Black	440	752	Black	315	461
American Indian	26	31	American Indian	16	21
Asian Pacific Islander	114	394	Asian Pacific Islander	66	174
Hispanic	269	429	Hispanic	163	252
Non-Hispanic	5,071	5,507	Non-Hispanic	3,407	3,577
	Estimated excess deaths	Percent difference in observed and expected deaths		Estimated excess deaths	Percent difference in observed and expected deaths
TOTAL	596	-10	TOTAL	258	-7
White	(0)	0	White	0	-0
Black	312	-41	Black	146	-32
American Indian	4	-15	American Indian	5	-23
Asian Pacific Islander	280	-71	Asian Pacific Islander	108	-62
Hispanic	160	-37	Hispanic	89	-35
Non-Hispanic	436	-8	Non-Hispanic	169	-5

Summary table of annual reductions "possible" for cancer (Method B)

Men			Women		
All cancers — Best group rates (varies by site)	Expected deaths	Observed deaths	**All cancers — Best group rates (varies by site)**	Expected deaths	Observed deaths
TOTAL	133,397	276,146	TOTAL	125,214	247,702
White	119,013	239,397	White	110,822	217,628
Black	10,942	32,505	Black	11,335	26,456
American Indian	643	753	American Indian	585	716
Asian Pacific Islander	2,799	3,492	Asian Pacific Islander	2,471	2,903
Hispanic	6,624	8,374	Hispanic	6,052	7,358
Non-Hispanic	126,773	267,772	Non-Hispanic	119,161	240,344
	Estimated excess deaths	Percent difference in observed and expected deaths		Estimated excess deaths	Percent difference in observed and expected deaths
TOTAL	142,749	-52	TOTAL	122,488	-49
White	120,383	-50	White	106,806	-49
Black	21,562	-66	Black	15,120	-57
American Indian	110	-15	American Indian	131	-18
Asian Pacific Islander	693	-20	Asian Pacific Islander	431	-15
Hispanic	1,750	-21	Hispanic	1,306	-18
Non-Hispanic	140,999	-53	Non-Hispanic	121,182	-50
Lung and bronchus — Best group rates (Hispanic)	Expected deaths	Observed deaths	**Lung and bronchus — Best group rates (Hispanic)**	Expected deaths	Observed deaths
TOTAL	40,971	91,673	TOTAL	19,699	54,951
White	36,643	79,943	White	17,526	49,416
Black	3,296	10,578	Black	1,725	4,890
American Indian	191	239	American Indian	86	149
Asian Pacific Islander	841	914	Asian Pacific Islander	362	495
Hispanic	1,947	1,947	Hispanic	886	886
Non-Hispanic	39,024	89,726	Non-Hispanic	18,813	54,065
	Estimated excess deaths	Percent difference in observed and expected deaths		Estimated excess deaths	Percent difference in observed and expected deaths
TOTAL	50,702	-55	TOTAL	35,252	-64
White	43,300	-54	White	31,890	-65
Black	7,281	-69	Black	3,165	-65
American Indian	48	-20	American Indian	63	-42
Asian Pacific Islander	73	-8	Asian Pacific Islander	133	-27
Hispanic	(0)	0	Hispanic	(0)	0
Non-Hispanic	50,702	-57	Non-Hispanic	35,252	-65

Breast
Best group rates (As Pacif Islander)

	Expected deaths	Observed deaths
TOTAL	18,236	43,513
White	15,917	38,045
Black	1,783	4,932
American Indian	98	98
Asian Pacific Islander	438	438
Hispanic	1,017	1,328
Non-Hispanic	17,219	42,184

	Estimated excess deaths	Percent difference in observed and expected deaths
TOTAL	25,277	-58
White	22,128	-58
Black	3,149	-64
American Indian	(0)	0
Asian Pacific Islander	0	-0
Hispanic	311	-23
Non-Hispanic	24,966	-59

Colon/rectum
Best group rates (Amer Indian)

	Expected deaths	Observed deaths
TOTAL	13,258	28,310
White	11,805	24,974
Black	1,100	2,910
American Indian	65	66
Asian Pacific Islander	288	360
Hispanic	676	814
Non-Hispanic	12,582	27,495

	Estimated excess deaths	Percent difference in observed and expected deaths
TOTAL	15,052	-53
White	13,169	-53
Black	1,811	-62
American Indian	0	-0
Asian Pacific Islander	72	-20
Hispanic	138	-17
Non-Hispanic	14,914	-54

Colon/rectum
Best group rates (Hispanic)

	Expected deaths	Observed deaths
TOTAL	15,954	28,919
White	14,215	25,303
Black	1,386	3,244
American Indian	69	71
Asian Pacific Islander	284	302
Hispanic	709	709
Non-Hispanic	15,245	28,210

	Estimated excess deaths	Percent difference in observed and expected deaths
TOTAL	12,964	-45
White	11,088	-44
Black	1,857	-57
American Indian	2	-2
Asian Pacific Islander	17	-6
Hispanic	(0)	0
Non-Hispanic	12,964	-46

Pancreas

Best group rates (Amer Indian)

	Expected deaths	Observed deaths
TOTAL	5,504	12,610
White	4,910	10,951
Black	450	1,449
American Indian	27	27
Asian Pacific Islander	117	183
Hispanic	273	440
Non-Hispanic	5,232	12,169

	Estimated excess deaths	Percent difference in observed and expected deaths
TOTAL	7,105	-56
White	6,041	-55
Black	999	-69
American Indian	0	-0
Asian Pacific Islander	65	-36
Hispanic	167	-38
Non-Hispanic	6,938	-57

Pancreas

Best group rates (Amer Indian)

	Expected deaths	Observed deaths
TOTAL	8,168	13,512
White	7,290	11,664
Black	701	1,650
American Indian	34	34
Asian Pacific Islander	142	163
Hispanic	353	441
Non-Hispanic	7,815	13,071

	Estimated excess deaths	Percent difference in observed and expected deaths
TOTAL	5,344	-40
White	4,374	-37
Black	950	-58
American Indian	0	-0
Asian Pacific Islander	20	-13
Hispanic	88	-20
Non-Hispanic	5,255	-40

Ovary

Best group rates (As Pacif Islander)

	Expected deaths	Observed deaths
TOTAL	6,403	13,081
White	5,614	11,888
Black	611	1,012
American Indian	33	35
Asian Pacific Islander	146	146
Hispanic	341	413
Non-Hispanic	6,062	12,668

	Estimated excess deaths	Percent difference in observed and expected deaths
TOTAL	6,678	-51
White	6,275	-53
Black	401	-40
American Indian	2	-6
Asian Pacific Islander	(0)	0
Hispanic	72	-18
Non-Hispanic	6,605	-52

Stomach

Best group rates (White)

	Expected deaths	Observed deaths
TOTAL	7,329	8,198
White	6,539	6,540
Black	599	1,327
American Indian	35	38
Asian Pacific Islander	155	293
Hispanic	362	519
Non-Hispanic	6,967	7,679
	Estimated excess deaths	**Percent difference in observed and expected deaths**
TOTAL	869	-11
White	0	-0
Black	728	-55
American Indian	3	-8
Asian Pacific Islander	138	-47
Hispanic	157	-30
Non-Hispanic	712	-9

Stomach

Best group rates (White)

	Expected deaths	Observed deaths
TOTAL	5,004	5,634
White	4,463	4,463
Black	432	928
American Indian	21	25
Asian Pacific Islander	88	219
Hispanic	220	374
Non-Hispanic	4,784	5,260
	Estimated excess deaths	**Percent difference in observed and expected deaths**
TOTAL	630	-11
White	0	-0
Black	495	-53
American Indian	4	-14
Asian Pacific Islander	131	-60
Hispanic	154	-41
Non-Hispanic	476	-9

Cervix

Best group rates (White)

	Expected deaths	Observed deaths
TOTAL	3,976	4,578
White	3,438	3,439
Black	410	997
American Indian	23	34
Asian Pacific Islander	105	109
Hispanic	245	336
Non-Hispanic	3,731	4,242
	Estimated excess deaths	**Percent difference in observed and expected deaths**
TOTAL	602	-13
White	0	-0
Black	588	-59
American Indian	10	-30
Asian Pacific Islander	4	-4
Hispanic	91	-27
Non-Hispanic	511	-12

Kidney/renal/pel
Best group rates (As Pac Islander)

	Expected deaths	Observed deaths
TOTAL	2,433	6,350
White	2,163	5,715
Black	204	550
American Indian	12	31
Asian Pacific Islander	54	54
Hispanic	127	257
Non-Hispanic	2,306	6,093
	Estimated excess deaths	**Percent difference in observed and expected deaths**
TOTAL	3,917	-62
White	3,552	-62
Black	346	-63
American Indian	19	-61
Asian Pacific Islander	0	-0
Hispanic	130	-51
Non-Hispanic	3,786	-62

Kidney/renal/pel
Best group rates (As Pacif Islander)

	Expected deaths	Observed deaths
TOTAL	1,685	4,099
White	1,501	3,678
Black	146	369
American Indian	7	23
Asian Pacific Islander	30	30
Hispanic	75	150
Non-Hispanic	1,610	3,949
	Estimated excess deaths	**Percent difference in observed and expected deaths**
TOTAL	2,414	-59
White	2,177	-59
Black	222	-60
American Indian	15	-68
Asian Pacific Islander	0	-0
Hispanic	75	-50
Non-Hispanic	2,339	-59

Other
Best group (Asi or Pacif Islander)

	Expected deaths	Observed deaths
TOTAL	43,975	88,231
White	39,044	77,673
Black	3,738	9,352
American Indian	225	238
Asian Pacific Islander	968	968
Hispanic	2,363	3,026
Non-Hispanic	41,612	85,205
	Estimated excess deaths	**Percent difference in observed and expected deaths**
TOTAL	44,256	-50
White	38,629	-50
Black	5,614	-60
American Indian	13	-6
Asian Pacific Islander	0	-0
Hispanic	662	-22
Non-Hispanic	43,594	-51

Other
Best group rates (As Pacif Islander)

	Expected deaths	Observed deaths
TOTAL	42,373	75,355
White	37,556	66,372
Black	3,814	7,950
American Indian	196	225
Asian Pacific Islander	808	808
Hispanic	2,036	2,462
Non-Hispanic	40,337	72,893
	Estimated excess deaths	**Percent difference in observed and expected deaths**
TOTAL	32,981	-44
White	28,816	-43
Black	4,136	-52
American Indian	29	-13
Asian Pacific Islander	(0)	0
Hispanic	425	-17
Non-Hispanic	32,556	-45

Prostate

Best group rates (As Pacif Islander)

	Expected deaths	Observed deaths
TOTAL	14,221	34,070
White	12,826	28,261
Black	1,082	5,477
American Indian	59	78
Asian Pacific Islander	254	254
Hispanic	587	917
Non-Hispanic	13,634	33,153
	Estimated excess deaths	**Percent difference in observed and expected deaths**
TOTAL	19,849	-58
White	15,436	-55
Black	4,394	-80
American Indian	19	-24
Asian Pacific Islander	(0)	0
Hispanic	330	-36
Non-Hispanic	19,519	-59

Nasopharynx

Best group rates (Hispanic)

	Expected deaths	Observed deaths
TOTAL	299	450
White	264	312
Black	26	62
American Indian	2	6
Asian Pacific Islander	7	71
Hispanic	17	17
Non-Hispanic	282	433
	Estimated excess deaths	**Percent difference in observed and expected deaths**
TOTAL	151	-33
White	47	-15
Black	36	-58
American Indian	4	-71
Asian Pacific Islander	63	-90
		0
Hispanic	0	-0
Non-Hispanic	151	-35

Nasopharynx

Best group rates (Hispanic)

	Expected deaths	Observed deaths
TOTAL	145	233
White	128	186
Black	13	24
American Indian	1	2
Asian Pacific Islander	3	21
Hispanic	7	7
Non-Hispanic	137	226
	Estimated excess deaths	**Percent difference in observed and expected deaths**
TOTAL	88	-38
White	58	-31
Black	10	-44
American Indian	1	-66
Asian Pacific Islander	18	-86
Hispanic	0	-0
Non-Hispanic	88	-39

Liver & intrahepatic bile Best group rates (White)	Expected deaths	Observed deaths
TOTAL	5,340	5,936
White	4,759	4,759
Black	440	752
American Indian	26	31
Asian Pacific Islander	114	394
Hispanic	269	429
Non-Hispanic	5,071	5,507
	Estimated excess deaths	**Percent difference in observed and expected deaths**
TOTAL	596	-10
White	(0)	0
Black	312	-41
American Indian	4	-15
Asian Pacific Islander	280	-71
Hispanic	160	-37
Non-Hispanic	436	-8

Liver & intrahepatic bile Best group rates (White)	Expected deaths	Observed deaths
TOTAL	3,571	3,829
White	3,174	3,174
Black	315	461
American Indian	16	21
Asian Pacific Islander	66	174
Hispanic	163	252
Non-Hispanic	3,407	3,577
	Estimated excess deaths	**Percent difference in observed and expected deaths**
TOTAL	258	-7
White	0	-0
Black	146	-32
American Indian	5	-23
Asian Pacific Islander	108	-62
Hispanic	89	-35
Non-Hispanic	169	-5

Committee and Staff Biographies

M. Alfred Haynes, M.D., is an epidemiologist and community physician having recently retired as President and Dean of the Drew Postgraduate Medical School and Founding Director of the Drew-Meharry-Morehouse Consortium Cancer Center. In addition to his academic positions at Drew University and the Johns Hopkins University, Dr. Haynes has served as a medical officer in the U.S. Public Health Service on the Cheyenne River Indian Reservations. He has served on a number of national governmental committees for various agencies, including the National Center for Health Statistics; the Agency for International Development; the President's Committee on Health Education; the Epidemiology, Biostatistics and Bioengineering Cluster of the President's Panel of Biomedical Research; and others. Dr. Haynes also chaired the Board of Scientific Counselors of the Division of Cancer Prevention and Control of the National Cancer Institute and was a member of the Advisory Board of the Fogarty International Center. Dr. Haynes is a member of the Institute of Medicine, the Alpha Omega Alpha Honors Medical Society, and Past-President of the American College of Preventive Medicine.

Regina M. Benjamin, M.D., M.B.A., is a medical practitioner in rural Bayou La Batre, Alabama. She is also a clinical professor and serves as a preceptor for rural medical/family medicine clerkships at the University of Alabama-Birmingham and the University of South Alabama Medical Schools. Dr. Benjamin became the first Young Physician (under age 40) elected to the American Medical Association (AMA) Board of Trustees, as well as its first African-American woman. She also serves as President of the AMA Education and Research Foundation. Dr. Benjamin attended Morehouse School of Medicine and received her M.D. from the University of Alabama Birmingham and her M.B.A. degree from Tulane University. She is a Diplomat of the American Board of Family Practice, and a Fellow of the American Academy of Family Physicians, and is a member of the Institute of Medicine. She was appointed to the Clinical Laboratory Improvement Act Committee (CLIAC), and is a member of the Council on Graduate Medical Education (COGME).

Charles L. Bennett, M.D., Ph.D., is Associate Professor of Medicine at the Lakeside Veterans Administration Hospital, Senior Faculty Fellow at the Institute for Health Science Research and Policy Studies, and Chairman of the Health Policy Program for the Robert H. Lurie Cancer Center of Northwestern University (one of the 31 NCI designated comprehensive cancer centers in the United States). His research includes health outcomes, medical decision making, and health economy and financing. More recently, his research has focused on sociocultural barriers to health care, with studies evaluating the prevalence of low literacy among cancer patients who are of lower socioeconomic status. Dr. Bennett is a member of the Health Service Committee of the American Society of Clinical Oncology, the Optimization for Health Care of the American Society of Hematology, and the Outcomes Committee of the National Comprehensive Cancer Center Network. He has a particular interest in strategies to improve the enrollment and conduct of clinical trials for cancer patients.

Baruch S. Blumberg, M.D., Ph.D., is currently Distinguished Scientist at Fox Chase Cancer Center in Philadelphia, and University Professor of Medicine and Anthropology at the University of Pennsylvania. He was Master of Balliol College, Oxford University, from 1989 to 1994 and, prior to that, Associate Director for Clinical Research at Fox Chase from 1964. He was on the staff of the National Institutes of Health, Maryland, from 1957 to 1964. He earned an M.D. degree from the College of Physicians and Surgeons, Columbia University, and a Ph.D. in biochemistry from Oxford University. His research has covered many areas including clinical research, epidemiology, virology, genetics, and anthropology. He was awarded the Nobel Prize in 1976 for "discoveries concerning new mechanisms for the origin and dissemination of infectious diseases" and specifically for the discovery of the hepatitis B virus. In 1993, he was elected to the National Inventors Hall of Fame for the invention of the hepatitis B vaccine and the diagnostic test for hepatitis B. He has taught medical anthropology at the University of Pennsylvania and elsewhere, and has been a Visiting Professor in India (Bangalore); Singapore; University of Kentucky (Lexington); Indiana University (Bloomington); the University of Otago, Dunedin, New Zealand; and Stanford University in California. He is a member of the Institute of Medicine (IOM) and the National Academy of Sciences (NAS). He is currently a member on the Committee on Human Rights of the NAS, IOM, and National Academy of Engineering (NAE).

Moon S. Chen, Ph.D. M.P.H., is Professor and Chair, Division of Health Behavior and Health Promotion, School of Public Health at the Ohio State University's College of Medicine and Public Health. Dr. Chen's research interests are in cardiovascular and cancer health education and promotion, especially among Asian-American and other ethnic minority communities. He is a charter member of the editorial board for the *Journal of Cancer Education*, and founding editor-in-chief of the *Asian-American and Pacific Islander Journal of Health*. Dr. Chen has served as a consultant to the Ministry of Public Health of the People's Republic of China; the U.S. Centers for Disease Control; and National Institutes of Health; and State public health departments in Ohio, Michigan, Virginia, and Hawaii; and was a member of the USA delegation to the United Kingdom conference on Black and Ethnic Minority Health in London in 1997.

Gilbert Friedell, M.D., is Director for Cancer Control at the University of Kentucky Markey Cancer Center. In his present position, he conveys breast cancer information to the public and to health professionals through the Kentucky Cancer Program Outreach Division, the nationally praised Kentucky Cancer Registry, and the Region 9 Cancer Information Service for Kentucky, Tennessee, and Arkansas—all organizations he helped to create. Throughout his career, Dr. Friedell has put particular emphasis on reaching the medically underserved with outreach programs in which trained, low-income, community-based women encourage their peers to receive mammograms and other cancer screenings. For several years, he served on the National Cancer Institute's Breast Cancer Task Force, and from 1971 to 1983 he was the Director of the NCI National Bladder Cancer Project. He is currently a member of the U.S. Department of Health and Human Services' National Action Plan on Breast Cancer, the Kentucky Breast Cancer Advisory Committee, and chair of the Steering Committee of NCI's Appalachia Leadership Initiative on Cancer. Dr. Friedell graduated from the University of Minnesota Medical School and received his training in pathology in Boston. Among his many honors, Dr. Friedell recently received an Avon Breast Cancer Leadership Award for outstanding contributions to breast cancer education, outreach, patient advocacy, support services, and research, especially in medically underserved communities.

Anna R. Giuliano, Ph.D., is Assistant Professor, Department of Family and Community Medicine, Epidemiology Section; and Director, Minority Cancer Prevention and Control Program, Arizona Cancer Center, University of Arizona. She currently serves as Principal Investigator for several projects at the University of Arizona: Native Women's Healing Circle, Juntos Contra El Cancer (Community-Based Cancer Education Program), and Young Women's Health Study (Efforts of Smoking on Persistent HPV Infection). Dr. Giuliano is involved internationally as a consultant on nutritional issues in Haiti, Kenya, and Tajikistan. She has authored numerous articles for several national, as well as international, peer-reviewed journals. Dr. Giuliano received her Ph.D. in Nutritional Biochemistry from Tufts University.

James Wilburn Hampton, M.D., is Medical Director, Troy and Dollie Smith Cancer Center at Integris Baptist Medical Center in Oklahoma City and Clinical Professor of Medicine at the University of Oklahoma. He is a Chickasaw. Dr. Hampton's research interests have spanned physiology and pathophysiology of cancer; thrombosis, hemostasis; leukemia; multiple myeloma and lymphoma especially Waldenstroms macroglobulinemia. He has pioneered observations on epidemiology of cancer in all American Indians/Alaska Natives in the Twentieth Century. He chairs a Network for Cancer Control Research in this special population for the National Cancer Institute. He serves on the AMA Consortium on Minority Affairs Governing Committee, the American Cancer Society Task Force for Cancer in the Socioeconomic Disadvantaged, the Steering Committee of the Intercultural Cancer Council, and the Advisory Committee for the Armed Forces control of prostate cancer. Dr. Hampton's specialty is hematology/medical oncology and he is a member of the fifteen state American Oncology Resources, a private practice organization which conducts clinical investigation in cancer.

Victor A. McKusick, M.D., Sc.D., D. Med. Sci. (h.c.), F.A.C.P., F.R.C.P., is currently Professor of Medical Genetics at The Johns Hopkins University. Previously, he served as Director, Division of Medical Genetics, Dept. of Medicine, Johns Hopkins University School of Medicine, 1957–1973; William Osler Professor and Director, Dept. of Medicine, The Johns Hopkins University School of Medicine; and Physician-in-Chief, Johns Hopkins Hospital, 1973–1985. Among his other professional activities, he has served as editor-in-chief of the journal *Medicine* (1985 to present); founding editor (with F. H. Ruddle) of *Genomics* (international journal of gene mapping and nucleotide sequencing emphasizing analyses of the human and other complex genomes); and founder and president, the Human Genome Organizations (HUGO). He is a master of the American College of Physicians and a founding member of the American Board of Medical Genetics. His current research interests are in the cataloging of human genes and genetic disorders, including collation of information on the human gene map and on the nature of the basic defect in disorders, on the one hand, with information on the clinical natural history and genetic characteristics of the disorder on the other. He is a member of Phi Beta Kappa, Alpha Omega Alpha, Association of American Physicians (Kober medal, 1990), American Genetic Association (Honorary Life Member), American Society of Human Genetics (Pres., 1974; William A. Allan Award, 1977, excellence in education award, 1997), the National Academy of Sciences, 1973 (James Murray Luck Award, 1982) and American Philosophical Society (Benjamin Franklin medal, 1996). He has held numerous consultant appointments, and has received 18 honorary degrees and many awards including the Lasker Award for special achievement in medical research.

Sarah Moody-Thomas, Ph.D., is Associate Director of the Louisiana State University Medical Center (LSUMC), Stanley S. Scott Cancer Center. She is Professor in the Department of Psychiatry and Psychology at LSUMC and the University of New Orleans, respectively. Dr. Thomas came to LSUMC from the University of New Orleans, where she served as Professor and Chair of the Department of Psychology. She earned her B.S. from Southern University and her Ph.D. in Clinical Psychology, with a co-major in public administration, from the University of Georgia. Dr. Thomas's expertise includes school-based interventions (particularly smoking prevention for African-American adolescents), community outreach, health education, and clinical research recruitment. She is chairperson of the Louisiana Coalition of the National Black Leadership Initiative on Cancer, a member of the Board of Directors of the New Orleans Chapter of the Susan G. Komen Breast Cancer Foundation, and the Greater New Orleans Unit of the American Cancer Society. She has initiated and actively participated in local, regional, and national efforts to broaden the cadre of participants in all aspects of cancer clinical research.

Lawrence Miike, M.D., J.D., is Director of the Department of Health for the State of Hawaii. He serves as the chief health and environmental official for the state. Under Dr. Miike's direction are 13 community hospitals; emergency medical services systems; adult, adolescent and children's mental health programs; alcohol and substance abuse programs, environmental monitoring, regulation and hazard response; comprehensive public health services; and health promotion and disease prevention programs. Dr. Miike holds a degree in medicine from the University of California, San Francisco, and a law degree from the University of California, Los Angeles. His professional life has been spent shaping health policy, at both the national and state level. He worked for various agencies in Washington, D.C., to help shape policies on health care reform, medical malpractice, medical ethics, and cancer-testing techniques. Dr. Miike served on the staff of the National Center for Health Services Research, the Office of Technology Assessment, among other federal agencies.

Larry Norton, M.D., is Associate Professor of Oncology at Mount Sinai School of Medicine. He is also Head, Breast Disease Management Team at Memorial Sloan-Kettering Cancer Center and Chief, Breast Oncology Service at Memorial Hospital for Cancer and Allied Disease. Dr. Norton's expertise is in cell kinetics and bioelectrochemisty. His interests include treatment of human cancer, including theory of tumor growth kinetics, electrochemistry of tumors, and enhancing chemotherapy with induced currents. Dr. Norton is a member of the American Society of Clinical Oncology, American Association for Cancer Research, Cell Kinetics Society, and the New York Cancer Society. He received his AB degree from the University of Rochester and his M.D. degree from the College of Physicians and Surgeons, Columbia University.

Madison Powers, D. Phil., is Senior Research Scholar at the Kennedy Institute of Ethics and Associate Professor of Philosophy at Georgetown University. His academic interests are political, legal, and moral philosophy; distributive justice and resource allocation; concepts of privacy in law and morality; law, ethics, and health policy; and genetics and reproductive ethics. Dr. Powers has written extensively on ethical issues in genetic testing, human subjects research, and patient confidentiality. He received his B.A. and M.A. from Vanderbilt University, and D. Phil. from the University College, Oxford. Dr. Powers is a co-recipient of a Health Policy Investigator Award from the Robert Wood Johnson Foundation and a Publication Grant from the National Library of Medicine, and has served as a consultant to several advisory committees and boards of the National Institutes of Health (NIH).

Susan C. Scrimshaw, Ph.D., is Dean, School of Public Health, and Professor of Community Health Sciences and Anthropology, University of Illinois-Chicago. Previously, she served as Professor of Public Health and Anthropology at University of California, Los Angeles and Associate Dean for Academic Programs for the School of Public Health of UCLA. Dr. Scrimshaw is an anthropologist who is especially tuned to Hispanic and African American public health issues. Dr. Scrimshaw's research interests are cross-cultural work on health access; health behavior; improving pregnancy outcomes; rapid anthropological assessment; combining qualitative and quantitative methods; Latino culture in the U.S. and Latin America; women's health; and managing cultural diversity. Dr. Scrimshaw is a member of the Institute of Medicine (IOM).

Fernando Trevino, Ph.D., is Professor and Chair of the Department of Public Health and Preventive Medicine and Executive Director of the Graduate Program in Public Health at the University of North Texas Health Science Center at Fort Worth. Prior to accepting these positions, Dr. Trevino served as Executive Director of the American Public Health Association in Washington, D.C. He also served as the Executive Editor of the *American Journal of Public Health.* Dr. Trevino was Dean of the School of Health Professions and Professor of Health Administration at Southwest Texas State University. Dr. Trevino has served on numerous national committees and panels including the U.S. Preventive Services Task Force, the National Committee on Vital and Health Statistics and the Institute of Medicine's Access to Health Care Monitoring Panel. He holds a Ph.D. degree in Preventive Medicine and Community Health from the University of Texas Medical Branch at Galveston, an M.P.H. degree from the University of Texas School of Public Health and a B.S. degree in Psychology from the University of Houston. Dr. Trevino has published and lectured extensively on national statistical data policy and Mexican American and minority health issues.

INSTITUTE OF MEDICINE STAFF

Brian D. Smedley, Ph.D., is a Senior Program Officer in the Health Sciences Policy Division and is Study Director for the Cancer Research Among Minorities and the Medically Underserved study. Dr. Smedley came to the IOM from the American Psychological Association, where he worked on a wide range of social, health, and education policy topics in his capacity as Director for Public Interest Policy. Prior to working at the APA, Dr. Smedley served as a Congressional Science Fellow, sponsored by the American Association for the Advancement of Science, and as a postdoctoral research fellow in the Education Policy Division of the Educational Testing Service in Princeton, N.J. Smedley received an A.B. degree in Psychology and Social Relations from Harvard University, and M.A. and Ph.D. degrees in clinical psychology from the University of California, Los Angeles. Smedley's previous research includes studies of the academic and psychosocial adjustment of African-American students at predominantly White and Historically Black Colleges and Universities (HBCUs).

Yvette J. Benjamin, B.A., B.S., PA-C, M.P.H., is a Research Associate at the National Academy of Sciences, Institute of Medicine in the Division of Health Sciences Policy. She is a Physician Assistant, who completed her training at George Washington University, Washington, D.C., in 1986. Ms. Benjamin holds a B.A. in psychology from The University of the Incarnate Word in San Antonio, Texas, and a B.S. in biology, from George Washington University. In 1995 Ms. Benjamin received her MPH from the George Washington University, School of Public Health, with a concentration in health policy. Ms. Benjamin has had extensive experience both as a clinician and as a researcher. At the IOM since 1993, Ms. Benjamin has provided support for several studies including Xenograft Transplantation: Ethics and Public Policy, Military Nursing Research, the Future of Academic Health Centers, and Environmental Justice: Research, Education and Health Policy Needs.

Thelma L. Cox is Senior Project Assistant in the Division of Health Sciences Policy. During her eight years at the Institute of Medicine, she has also provided assistance to the Division of Health Care Services and the Division of Biobehavioral Sciences and Mental Disorders. Ms. Cox has worked on several IOM projects, including: Designing a Strategy for Quality Review and Assurance in Medicare; Evaluating the Artificial Heart Program of the National Heart, Lung, and Blood Institute; Advising the National Library of Medicine on Information Center Services in Technology Assessment and Health Services Research; Study of FDA Advisory Committees, Federal Regulation of Methadone Treatment; Legal and Ethical Issues Relating to the Inclusion of Women in Clinical Studies; Depressive Symptoms in Primary Care Patients: Implications for Prevention; Social and Behavioral Science Base for HIV/AIDS Prevention and Intervention; and Review of the Fialuridine (FIAU/FIAC) Clinical Trials. Ms. Cox has received the National Research Council Recognition Award and the IOM Staff Achievement Award.

Index